Essentials in Elbow Surgery

Samuel Antuña • Raúl Barco

Editors

Essentials in Elbow Surgery

A Comprehensive Approach
to Common Elbow Disorders

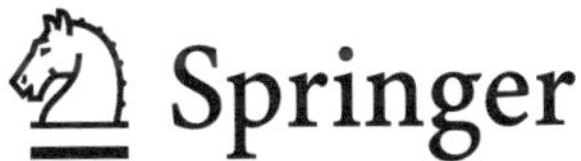

Editors
Samuel Antuña
Shoulder and Elbow Unit
Hospital Universitario La Paz
Madrid
Spain

Raúl Barco
Shoulder and Elbow Unit
Hospital Universitario La Paz
Madrid
Spain

ISBN 978-1-4471-7012-9   ISBN 978-1-4471-4625-4   (eBook)
DOI 10.1007/978-1-4471-4625-4
Springer London Heidelberg New York Dordrecht

Printed on acid-free paper

Springer is part of Springer Science+Business Media (www.springer.com)

To Ana and Elena
And to Carla, Adriana, Miguel, and Daniel
To our Parents, Teachers, and Colleagues

Foreword

We often refer to the elbow as the "joint in between." While this accurately reflects the anatomic connection of the shoulder and the hand, it is also true metaphorically as it represents a bit of a void in our knowledge of upper extremity pathology and treatment. We have numerous fellowships worldwide dealing with all aspects of the shoulder and of the hand. Our understanding of the elbow continues to be rudimentary by comparison. Thus, the effort of Doctors Antuña and Barco to address this deficiency is noteworthy. They have assembled experts from around the globe who are well trained in elbow pathology and are active as teachers and clinician/surgeons. The book has been very carefully designed to provide practical insights to the clinician regarding both diagnosis and management. Importantly, the book is organized and written from the perspective of the surgeon who may be less versed and less comfortable with elbow problems.

The content and organization of this textbook is at once simple but comprehensive, basic, but detailed. The contributions have offered the most current insight regarding not just the management but also a clear understanding of the pathoanatomy and its clinical relevance. The intent is to provide the busy and possibly less familiar clinician with a readily available, comprehensive, yet concise guide to the management of conditions, some of which are seen frequently, and others may not be seen on a daily basis by even well-trained orthopedic surgeons. The content is comprehensive in that it includes the management of elbow trauma and the recognition and proper care of soft tissue- and sports-type injuries and pathology, and finally, a detailed treatment of reconstructive surgery including joint replacement is provided. Thus, this should find a needed position in the surgeon's library who deals with elbow problems.

On a personal note, I am particularly proud of this effort since the majority of the contributors are well known to me having training to some extent at the Mayo Clinic. I am proud of their accomplishments as reflected by their contribution to this volume.

Doctors Antuña and Barco are to be commended for their efforts to develop and publish this much needed text. I consider this to be an authoritative statement regarding current concepts in management of elbow problems.

Bernard F. Morrey
Professor of Orthopedics, Mayo Clinic, Rochester, MN
Professor of Orthopedics, University of Texas Health Science Center,
San Antonio, TX

Preface

The book you are about to read has been written to help you understand and treat common elbow problems. We do not expect you to be an expert elbow surgeon when you finish it; however, you will be a knowledgeable orthopedic surgeon on the daily acute and chronic elbow problems that you are routinely encountering in your practice. If you go through the nine chapters in detail and follow the indications, we are quite sure you will be more confident in taking care of difficult fractures around the elbow, you will be able to dilucidate the source of the pain, and you will have solid guidelines to plan the best treatment.

When we thought about this project, our idea was very simple. Nowadays, there are a few very good and comprehensive books available on elbow surgery. Although they are useful to obtain discrete information about specific topics, they may be too large to be user friendly for a general orthopedic surgeon. The increasing interest among young surgeons on elbow surgery is remarkable. It has been our experience throughout the years, teaching our residents and visitors, that there is a real demand for a less extensive book that is easy to read, with practical information about the most commonly encountered problems. This text would be enough to understand the common elbow practice for a general orthopedic surgeon and a guide to learn basic elbow surgery during training.

By far, the number one highlight of this text is the list of contributors. We are deeply in debt with all of them. They are among the best elbow surgeons of the world, very well known for their expertise and dedication to teaching and science. This is their book. All have made a generous effort in writing chapters with a homogenous style and consistent information. This information is based on their clinical experience, and this is really the value of *Essentials in Elbow Surgery*.

Finally, we are grateful to our patients and all our colleagues in the Hospital Universitario La Paz. We have built a clinical practice based on their confidence. Without the generosity of our partners sending patients to us, and the trust of these patients in our capabilities and dedication, we could not enrich our expertise in this field. We hope this book will help many other patients around the world.

Madrid, Spain   Samuel Antuña
Madrid, Spain   Raúl Barco

Contents

Contributors

Samuel Antuña, MD, PhD, FEBOT Shoulder and Elbow Unit, Department of Orthopaedic Surgery and Traumatology, Hospital Universitario La Paz, Madrid, Spain

George S. Athwal, MD, FRCSC HULC, St. Joseph's Health Care, London, ON, Canada

José R. Ballesteros, MD, FEBOT Department of Orthopaedic Surgery, Hospital Clínic de Barcelona, Barcelona, Spain

Raúl Barco, MD, PhD, FEBOT Shoulder and Elbow Unit, Department of Orthopaedic Surgery and Traumatology, Hospital Universitario La Paz, Hospital Madrid Norte Sanchinarro, Madrid, Spain

Theodore A. Blaine, MD, MA, AB Department of Orthopaedics and Rehabilitation, Yale School of Medicine, New Haven, CT, USA

Nicolas Bonnevialle, MD, PhD Orthopaedic and Traumatology Department, University Hospital Toulouse, Toulouse, France

Parham Daneshvar, MD Department of Orthopedic Surgery, University of British Columbia/Providence Health Care, Vancouver, BC, Canada

Bryant Ho, MD Department of Orthopaedic Surgery, Northwestern University, Chicago, IL, USA

Department of Orthopaedic Surgery, Northwestern University, Feinberg School of Medicine, Chicago, IL, USA

Opeyemi E. Lamikanra, MD Department of Orthopaedics and Rehabilitation, Yale University School of Medicine, New Haven, CT, USA

Manuel Llusá, MD, PhD Department of Orthopaedic Surgery, Department of Anatomy, Hospital Universitario Vall d'Hebrón, University of Barcelona, Barcelona, Spain

Pierre Mansat, MD, PhD Orthopaedic and Traumatology Department, University Hospital Toulouse, Toulouse, France

Guido Marra Department of Orthopaedic Surgery, Northwestern University, Feinberg School of Medicine, Chicago, IL, USA

J. Whitcomb Pollock, MD, MSc, FRCSC Department of Surgery,
The Ottawa Hospital, The University of Ottawa, Ottawa, ON, Canada

Joaquin Sanchez-Sotelo, MD, PhD Department of Orthopedic Surgery,
Mayo Clinic, Rochester, MN, USA

David Stanley, MB BS BSc (Hons) FRCS Orthopaedic Department,
Sheffield Teaching Hospitals NHS Foundation Trust, Sheffield, South
Yorkshire, UK

Charlie Talbot, MBChB MSc(Eng) FRCS (Tr/Orth) Department of
Orthopaedic Surgery, Harrogate & District NHS Foundation Trust,
Harrogate, North Yorkshire, UK

Paul M. Tomaszewski, MD, MS Department of Orthopaedics and
Rehabilitation, Yale University School of Medicine, New Haven, CT, USA

Matthias Vanhees, MD Orthopedic and Traumatology, AZ Monica/MoRe
Foundation, Antwerp, Belgium

Roger P. van Riet, MD, PhD Orthopedics and Traumatology, AZ Monica/
MoRe Foundation, Antwerp, Belgium

Orthopedics and Traumatology, Erasme University Hospital Brussels,
Brussels, Belgium

Frederik Verstreken, MD Orthopedic and Traumatology, AZ Monica/
MoRe Foundation, Antwerp, Belgium

Orthopedic and Traumatology, University Hospital Antwerp,
Antwerp, Belgium

Alem Yacob, MD, MSc Department of Orthopaedics and Rehabilitation,
Yale University School of Medicine, New Haven, CT, USA

Applied Anatomy and Surgical Approaches to the Elbow

1

Raúl Barco, José R. Ballesteros, Manuel Llusá, and Samuel Antuña

Abstract

Knowledge of the anatomy and surgical approaches is crucial to develop a surgical strategy while minimizing complications. The most widely used approaches of the elbow will be reviewed with an emphasis on how to extend the approaches if so needed and according to which exposures are best used for the most common elbow pathologies. Key aspects of neurovascular relationships are discussed to protect them during elbow surgery.

Keywords

Surgical approaches • Anatomy • Exposure

R. Barco, MD, PhD, FEBOT (✉)
Shoulder and Elbow Unit, Department of Orthopaedic
Surgery and Traumatology, Hospital Universitario La Paz,
Hospital Madrid Norte Sanchinarro,
Paseo de la Castellana 261, Madrid 28046, Spain
e-mail: raulbarco@hotmail.com

J.R. Ballesteros, MD, FEBOT
Department of Orthopaedic Surgery, Hospital Clínic
de Barcelona, Villarroel 170, Barcelona 08036, Spain
e-mail: jrballes@clinic.ub.es

M. Llusá, MD, PhD
Department of Orthopaedic Surgery,
Department of Anatomy, Hospital Universitario
Vall d'Hebrón, University of Barcelona,
P. de la Vall d'Hebron, 119-129,
Barcelona 08035, Spain
e-mail: mllusa@ub.edu

S. Antuña, MD, PhD, FEBOT
Shoulder and Elbow Unit, Department of Orthopaedic
Surgery and Traumatology, Hospital Universitario La Paz,
Paseo de la Castellana 261, Madrid 28046, Spain
e-mail: santuna@asturias.com

Introduction

Detailed knowledge of elbow anatomy is crucial to understand and treat the spectrum of pathologies that affect this joint. Three-dimensional recognition of anatomy is probably more important in the elbow than in other joints due to the amount of neurovascular structures that are in close vicinity in a very small area that includes three joints. Despite the large number of approaches described in the elbow literature, only a few should be mastered in clinical practice. In this chapter, we will cover the approaches required to treat the most common problems encountered in elbow surgery, with an emphasis being made on how to extend the planned approach when an unexpected finding arises intraoperatively. We will exclude arthroscopic approaches that will be covered in another chapter.

S. Antuña, R. Barco (eds.), *Essentials in Elbow Surgery*,
DOI 10.1007/978-1-4471-4625-4_1, © Springer-Verlag London 2014

General Principles

Probably, the best starting point for a successful surgery lies in the correct analysis of the injury. This will necessarily lead to a surgical plan, which will include exposure, expected and potentially unexpected findings and their treatment. Unexpected findings may or may not require a separate exposure [1].

Previous scars must be taken into account. If the previous scar is mobile and non-adherent to deep tissues, it may be obviated, but it is probably better if it can be included in the new surgical plan. When a separate incision must be made, an appropriate skin bridge must be respected to avoid skin ischemia. Full-thickness subcutaneous flaps are favoured because they respect the skin circulation.

Prior operative notes are very helpful but seldom available. They are especially useful when approaching the medial side of the elbow regarding previous transposition of the ulnar nerve. Superficial nerves are always severed to some extent but care to protect them must be exercised, specifically in the medial side of the elbow where they can lead to painful neuromas.

Whenever possible, internervous anatomical planes should be used because they are safer, cause less bleeding and are probably less painful. A tourniquet is probably recommended for all procedures because dissection is easier, surgery is more precise and hematomas are avoided. Inflammation and bleeding can be linked to an increased risk of stiffness and precise, careful surgery may limit this risk. The use of dressings, splints, cold therapy and elevation may be used accordingly to the pathology as may minimize bleeding and inflammation.

Approaches

Throughout the years, many approaches and modifications have been developed in elbow surgery. In clinical practice, however, only a few of these are really required to perform the most common surgical procedures to the elbow (Tables 1.1, 1.2, and 1.3). We tend to favour surgical approaches that are versatile for the whole spectrum of elbow pathology and these will be included in this chapter; more specific approaches will be only referenced. We will present the surgical approaches according to the pathology for which they are being used.

Table 1.1 Posterior approaches

Approach	Indication	Extension	Commentary	Nerves in danger
Alonso-Llames [2]	Distal humerus fractures (extra-articular)	Proximal with protection of radial nerve. Distal through ECU-anconeus interval	Easy conversion to olecranon osteotomy	Ulnar nerve, radial nerve
Triceps-splitting [3, 4, 6]	Distal humeral fractures, total elbow arthroplasty	Proximally limited by the radial nerve	May be performed in the midline or slightly medially	Ulnar nerve, radial nerve
Olecranon osteotomy [7]	Distal humeral fractures	Proximally until radial nerve	Fixation with multiple options	Ulnar nerve
Bryan-Morrey [5]	Elbow arthroplasty, stiffness	Proximally medial (to triceps) and distally between ECU and FCU	Must protect the ulnar nerve, especially during dislocation of the joint	Ulnar nerve

Table 1.2 Lateral approaches

Approach	Indication	Extension	Commentary	Nerves in danger
Kocher [9]	Radiocapitellar fractures, lateral instability	Proximal and distal Mayo-modified Kocher approach includes detachment of 1/3 triceps tendon	Limited part of the Kocher may be used	Radial nerve in proximal extension
Kaplan [8]	Radial head fractures	Proximally	Limited indications	PIN
Column procedure [13]	Elbow stiffness	Distal extension through EDC-ECR interval		PIN

Table 1.3 Medial approaches

Approach	Indication	Extension	Commentary	Nerves in danger
Over the top [14]	Elbow stiffness Coronoid fracture fixation	Proximal		Ulnar and median nerve
FCU approach	Elbow stiffness, medial collateral ligament repair, coronoid fracture fixation	Proximally and distally (ulnar nerve)	May be performed through a split in the humeral head, through the interval between the ulnar and humeral heads or detaching both heads of the FCU	Ulnar nerve

Distal Humerus Fractures

Any approach to the distal humerus must balance how to manage the triceps and how to gain the maximum access to the fracture. The available approaches include [2–6]:

- The bilaterotricipital approach (Alonso-Llames approach, triceps on)
- The transtricipital approaches, with the incision through the midline (Campbell) or slightly medial to the midline (Stanley/Shahane)
- Olecranon osteotomy
- The triceps-reflecting approaches: Bryan-Morrey or detachment of the triceps-anconeus insertion complex distally (TRAP procedure)

Leaving the triceps attachment intact will obviously reduce the complications associated with an olecranon osteotomy or triceps detachment. There is a tendency to use an Alonso-Llames approach for the more simple fractures, with minimal involvement of the joint surface, and an olecranon osteotomy for the more complex fractures with intraarticular extension. Fixation of the olecranon osteotomy may be performed with tension-band wire fixation, intramedullary screw or nail or a plate.

Complex articular fractures of the capitellum and trochlea may probably benefit from an olecranon osteotomy because it allows the best joint exposure. However, the most simple fractures of the capitellum may be approached through an arthroscopic approach or a modified Kocher approach with slight proximal extension.

When we are fixing a distal humerus fracture with diaphyseal extension, the approach needs to be extended proximally in order to apply longer plates. Under these circumstances, the surgeon will need to dissect the radial nerve laterally and posteriorly and the ulnar nerve medially.

Depending on the type and location of the distal humerus fracture, the ulnar nerve may be left alone or, more commonly, identified and protected throughout the procedure. The decision to transpose the nerve anteriorly at the end of the procedure is controversial. However, if the nerve has any tendency to subluxate anteriorly or if it lies directly on top of the medial plate, we do not hesitate to transpose it anteriorly into a subcutaneous pocket.

The Alonso-Llames Approach (Bilaterotricipital Approach)

This is an approach first described for use in treatment of paediatric supracondylar fractures of the humerus. Its main advantage is that it leaves the triceps intact. The surgeon can work through either side of the muscle belly and there is no need to protect the extensor mechanism postoperatively [2].

A posterior skin incision is used and full-thickness subcutaneous flaps are developed. Once identified, the medial and lateral borders of the triceps are incised and dissected free from the posterior part of the humerus. Ulnar nerve dissection and protection are recommended during the approach and during any manipulation of the forearm to avoid traction injuries to the nerve (Fig. 1.1). The radial nerve may need to be dissected if the exposure has to be extended proximally. The identification of the posterior antebrachial cutaneous nerve (a branch of the radial nerve) is usually more distal and can guide us in the localization of the radial nerve proximally.

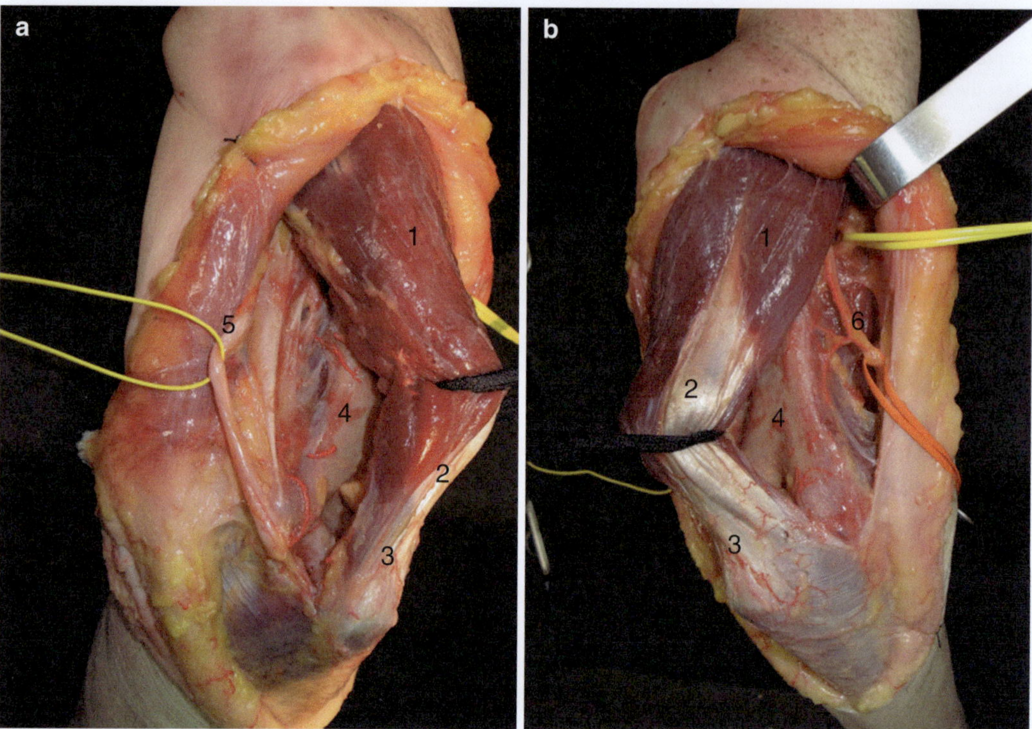

Fig. 1.1 The Alonso-Llames approach. Bilaterotricipital approach allows access to both sides of the distal humerus, preserving the triceps insertion. (**a**) Ulnar nerve dissection and protection are recommended. (**b**) Radial nerve crosses the humerus in the posterolateral proximal portion at the level of the musculotendinous junction of the triceps, just before perforating the intermuscular septum to run below *brachioradialis* muscle. *1* Triceps muscle, *2* triceps superficial aponeurosis, *3* triceps tendon, *4* distal humerus, *5* ulnar nerve, *6* radial nerve

The distal exposure achieved with this approach is limited, so it is not suitable for complex articular fractures. An extension of this approach laterally through the Kocher interval (between ECU and anconeus) has been described to increase the distal exposure [7]. Proximally, the radial nerve crosses the humerus from posteromedial to posterolateral approximately at the level of the musculotendinous junction of the triceps.

Posterior Triceps-Splitting Approaches

Campbell described a simple exposure that can be extended to the level of the radial nerve proximally and along the ulna distally [3]. The triceps tendon and muscle are incised on its midline exposing the humerus and dissecting each half of the triceps to either side (Fig. 1.2). Ulnar nerve location and protection are advised. Distally, the incision runs over the olecranon and separates the anconeus laterally and the flexor carpi ulnaris medially. Access to the posterior and posterolateral aspect of the humerus is readily available but positioning of true lateral plates can be cumbersome because the divided triceps difficults the correct angulation of the drill and screw insertion. Meticulous closure of the triceps with side-to-side sutures and, probably, transosseous sutures at the level of the aponeurosis insertion is recommended [4, 5].

Olecranon Osteotomy

This is probably the most utilized approach to treat distal humerus fractures because it provides great access to the articular surface and the columns [7]. The chevron osteotomy is favoured

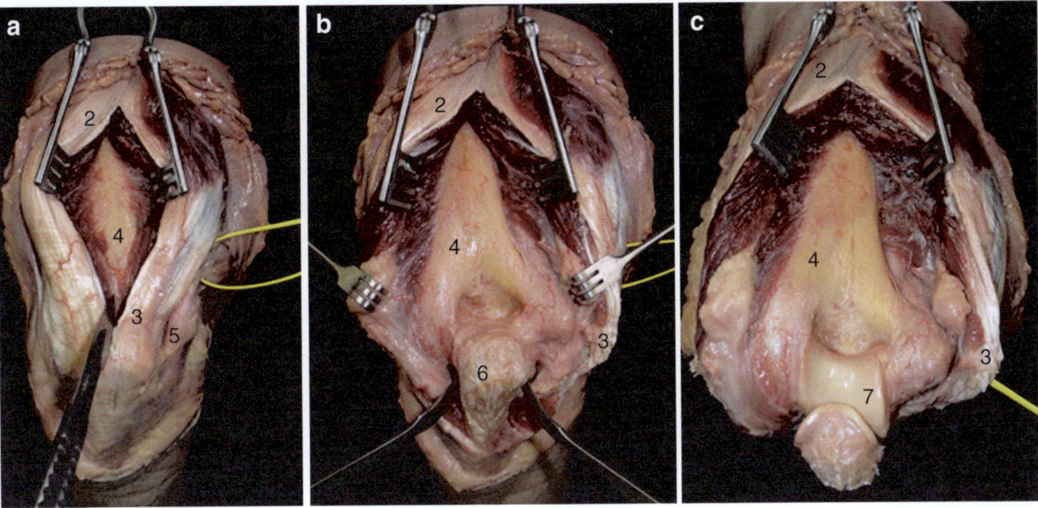

Fig 1.2 The Campbell approach. Posterior triceps-splitting approach through midline triceps tendon. (**a**) After ulnar nerve location and protection, a longitudinal incision in the superficial aponeurosis of the triceps tendon and muscle is performed. (**b**) Exposition of the olecranon retracting the *anconeus* muscle laterally and the flexor carpi ulnaris muscle medially. (**c**) Flexion of the elbow joint permits a better exposure of the distal humerus. *1* Triceps muscle, *2* triceps superficial aponeurosis, *3* triceps tendon, *4* distal humerus, *5* ulnar nerve, *6* olecranon, *7* trochlea

over transverse osteotomy because of added intrinsic stability. The main disadvantage of this approach is the fixation method for the osteotomy, which frequently needs additional surgery to remove the osteosynthesis due to mobilization and secondary irritation.

A posterior skin incision is used and dissection to the triceps aponeurosis and olecranon is performed preserving thick fasciocutaneous flaps. Preparing the final fixation method may be performed at this moment or can be done at the end of the procedure. The ulnar nerve should be located and protected. The joint is opened laterally and is protected with a sponge when performing the osteotomy (Fig. 1.3).

A distal chevron is made at the level of the bare spot of the greater sigmoid notch of the ulna. The cut is started with a saw and finished with an osteotome. The proximal olecranon and tendon are retracted proximally and separated from capsular attachments and collateral ligaments. This exposure may be continued proximally using the bilaterotricipital approach described previously. At the end of the procedure, the olecranon is reduced and fixed with a cerclage with K-wires, a lag screw, an intramedullary nail or a plate.

In an attempt to avoid denervation of the anconeus, some authors favour dissecting the anconeus distal the ulna without detaching it from the triceps to preserve its innervation. At the end of the procedure, it is sutured back to the anconeus and flexor carpi ulnaris.

Distal Humerus Nonunions

When approaching distal humeral nonunions, the decision on whether an osteosynthesis with bone graft or an arthroplasty is required must be made based on the amount and quality of distal bone stock and the status of the articular surface.

If fixation is elected, an Alonso-Llames approach is preferred if there is no joint incongruity or malalignment. Otherwise, an olecranon osteotomy is a better option. If the objective of the surgery is removing the distal humerus and implanting a linked elbow arthroplasty, this is

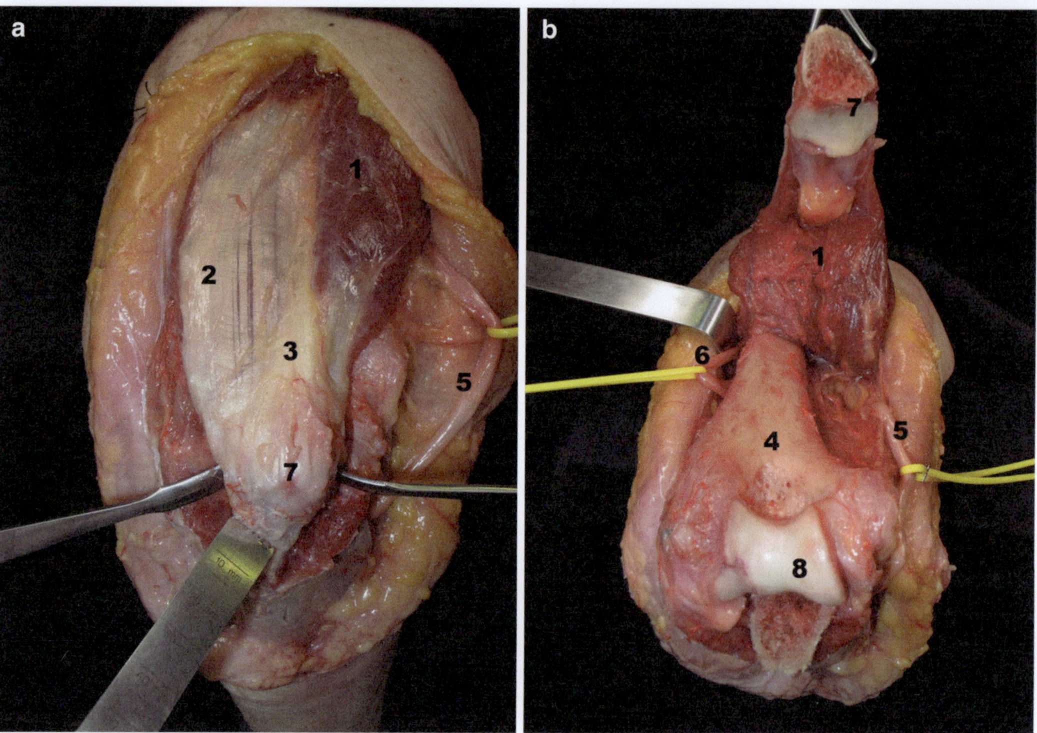

Fig. 1.3 The olecranon osteotomy. (**a**) Chevron osteotomy of the olecranon through the bare area which is localized after opening the joint at both sides of the olecranon. (**b**) Retracting the olecranon osteotomy and triceps muscle proximally gives us a great access to all the articular surface and columns of the distal humerus. Special attention should be paid to the ulnar and radial nerve. *1* Triceps muscle, *2* triceps superficial aponeurosis, *3* triceps tendon, *4* distal humerus, *5* ulnar nerve, *6* radial nerve, *7* olecranon, *8* trochlea

ideally done without sacrificing the extensor mechanism by using an Alonso-Llames approach.

There are probably cases where the final decision must be taken intraoperatively. In these cases, if there is joint incongruity and malalignment, a Bryan-Morrey approach may be preferred (see approach under total elbow arthroplasty indication). Otherwise, a bilaterotricipital approach is our first choice.

Fractures of the Radial Head and Capitellum: The Simple Case

Access to the lateral aspect of the elbow can be done through a lateral direct skin incision or with a posterior "universal" skin incision and elevation of a thick fasciocutaneous flap until the epicondyle is reached. The surgeon must make the choice based on the presence of associated injuries that might need to be treated also.

Most radial head fractures can be treated through a Kaplan or a limited Kocher exposure with a direct lateral skin incision [8, 9]. More complex cases may need a posterior skin incision.

Capitellar fractures need to be carefully assessed to rule out significant posterior comminution and extension into the trochlea, as these findings are important to elect the optimal approach. If a simple capitellar fracture is observed, this may be a good indication for arthroscopic-assisted fixation. If not feasible or the surgeon does not have experience with elbow arthroscopy, a Kocher approach provides the best access to fix these injuries.

Kaplan Approach

This approach is mostly used for isolated fractures of the radial head, specifically those involving the anterior half, without associated injury to the lateral collateral ligament complex leading to instability [8]. A 4 cm skin incision extending

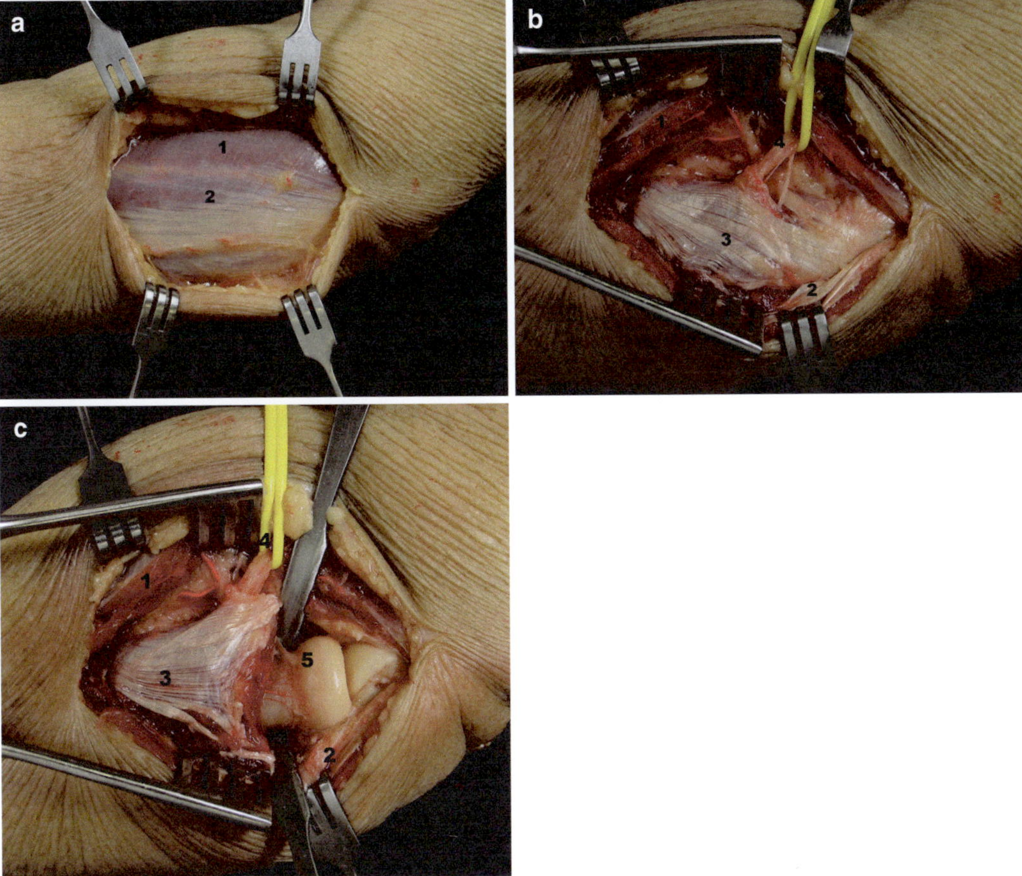

Fig. 1.4 The Kaplan approach. (**a**) Superficial view of the proximal forearm. The incision is in line with the interval between the *extensor carpi radialis brevis* muscle and the *extensor digitorum* muscle. (**b**) It is necessary to elevate and retract this muscle in order to show the *supinator* muscle. Localize the key structure of the area, the radial nerve. With forearm pronation, the posterior interosseous nerve moves medially from the operative field. (**c**) Incise the annular ligament, the joint capsule and the proximal origin of the *supinator* muscle, to expose the *capitellum* and the radial head. *1 Extensor carpi radialis brevis* muscle, *2 extensor digitorum* muscle, *3 supinator* muscle, *4* radial nerve, posterior interosseous nerve, *5* radial head

from the lateral epicondyle towards the Lister's tubercle of the distal radius is performed and the superficial interval between the extensor carpi radialis longus and the extensor digitorum muscle is developed (Fig. 1.4).

On deep dissection, we need to identify and develop the interval between extensor carpi radialis brevis (ECRB) and the supinator. The fibres of the supinator muscle are oblique to the fibres of the ECRB. Access to the radial head is granted by partially detaching the proximal aspect of the origin of the supinator. The capsule is underneath this plane and is incised longitudinally to access the radial head. The posterior interosseous nerve is in close vicinity. Working with the forearm in pronation and avoiding Hohmann's retractors on the neck of the radius may protect the nerve [10].

Kocher Approach

The Kocher approach utilizes the interval between the anconeus and the extensor carpi ulnaris [9]. It is versatile because it can be extended proximally and safe because the ECU is protecting the radial nerve. However, in this approach, care must be taken to identify, preserve or repair, if necessary, the lateral ligamentous complex. It is the preferred approach for radial head fractures associated with elbow instability and for capitellar fractures without significant comminution or medial extension.

The interval between the anconeus and the ECU can be identified by subtle palpation: by moving your finger from posterior to anterior, you can feel the anterior margin of the anconeus where the interval is located. Additionally, a thin strip of fat is usually present in this interval. It is better defined distally, as more proximally the fascia of both muscles coalesces towards the insertion.

The lateral capsule and ligaments are identified and incised to enter the joint. The lateral collateral ligament originates from the lateral epicondyle and inserts in the *crista supinatoris* of the ulna. These fibres must be recognized and protected when opening the capsule. It is usually safe to open the capsule just anterior to the ligament if it is intact (Fig. 1.5). If the ligament is torn in the context of a fracture dislocation, the proximal stump of the ligament should be dissected and tagged for final reattachment at the end of the operation.

In cases of epicondylar fractures, this approach may not need to be performed and simple reduction through a lateral skin incision may suffice. However, in cases of capitellar fractures or fractures extending into the metaphysis, the Kocher approach may need to be extended proximally to improve visualization of the reduction and orientation of the screws, especially if they are inserted from anterior to posterior (Fig. 1.6). In cases of posterior to anterior screw fixation, the anconeus and the triceps have to be mobilized medially to gain proper access for screw insertion.

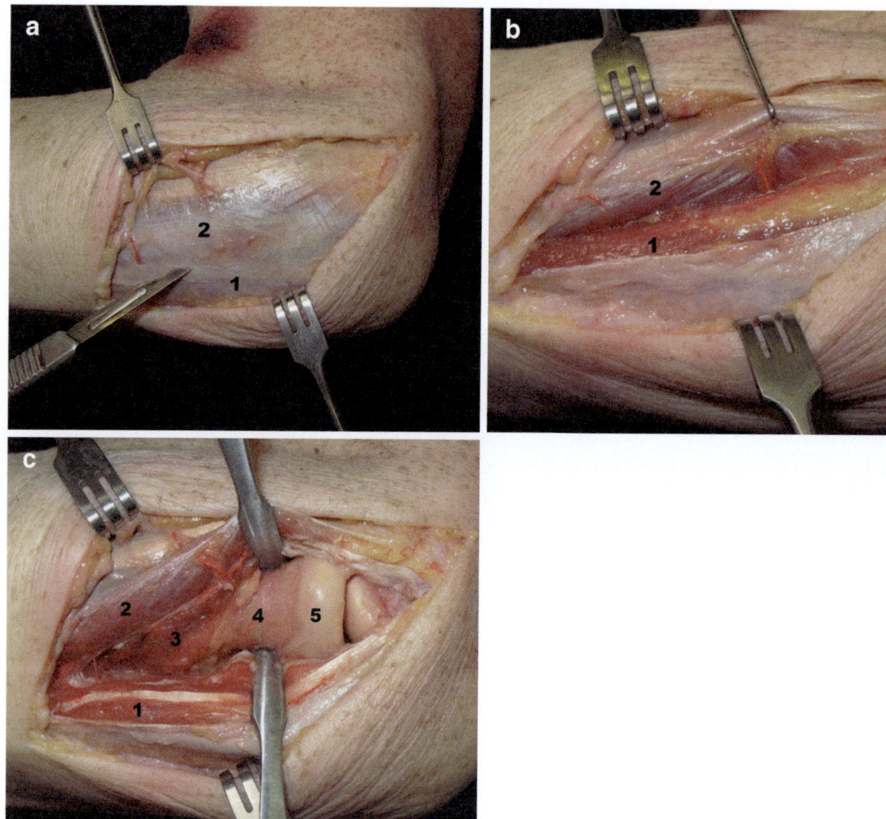

Fig. 1.5 The Kocher approach. (**a**) Localize the "white line" and small perforator arteries to identify the interval between the *anconeus* and the *extensor carpi ulnaris* (ECU) muscle. It is easier to define this interval in the distal part of the approach. (**b**) Incision of the superficial aponeurosis and retraction of both muscles, *anconeus* and ECU muscles. (**c**) Open the capsule just anterior to the lateral ulnar collateral ligament. Exposition of the neck and the head of the radius. *1 Anconeus* muscle, *2 ECU* muscle, *3 supinator* muscle, *4* neck of the radius, *5* head of the radius

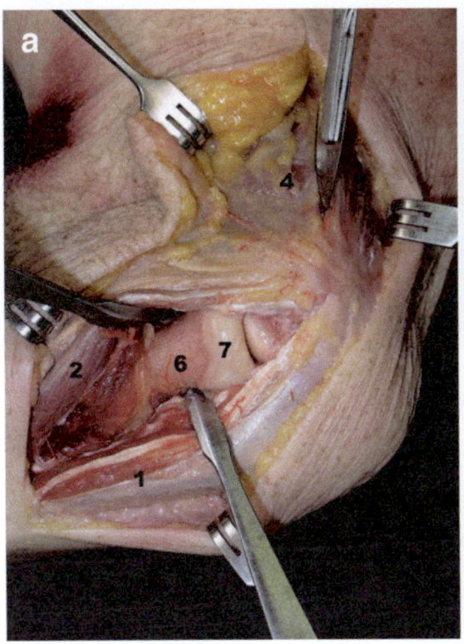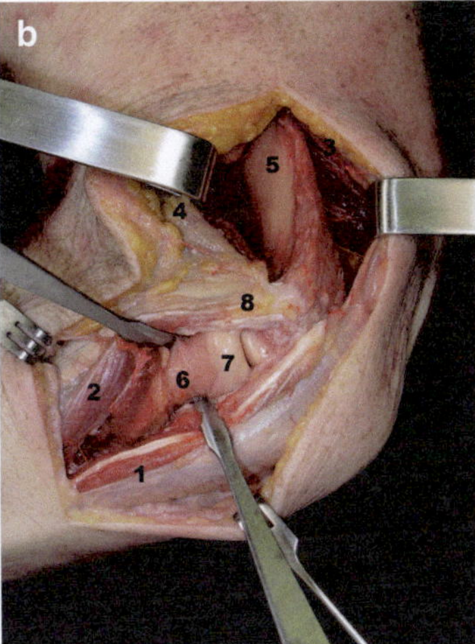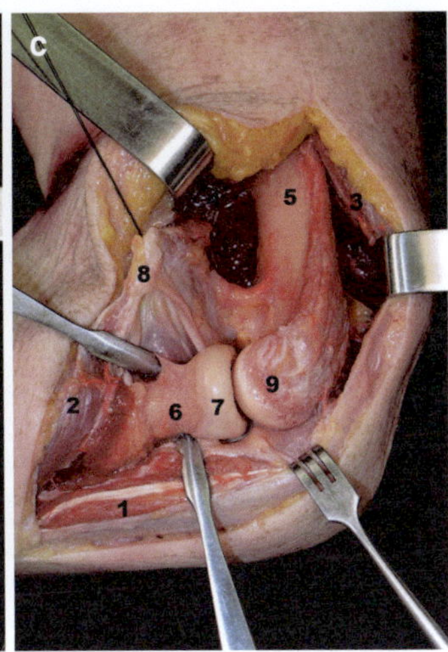

Fig. 1.6 The extended Kocher approach. (**a**) Proximal extension of the Kocher approach. Incision between the triceps muscle and the supraepicondylar origin of the *brachioradialis* (BR) and the *extensor carpi radialis longus* (ECRL) muscles. (**b**) Retraction of these muscles gives access to the lateral column of the distal humerus. (**c**) Detaching the lateral collateral ligament and the common origin of the extensor muscles gives access to the radiocapitellar joint. *1 Anconeus* muscle, *2 extensor carpi ulnaris* muscle, *3* triceps muscle, *4* BR-ECRL muscles, *5* lateral column of the distal humerus, *6* neck of the radius, *7* head of the radius, *8* common origin of the extensor muscles, *9* capitellum

Fractures of the Radial Head and Capitellum: The Complex Case

Usually, complex fractures of the radial head and distal articular humeral fractures include an increased number of fracture fragments, metaphyseal bone impaction and associated ligamentous and bony injuries that may difficult fracture reduction, fixation, stability and, hence, prognosis. Recognition of all the associated injuries is critical to understand the mechanism of injury and treat them accordingly.

Instead of using a direct lateral incision, we usually favour performing a midline posterior skin incision that allows access to the lateral and medial sides. There are, however, surgeons who prefer performing separate lateral and medial incisions.

Complex radial head fractures may need an associated lateral collateral ligament and extensor muscle repair and this is easily accessed through a Kocher approach rather than a Kaplan approach. Dissection must avoid extending the original damage to the ligaments. Ligament reconstruction may be performed through bone tunnels or with the aid of an anchor. If there is an associated coronoid fracture (terrible triad injury), the repair should follow an inside-out repair, starting with the coronoid and finishing with the ligament repair. The coronoid is easily accessed through the joint if a radial head resection is performed before the prosthesis is implanted. In terrible triad cases where the radial head has a simple fracture pattern and only needs to be fixed, access to the coronoid is performed before fixation of the radial head by extending the Kocher approach proximally, detaching the extensors from the humerus and elevating the anterior capsule.

Complex capitellar fractures with medial extension can be fixed through a Kocher approach if there is no severe comminution. Should the fracture fixation become difficult, it is reasonable to detach the lateral collateral ligament to enlarge the approach and reattach it at the end of the procedure. Occasionally, the fracture line affects the lateral epicondyle and the repair can be done by elevating this fragment and reflecting the lateral ligament complex with it.

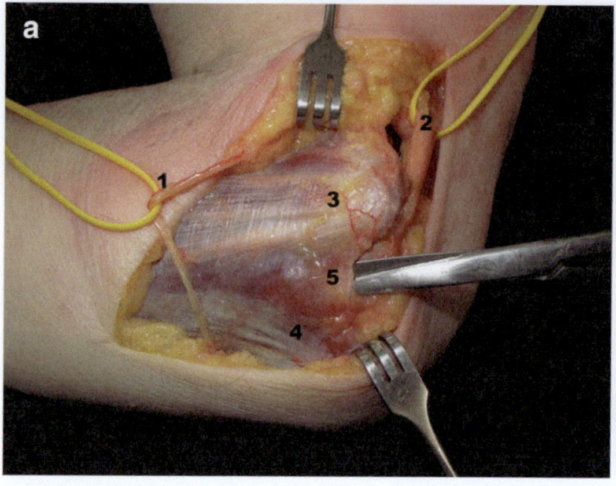
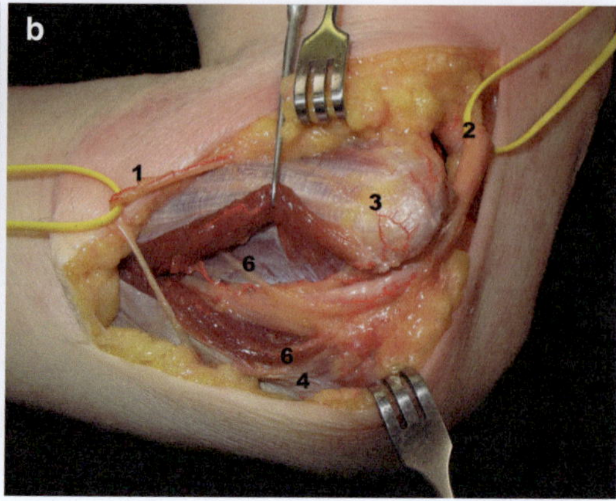

Fig. 1.7 The FCU interval approach. (**a**) Identification and protection of the *medial antebrachial cutaneous nerve* (MABCN). Identify and protect the ulnar nerve which lies in the proximal interval between the humeral and ulnar heads of the *flexor carpi ulnaris* (FCU), and after, identify and protect the ulnar nerve. (**b**) Splitting and retraction of this interval protecting the innervation of the humeral and ulnar head of the FCU muscle. *1* MABC nerve, *2* ulnar nerve, *3* humeral head of the FCU muscle, *4* ulnar head of the FCU, *5* FCU interval (arcade of Osborne)

Fractures of the Coronoid and Epitrochlea

A posterior midline skin incision is preferred to gain access to the medial aspect of the elbow as it reduces the risk of damaging the medial antebrachial cutaneous nerve (MABCN). If a midline skin incision is used, identification and protection of this nerve must be provided, especially in the distal part of the incision where the nerve usually arborizes. Injury to this nerve may lead to painful neuromas.

The ulnar nerve must be identified and protected. Decompression in the ulnar tunnel is occasionally needed in some epitrochlear fractures and fractures of the coronoid that include the anteromedial facet or when they need plate fixation.

Anteromedial coronoid fractures in the context of posteromedial varus instability may involve a very small fragment, precluding safe fixation. This situation must be anticipated preoperatively to avoid a difficult unnecessary dissection. Applying a lateral external fixator to avoid varus moment of the arm associated to a lateral ligament reconstruction is a better option for these cases.

When there is a large fracture fragment, reduction and internal fixation with screws with or without buttressing plates is required.

FCU Interval Approach

This approach uses the interval between the humeral and the ulnar heads of the FCU. The ulnar nerve lies in this interval and has a direct relationship with the medial collateral ligament. Identification and proper protection of the nerve are necessary. In some cases, the ulnar nerve needs to be fully mobilized to work safely. At the end of the procedure, the nerve can be left in place or transposed anteriorly depending on its tendency to subluxate and its position related to metallic implants (Fig. 1.7).

To gain exposure into the joint, the sublime tubercle is located by palpation. The humeral head of the FCU is split in line with its fibres 1 cm distally to the sublime tubercle and dissected to bone [11]. With a scalpel blade placed parallel to the bone, we progress proximally as we encounter the sublime tubercle leaving the MCL insertion below the scalpel blade and the FCU above it. The brachialis muscle will be seen in the deep aspect of this exposure with its fibres inserting distally to the coronoid with an angulation of 60°. We direct the dissection towards the epicondyle and progress until the capsule is observed (Fig. 1.8). The capsule is incised in line with the MCL and just anterior to it, exposing the ulnohumeral joint and extending the approach proximally by elevating the capsule up to the medial epicondyle.

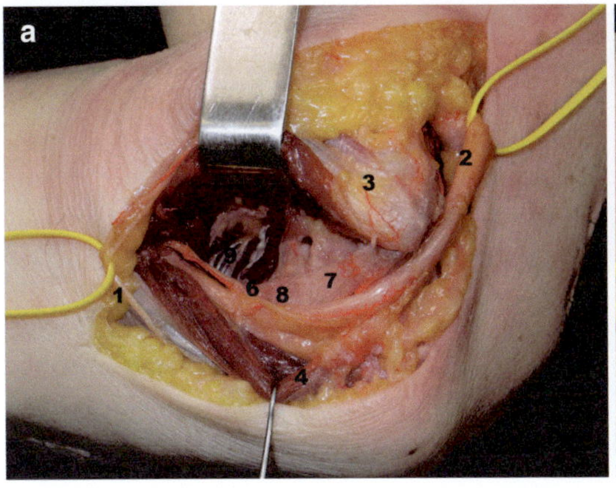
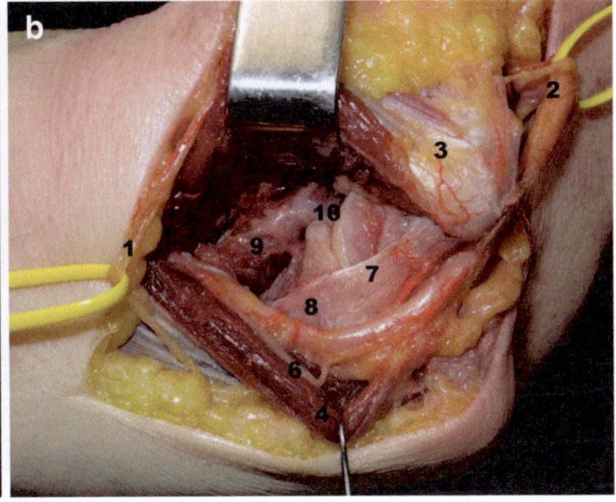

Fig. 1.8 (**a**) In the deep part of the approach, the medial collateral ligament, coronoid process and *brachialis* muscle can be seen. (**b**) Incision of the capsule anterior to the medial collateral ligament. Identification of the *sublime* tubercle, ulnohumeral joint line and *brachialis* muscle. *1* MABC nerve, *2* ulnar nerve, *3* humeral head of the FCU, *4* ulnar head of the FCU muscle, *5* FCU interval (arcade of Osborne), *6* motor branches to humeral and ulnar heads of the FCU muscle, *7* medial collateral ligament, *8* *sublimis* tubercle, *9* *brachialis* muscle, *10* ulnohumeral joint line

Tip fractures are readily visible. Anteromedial fractures can be found just underneath the most anterior part of the MCL. If the exposure needs to be extended distally, the brachialis and the FCU are dissected from the ulna, protecting the ulnar nerve and its branches. For some tip fractures, a medial "over-the-top" procedure may be preferred (see next section).

Stiffness

Nowadays, simple elbow stiffness and the majority of patients with primary osteoarthritis are effectively treated with arthroscopic techniques. Nevertheless, in our practice, there are still a few indications for an open approach. The election of the most appropriate surgical procedure in a stiff elbow is based on the state of the articular cartilage and the location of the pathology.

When we are treating a patient with a stiff elbow, we consider the ulnar nerve as part of the pathology. The nerve should be addressed whenever preoperative ulnar nerve symptoms are present or when there is limited preoperative flexion.

Open capsular release may be performed through the lateral column approach or medially through the over-the-top approach. Distraction-interposition arthroplasty is usually performed through a Mayo-modified Kocher posterolateral triceps-sparing approach.

Column Procedure

A direct lateral skin incision is performed extending 6 cm from the lateral epicondyle proximally. This approach could be considered the proximal extension of a Kocher approach [13]. Dissection is started proximally, detaching the brachioradialis anteriorly and the triceps posteriorly from the supracondylar ridge. Identification of the plane between the anterior capsule and brachialis and the triceps and posterior capsule is critical. Full dissection of these planes is recommended prior to excision of the capsule (Fig. 1.9). When the ulnar nerve needs to be addressed, a posterior skin incision is preferred because it allows simultaneous access to the medial aspect of the elbow – to decompress the nerve and excise the posterior band of the MCL – and to the lateral column, to perform the capsulectomy.

"Over-the-Top" Procedure

Originally described for releasing elbow contractures, its main advantage is that it addresses both the elbow contracture and the ulnar nerve [14]. We prefer to use a posterior midline incision but a medial skin incision may be used if the MABCN is protected.

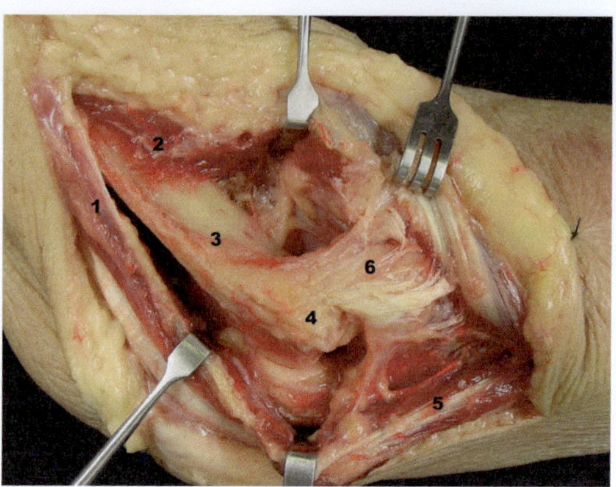

Fig. 1.9 The column procedure showed as a proximal extension of Kocher approach by elevating the *brachioradialis* and triceps muscles. Identification and dissection of the capsule are important. The lateral collateral ligament is preserved. For simple elbow stiffness, only the superior part of the approach, above the lateral epicondyle, is used. *1* Triceps muscle, *2 brachioradialis* muscle, *3* humerus, *4* lateral epicondyle, *5 anconeus* muscle, *6* common extensor muscles and lateral collateral ligament origin

The rationale of this approach is similar to the column procedure. An incision of the supracondylar ridge is started around 5 cm proximally to the medial epicondyle and continued distally leaving the brachialis anteriorly and the triceps posteriorly. The anterior dissection runs through the pronator teres and the common flexor tendon leaving a part of fascia attached to the ridge to facilitate later closure. The plane between the brachialis and the capsule is found and developed using a periosteal elevator. Careful dissection must be performed because of the vicinity of the median nerve and the brachial arteriovenous bundle (Fig. 1.10). Posteriorly, the triceps is elevated from the capsule while the ulnar nerve is protected anteriorly. The posterior capsule is excised and the posterior band of the MCL is divided in cases with severe loss of flexion.

Mayo-Modified Kocher Posterolateral Triceps-Sparing Approach

A midline posterior skin incision is preferred. A Kocher approach is performed using the interval between the anconeus and the extensor carpi ulnaris and is extended proximally to divide the extensor muscles and brachioradialis anteriorly and the triceps posteriorly [12]. The ulnar nerve should be released and protected, especially during the dislocation manoeuvre (Fig. 1.11).

The triceps and anconeus should be released from lateral to medial until the triceps tendon is able to flip over. This usually implies careful elevation of no more than half of the triceps attachments from the olecranon.

The lateral ligament is released proximally from the epicondyle and the elbow is dislocated to gain access to the articular surface. The cartilage is debrided and the graft is interposed and left in place with transosseous sutures. Lateral ligament repair with or without adjuvant ligamentous augmentation is performed.

Ligamentous Reconstruction

Lateral ligamentous reconstruction may be approached through a limited lateral incision and a Kocher approach (Fig. 1.5). Enough exposure of the crista supinatoris is necessary to perform the bone tunnels and pass the tendinous graft. Proximally, we favour using the docking technique but fixation may be done through bone tunnels ("yoke stitch") or with an interference screw.

Medial ligamentous reconstruction has evolved from extensive approaches to more limited ones. The location and configuration of bone tunnels have also been substantially modified. All these modifications have been directed to avoid complications related to the ulnar nerve.

A limited transmuscular approach through the humeral head of the FCU is performed just anterior to the MCL [11]. The dissection is continued proximally sliding the surgical blade on top of the MCL up to the medial epicondyle where the graft is fixed proximally (see Fig. 1.7). There are many different options available to fix the graft distally and proximally. However, when fixing the graft proximally, care must be taken to avoid injuring the ulnar nerve.

Distal Biceps Repair

Distal biceps repair may be done through a double or a single anterior skin incision. Overall, the rate of complications is similar between both approaches, but the anterior single incision has been associated with a higher rate of lateral antebrachial cutaneous nerve (LABCN)

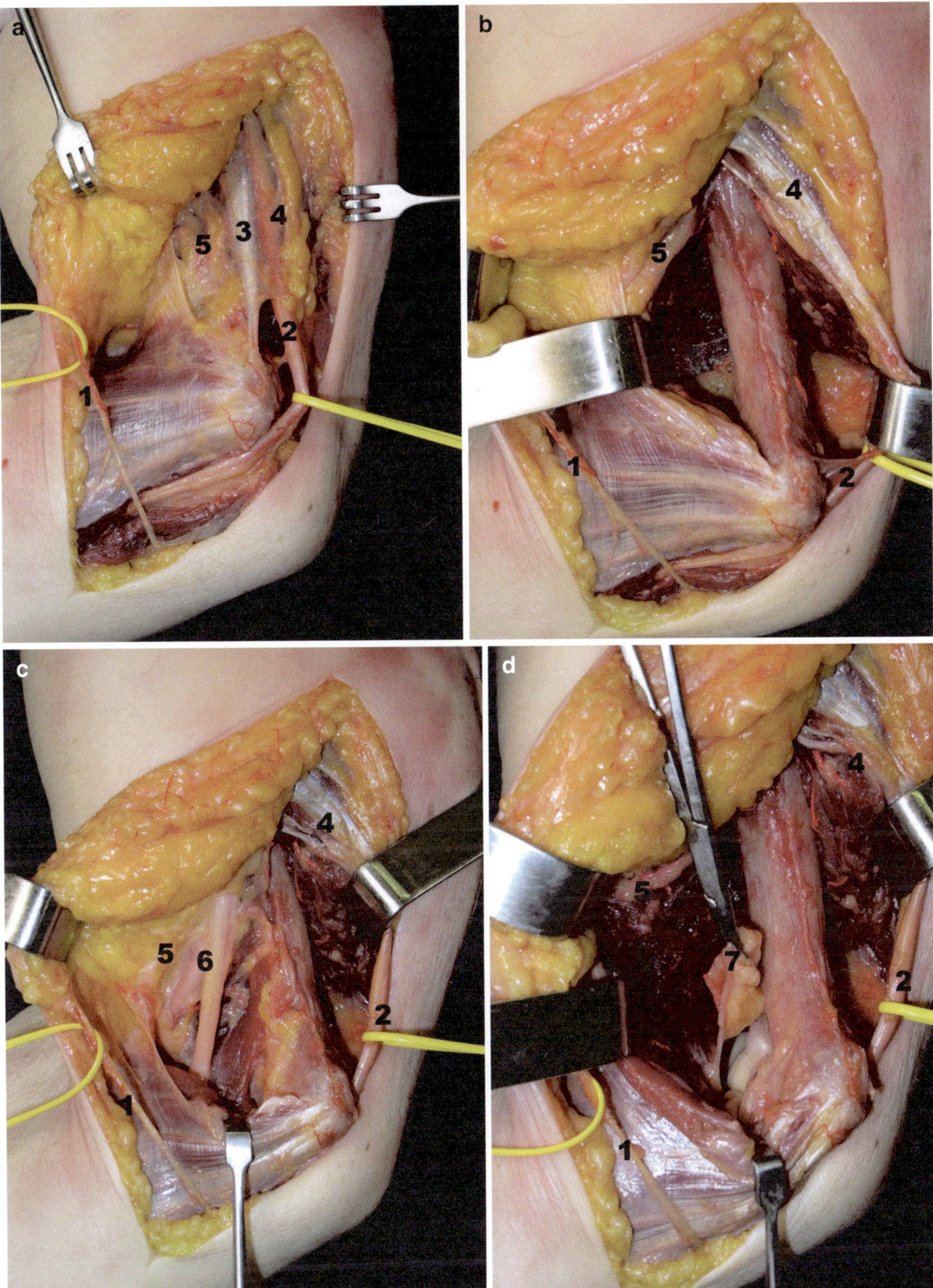

Fig. 1.10 The "over-the-top" approach. (**a**) Identification and protection of the *medial antebrachial cutaneous nerve* (MABCN) and ulnar nerve. Localize the medial intermuscular septum proximally, between the triceps and *brachialis* muscles. (**b**) Deepening the intermuscular interval gives access to the distal humerus and proximal elbow joint. (**c**) Distally, the surgical approach runs through *pronator teres* muscle and common flexor tendon. Be careful with the neurovascular bundle (brachial vessels and median nerve). (**d**) This is a wide exposure that gives access to the elbow joint anteriorly and posteriorly. *1 Medial antebrachial cutaneous nerve* (MABCN), *2* ulnar nerve, *3* intermuscular septum; *4* triceps muscle, *5 brachialis* muscle, *6* neurovascular bundle, *7* joint capsule

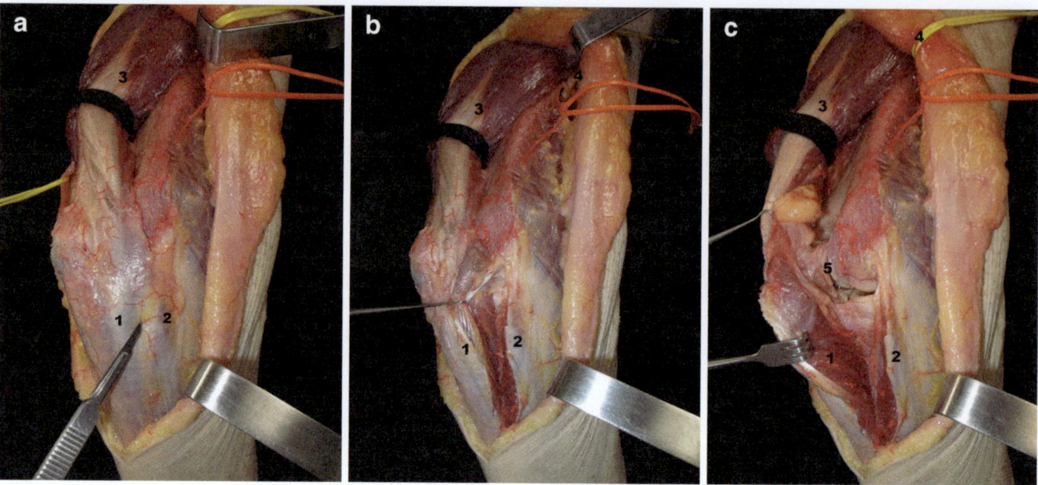

Fig. 1.11 The Mayo-modified Kocher posterolateral approach. (**a**) Midline posterior skin incision. Distally localize the Kocher interval (between *anconeus* and *extensor carpi ulnaris* muscles). (**b**) Approach through the Kocher interval. Proximally develop the interval between triceps muscle and lateral intermuscular septum. Note the continuity between the *vastus medialis* and *anconeus* muscles (both muscles share the same motor branch). (**c**) Deepen the approach to gain access to the elbow joint. Note the location of the ulnar nerve proximally. *1 Anconeus* muscle, *2 extensor carpi ulnaris* muscle, *3* triceps muscle, *4* radial nerve, *5* elbow joint

neuropraxia. On the other hand, the double incision has a higher risk of heterotopic ossification. Complications are greatly reduced if surgery is performed promptly.

Single Incision Approach

A transverse skin incision 4 cm distal to the anterior elbow crease is performed. Protection of the LABCN is mandatory but full dissection is probably not necessary (Fig. 1.12) [15]. Milking the biceps muscle belly usually delivers the tendon into the wound.

There are many different methods of repair of the distal biceps but all include grasping the tendon with a self-reinforcing suture and performing a tunnel on the radial tuberosity where the tendon is introduced.

The risk of radial nerve palsy is related to the position of retractors over the radial tuberosity to improve visualization or when the drilling on the radial tuberosity is performed. This risk may be reduced by retracting with a Farabeuf-type retractor and by angling the drill 30° medially.

Recurrent radial vessels typically have to be identified and ligated to avoid hematomas that can increase the incidence of heterotopic ossification.

Two-Incision Approach

When performing a two-incision technique in the acute setting, the tract of the tendon from the anterior incision to the radial tuberosity may be easily identified. A long curved haemostat is used to penetrate the interosseous membrane around the radial tuberosity, trying to stay away from the ulna, as this will diminish the rate of heterotopic ossification [12]. The haemostat is then advanced through the extensor carpi ulnaris, tenting the skin on the posterolateral aspect of the proximal forearm, indicating the site of the skin incision for the posterior approach.

Total Elbow Arthroplasty

Indications for total elbow arthroplasty include distal humeral fractures, nonunions, inflammatory arthropathies and posttraumatic osteoarthritis. As a principle, an Alonso-Llames approach should be used whenever possible because it obviates the complications associated with the triceps. The main limitation of this approach is that it provides less exposure than the Bryan-Morrey approach [5]. Other useful approaches go through the triceps tendon and have been previously described.

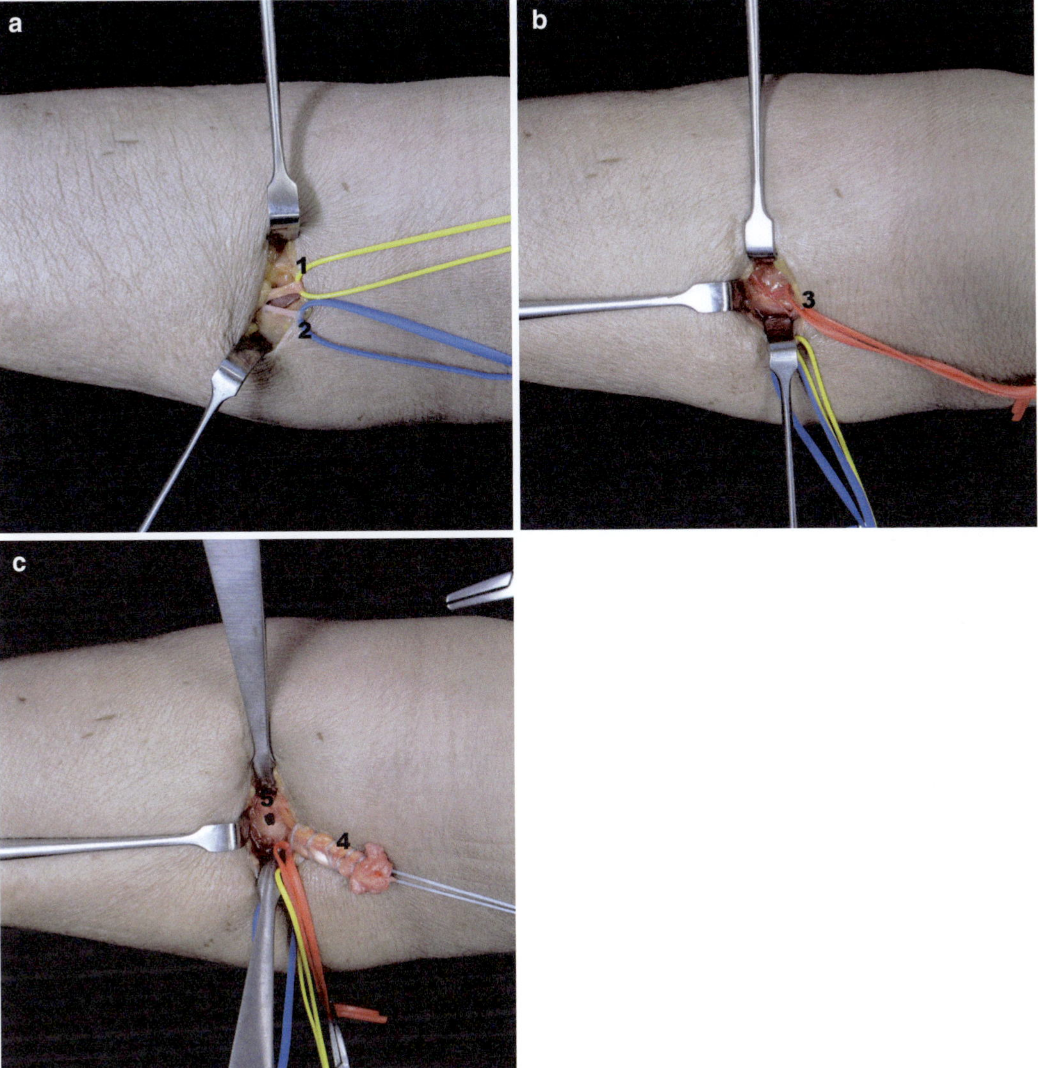

Fig. 1.12 The anterior approach for distal biceps insertion. Close-up of the anterior aspect of the elbow; hand is on your left and shoulder on your right. (**a**) Transverse incision and identification of the *lateral antebrachial cutaneous nerve* (LABCN) and cephalic vein. (**b**) Deepen the plane between the mobile wad of Henry and biceps-brachialis muscles and identify and ligate if necessary the recurrent radial vessels. At the bottom of this interval is the radial nerve that should be preserved. (**c**) Grasping suture of the distal biceps tendon and tunnel on the radial tuberosity. *1* LACB nerve, *2* cephalic vein, *3* recurrent radial vessels, *4* distal biceps tendon, *5* radial tuberosity

Bryan-Morrey Approach

A long posterior skin incision is performed just slightly lateral to the tip of the olecranon. After elevating the cutaneous flaps, the ulnar nerve is dissected and protected throughout the procedure, especially with the dislocation manoeuvre performed. At the end of the procedure, it is usually transposed anteriorly into a subcutaneous pouch.

The triceps is released from the entire posterior aspect of the distal humerus (Fig. 1.13). The forearm fascia and ulnar periosteum are elevated from the medial margin of the ulna. The triceps tendon is carefully detached from the tip of the olecranon by sharp dissection of Sharpey's fibres. The lateral margin of the proximal ulna is then identified and the anconeus is elevated from its ulnar bed. Finally, the extensor mechanism is reflected laterally from the margin of the lateral epicondyle.

Reconstruction of the extensor mechanism is an integral part of the procedure and it includes

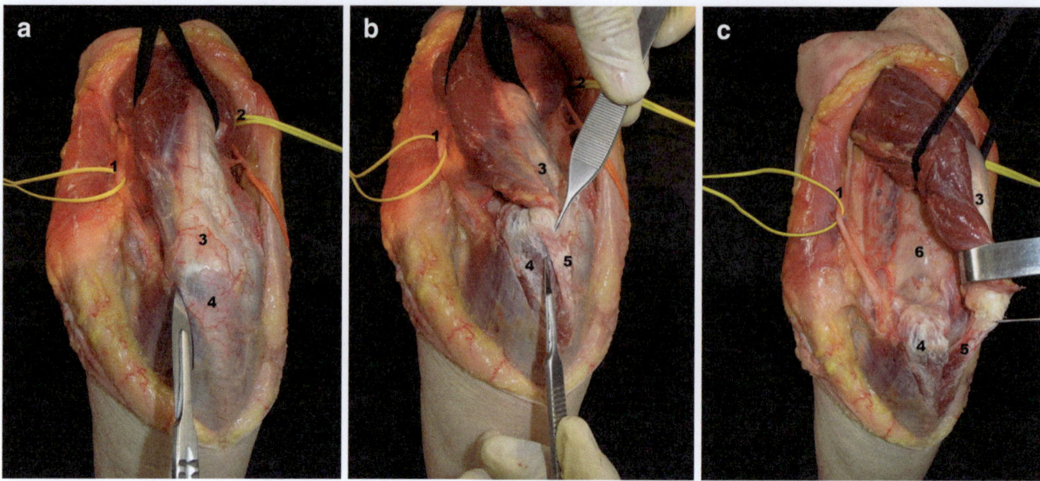

Fig. 1.13 The Bryan-Morrey approach. Triceps tendon should be everted from medial to lateral. (**a**) Posterior midline incision. The first step is identification of the ulnar nerve and the medial border of triceps. Identification of the radial nerve in the upper part of the lateral area is rarely needed. (**b**) Detachment of the triceps tendon from the olecranon. (**c**) Laterally, the *anconeus* muscle is elevated from the ulna and the whole extensor mechanism is reflected laterally. *1* Ulnar nerve, *2* radial nerve, *3* triceps tendon, *4* olecranon, *5* *anconeus* muscle, *6* distal humerus

performing two oblique and one transverse bone tunnels in the olecranon. A Krackow stitch is passed through the triceps tendon and then passed in a criss-cross manner through the proximal ulna. Postoperative protection of extension against resistance is recommended.

Conclusion

A thorough knowledge of the anatomical structures is key to perform a safe approach and is critical in the success for the different procedures performed in the elbow. An emphasis on the location of neurovascular structures in relation with the approach has been made because these are the most disastrous complications in elbow surgery. Following the surgical principles outlined at the beginning of the chapter will probably help the surgeon to perform effective elbow surgery while minimizing complications.

References

1. Harty M, Joyce III JJ. Surgical approaches to the elbow. J Bone Joint Surg Am. 1964;46:1598–606.
2. Alonso-Llames M. Bilaterotricipital approach to the elbow. Acta Orthop Scand. 1972;43:479–90.
3. Campbell WC. Incision for exposure of the elbow joint. Am J Surg. 1932;15:65–7.
4. Shahane SA, Stanley D. A posterior approach to the elbow joint. J Bone Joint Surg Br. 2000;81:1020–2.
5. Bryan RS, Morrey BF. Extensive posterior exposure of the elbow: a triceps sparing approach. Clin Orthop Relat Res. 1982;166:188–92.
6. O'Driscoll SW. The triceps-reflecting anconeus pedicle (TRAP) approach for distal humeral fractures and nonunions. Orthop Clin North Am. 2000;31(1):91–101.
7. MacAusland WR. Ankylosis of the elbow, with report of four cases treated by arthroplasty. JAMA. 1915;64:312–8.
8. Kaplan EB. Surgical approaches to the proximal end of the radius and its use in fractures of the head and neck of the radius. J Bone Joint Surg. 1941;23:86.
9. Kocher T. Text-book of operative surgery. 3rd ed. London: Adam and Charles Black; 1911. p. 313–8.
10. Strachan JH, Ellis BW. Vulnerability of the posterior interosseous nerve during radial head resection. J Bone Joint Surg. 1971;53B:320–3.
11. Dines JS, ElAttrache NS, Conway JE, Smith W, Ahmad CS. Clinical outcomes of the DANE TJ technique to treat ulnar collateral ligament insufficiency of the elbow. Am J Sports Med. 2007;35(12):2039–44.
12. Morrey BF. Surgical exposures. In: The Shoulder and its disorders. 3rd ed. Philadelphia, W.B. Saunders; 2000. p. 109–134.
13. Mansat P, Morrey BF. The Column Procedure: a limited lateral approach for extrinsic contracture of the elbow. J Bone Joint Surg Am. 1998;80:1603–15.
14. Kasparyan NG, Hotchkiss RN. Dynamic skeletal fixation in the upper extremity. Hand Clin. 1997;13:643–63.
15. Henry AK. Extensile exposure. 2nd ed. Edinburgh and London: E & S Livingstone; 1966. p. 113–115s.

Lateral Elbow Pain

Samuel Antuña and Raúl Barco

Abstract

Lateral elbow pain is one of the most common sources of medical consultation for elbow disorders. The aetiology of lateral elbow pain is reviewed with an emphasis on the differential diagnosis including key aspects of clinical examination and imaging for lateral epicondylitis, plica, osteochondritis dissecans, radiocapitellar arthritis and posterolateral rotatory instability. Nonoperative and operative treatment of lateral elbow pain is discussed.

Keywords

Lateral elbow pain • Diagnosis • Treatment

Epidemiology

Pain on the lateral aspect of the elbow is probably the most common reason for consultation in patients with non-traumatic elbow pain. Although the majority of patients are categorized as having tendinous problems, there are many other pathologic conditions that mimic lateral epicondylitis (LE). Lateral elbow pain accounts for 5–7/1,000 visits to a general practitioner, affecting equally middle-age males and females [1]. It is quite prevalent among racket sport players, but is also common in work-related problems. Orthopaedic surgeons will face throughout their career many patients with lateral elbow pain. It is therefore desirable to be capable of identifying the aetiology of the pain in order to indicate the most appropriate treatment.

S. Antuña, MD, PhD, FEBOT (✉)
Shoulder and Elbow Unit,
Department of Orthopaedic Surgery
and Traumatology, Hospital Universitario La Paz,
Castellana 261, Madrid 28046, Spain
e-mail: santuna@asturias.com

R. Barco, MD, PhD, FEBOT
Shoulder and Elbow Unit,
Department of Orthopaedic Surgery
and Traumatology, Hospital Universitario La Paz,
Hospital Madrid Norte Sanchinarro,
Paseo de la Castellana 261, Madrid 28046, Spain
e-mail: raulbarco@hotmail.com

The Problem

When interviewing a patient with elbow pain referred to the lateral aspect of the joint, there are three main questions that should be raised to make an initial approach to the most probable cause. We need to know if there is a history of trauma to the

S. Antuña, R. Barco (eds.), *Essentials in Elbow Surgery,*
DOI 10.1007/978-1-4471-4625-4_2, © Springer-Verlag London 2014

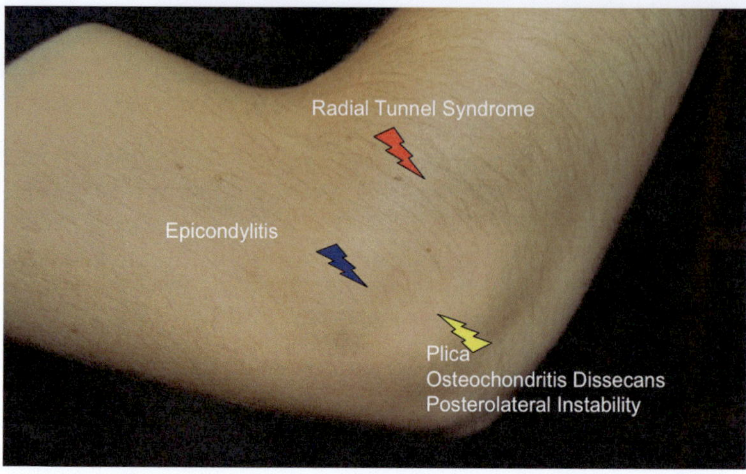

Fig. 2.1 Categorization of lateral elbow pain is initially done according to its location

elbow: If the patient refers a major traumatic event as an elbow dislocation or radial head fracture, we should probably focus more on intraarticular problems as instability, osteochondral damage or a plica; minor, repetitive strains should make us think on the possibility of LE or radial tunnel syndrome (RTS). Secondly, we need to know the age of the patient; young patients with elbow pain should make us think about osteochondritis dissecans (OD) or plica; middle-age population more commonly have tendinous problems or radial nerve compression, especially if they relate a history of repetitive prono-supination movements or continuous strains to the wrist extensors. Finally the third question is where they feel the pain: whether it is on the lateral epicondyle, suggesting LE; posterior to it, suggesting a plica or OD; or inferior to it, suggesting RTS (Fig. 2.1).

Patient Workup

Clinical Exam

After the initial interview with the patient, we should perform a detailed physical exam. Pain with palpation just slightly anterior and superior to the most prominent part of the lateral epicondyle is almost exclusive of LE. If pain is elicited more posteriorly and distally, at the level of the radiocapitellar joint, it could be caused by an osteochondral lesion – which would be identified

by palpating the posterior part of the capitellum, just proximal to the radial head – or by synovial plica if the pain is referred at the joint level. Instability does not cause pain on palpation, and it should be examined by provocative manoeuvres. Pain distal to the epicondyle, at the level of the supinator muscle, just anterior to the mobile wad of the brachioradialis, is very suggestive of RTS.

There are several clinical tests that have proved to be useful for the clinical workup of lateral elbow pain. If we ask the patient to extend the wrist against resistance with the elbow flexed to 90°, it may cause mild pain on the extensor carpi radialis brevis (ECRB) insertion when there is LE; however, if we repeat this manoeuvre with the elbow fully extended, it is invariably positive when there is LE. This simple test has been extremely useful in our practice to differentiate LE from other diagnosis (Fig. 2.2). Pain over the lateral epicondyle with resisted extension of the third finger may also be positive with LE, indicating extension of the degenerative process in to the extensor digitorum communis.

The flexion-pronation test was described to detect entrapping synovial plica into the radiocapitellar joint [2]. It is positive if a snap is reproduced by passively flexing a pronated arm in the range of 90–110° of flexion (Fig. 2.3).

The active radiocapitellar compression test was described to detect intraarticular pathology compatible with OD [3]. The patient makes active prono-supination movements while axially loading the arm (Fig. 2.4). It is positive if the

Fig. 2.2 If lateral elbow pain is caused by lateral epicondylitis (LE), the comparative test of resisted wrist extension with the elbow flexed 90° (**a**) and fully extended (**b**) is very useful. Patients with LE have significantly more intense pain anterior to the lateral epicondyle when the manoeuvre is done with the elbow extended

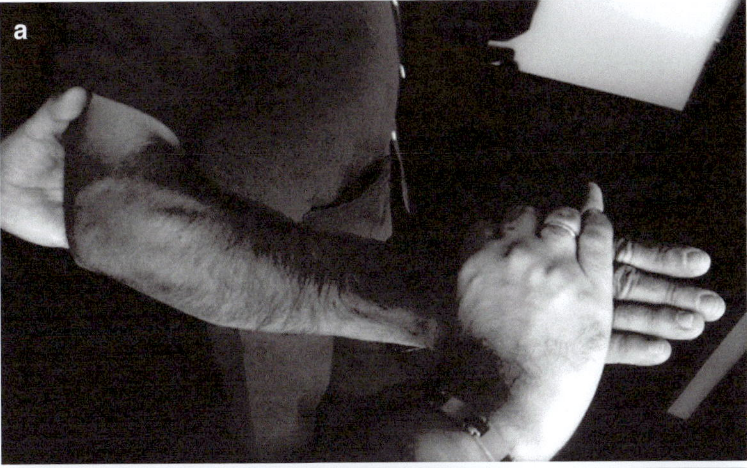

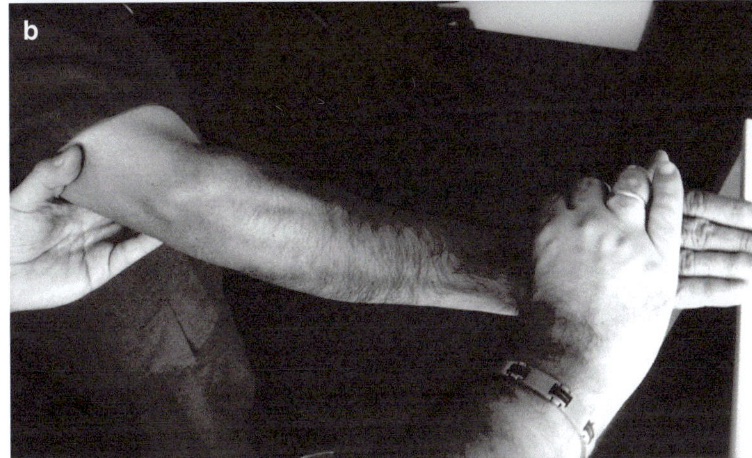

Fig. 2.3 The flexion-pronation test is positive if the symptoms are reproduced even without a snapping. The forearm is maximally pronated and passively flexed to 90–110°. The snapping can be felt during this limited range of motion

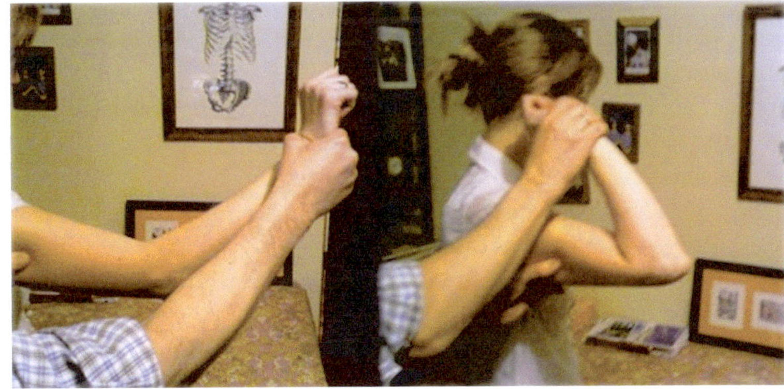

patient experiences pain over the posterior and lateral aspect of the elbow.

In order to rule out a RTS, there are several manoeuvres that can be done, although they have not shown high sensitivity and specificity. The radial tunnel compression test is performed by palpating the anterior aspect of the radial neck in the area where the radial nerve enters the arcade of Frohse, just anterior to the mobile wad [4]. If patient experiences pain, especially if there is no

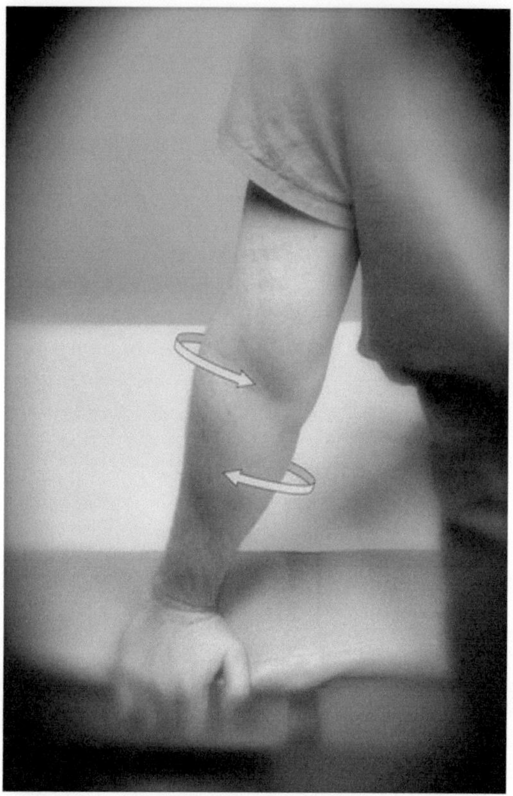

Fig. 2.4 The radiocapitellar compression test for osteochondritis dissecans. The patient pronates and supinates the forearm (*curved arrows*) in full extension causing compression at the radiocapitellar joint. The test is positive if there is reproduction of patient's symptoms

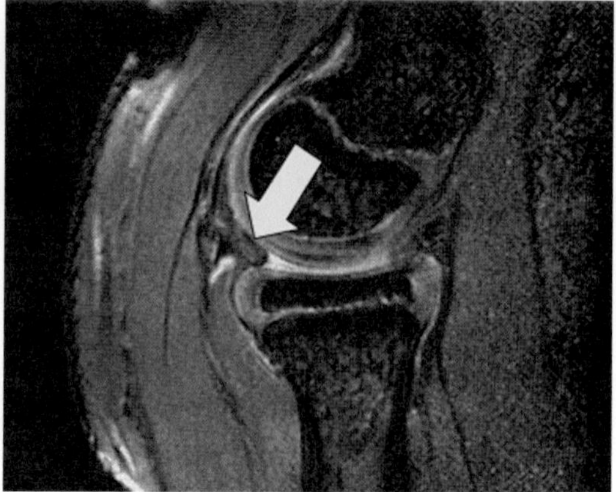

Fig. 2.5 MRI of a patient with a synovial fold entrapping into the radiocapitellar joint (*arrow*)

the ECRB. If the X-rays are normal and the clinical exam orients towards LE, no more radiographic studies should probably be made. Ultrasound or MRI does not add very much information when LE is suspected. If, however, the diagnosis is unclear, and the physician is unsure on what is causing pain, an MRI of the elbow would help excluding other cause of RTS as tumours or ganglions [6]. High-resolution MRI can be useful to detect radiocapitellar plica [7] (Fig. 2.5).

pain on the contralateral side, the test is considered positive. When there is pain with resisted forearm supination with the elbow extended, it may also be suggestive of RTS.

It is important to know that some patients will present with a non-conclusive clinical exam. It is also possible to see patients with symptoms compatible with two different entities. In fact, although it is very rarely seen, two pathologic processes may be present at the same time, as it occurs with lateral LE and RTS or LE with a plica [5].

Imaging

Simple radiographs of the elbow should be done to exclude the presence of radiocapitellar arthritis, OD or calcification on the proximal insertion of

Lateral Epicondylitis

Indications

LE is the most common cause of lateral elbow pain. The great majority of patients get better over time and do not need aggressive treatments. Oral medication and physiotherapy can help, but they have failed to prove clear benefit [8]. If pain persists beyond 3 months or the patient pursues a quicker recovery, we offer an injection of platelet-rich plasma. The studies available with this form of treatment have shown promising results [9, 10]. If this option does not solve the problem, surgical treatment is offered, although usually never before 6 months. Our preferred surgical treatment is arthroscopic debridement. Other surgical options are also valid, but no technique has demonstrated to be better than the others [11–13].

Surgical Technique

Arthroscopic release of LE implies resection of the degenerated tendon, usually only the ECRB and the adjacent capsule, which usually is tethered. Care must be taken not to debride posteriorly to the anterior third of the radial head, to avoid damage to the lateral collateral ligament.

Results and Complications

A patient with clinical diagnosis of LE will get better usually in 3 or 4 months with conservative measures. If the tendon fails to heal and becomes degenerated, the pain may persist and surgical debridement will be necessary [14]. The outcome of arthroscopic debridement is very good. Bad results are linked to wrong diagnosis, worker compensation or poor technique [13].

Chronic Lateral Instability

Indications

Lateral instability is a rare cause of lateral elbow pain, but it is quite important to acknowledge the possibility of developing iatrogenic instability after surgical treatment of LE [15]. This topic is well covered in Chap. 7. Patients with instability will present with a history of a major or minor traumatic event, or a previous surgical intervention on the lateral aspect of the elbow. They complain of non-specific pain, inability to perform tasks that involve extension and supination of the elbow and maybe catching and locking. Clinical exam is very specific and tries to reproduce the instability. Unfortunately if posterolateral instability is confirmed, the patient will need an operative intervention to reconstruct the ligaments.

Surgical Technique

When posterolateral rotatory instability is confirmed, reconstruction of the lateral ligament complex will be necessary. Our preferred method of reconstruction is the docking technique with triceps fascia or a semitendinosus allograft.

Results and Complications

The outcome of lateral instability surgery depends on the coexistence of intraarticular damage and associated injuries. If the elbow is unstable after LE treatment, reconstruction is usually very successful. If the patient had previous damage to the cartilage or fractures, the prognosis worsens [16].

Radial Tunnel Syndrome

Indications

Patients with RTS typically present with pain distal to the lateral epicondyle in the region of the mobile wad. It is usually a burning discomfort that increases after tasks that include wrist extension and forearm rotation. Pain is present at night and at rest. It is caused by irritation of the posterior interosseous nerve as it enters the arcade of Frohse on the supinator. There is no associated motor deficiency [4]. The most common reason is entrapment of the nerve due to muscle hypertrophy or due to inflammation and subsequent fibrosis of the proximal edge of the muscle (Fig. 2.6). Very uncommonly it may be caused by a mass. Other possible areas of compression are the proximal end of the ECRB (coexisting with LE) or the radial recurrent vessels [17]. Electromyography and nerve conduction studies are most commonly negative in this condition and do not help much in establishing the diagnosis. A trial injection of local anaesthetic may be used to see if symptoms resolve.

As it occurs with LE, the vast majority of patients get better with conservative treatment aimed to reduce the contracture of the supinator by massage, avoiding repetitive forearm rotational movements and local and systemic anti-inflammatory measures [18]. If there are no work compensation issues, and the patient does not improve after a reasonable time of 3–6 months, it may be wise to surgically explore the

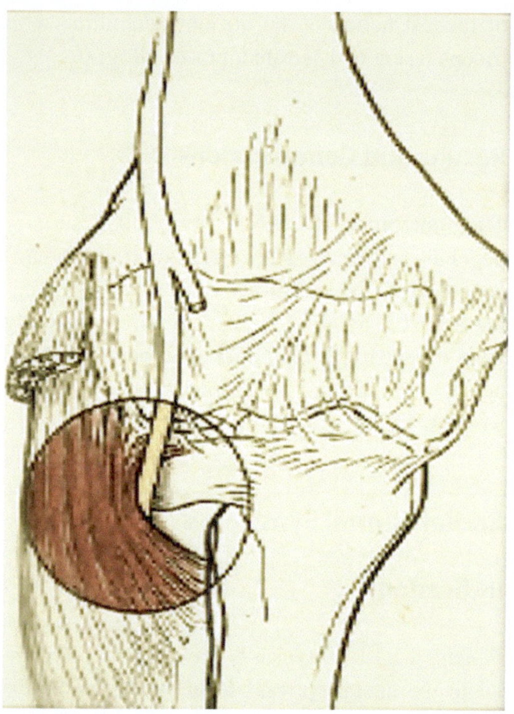

Fig. 2.6 The radial nerve entering the supinator. This is the most common site for nerve compression

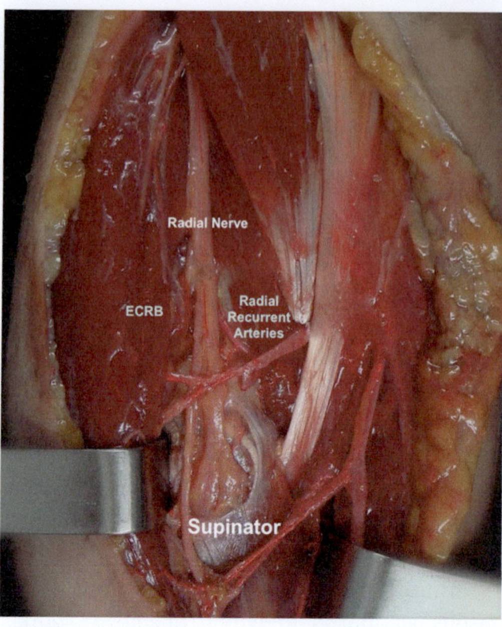

Fig. 2.7 Anatomical preparation showing the potential areas of compression of the nerve leading to radial tunnel syndrome

nerve and release the proximal part of the supinator. Obviously if the imaging test shows an anatomical abnormality or mass, it should be corrected.

Surgical Technique

The surgical procedure involves releasing the radial nerve from the origin of the ECRB to the distal end of the supinator. This is best performed through an anterior approach of Henry, which allows complete dissection of the radial nerve addressing all possible areas of compression (Fig. 2.7).

Results and Complications

Conservative treatment of RTS with splinting and physiotherapy usually leads to resolution of symptoms. Very rarely patients do not get better and surgical intervention may be the last option.

In the past it was thought that this condition coexisted with LE very often [17]. However, this is not our experience, and it may well be that it has been over-diagnosed. In fact it is an infrequent diagnosis in our practice. The results of operative treatment depend on the presence of additional symptoms or confusing diagnoses. If the patient is not worker compensation, and the diagnosis is clear, usually the patients get better. They also get better if the nerve compression is due to a ganglion or a tumour. However, the outcome might be unpredictable if this operation is performed for idiopathic RTS in a manual worker with concomitant LE. Most reports give no more than a 70 % probability of improving [19, 20].

Plica Syndrome

Indications

The presence of a radiocapitellar synovial fold has been recognized for many years. The fact that the plica may be a cause of elbow pain was confirmed by several studies that showed improvement of lateral elbow pain after plica excision [21, 22]. As it occurs with RTS and LE, it has been said that plica and LE commonly coexist. Our experience is that they do not. Moreover, pain coming from a plica usually follows a minor trauma to the elbow and sometimes can be seen after undisplaced radial head fractures. Under those circumstances, the plica may become inflamed and thickened, entrapping into the radiocapitellar joint and causing reactive synovitis. Patients have pain posterolateral to the lateral epicondyle, which can be reproduced by palpating the radiohumeral space laterally and posteriorly. Occasionally they refer a clicking or catching sensation with flexion of the elbow. The flexion-pronation test may be useful, but is not always positive [2]. The diagnosis should be made by exclusion because imaging studies are not sensitive to detect this entity [23]. Therefore, if a patient has continuous pain that is not due to LE or RTS, and has the history compatible with plica, an arthroscopic examination may be warranted [24–26].

Surgical Technique

Arthroscopic excision of the plica, if performed properly, resolves the symptoms. From the anteromedial portal, the radial head is examined and an area of synovitis is normally found with a fold overhanging the radial head (Fig. 2.8). Removal of the plica should be completed by entering the elbow through the posterolateral portal and excision of the posterior extension of the synovial fold. Failing to do this posterior resection is one of the most common reasons for lack of improvement in these patients.

Results and Complications

The reported results of radiocapitellar plica excision are presented in Table 2.1. If the diagnosis is correct, the procedure solves the problem. Reasons for failure are inappropriate resection, confusing diagnosis and worker-compensation issues.

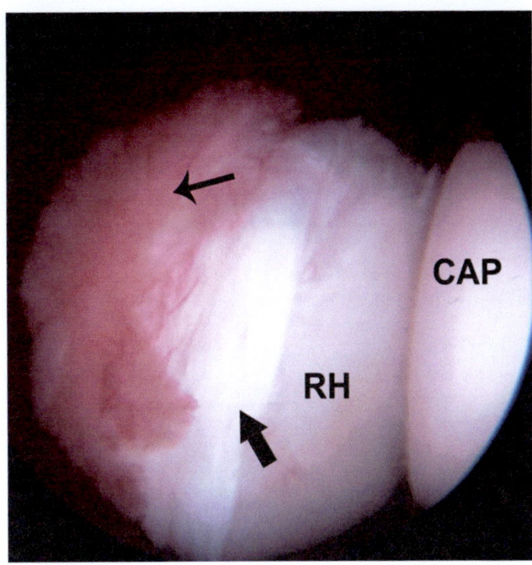

Fig. 2.8 Arthroscopic view of a synovial plica over the radial head with a surrounding area of synovitis *RH* radial head, *CAP* capitellum

Osteochondritis Dissecans

Indications

OD is not a common diagnosis in the elbow. It is seen in adolescents and young adults. It must be differentiated from Panner's disease, which is a growth disorder with avascular necrosis of the lateral condyle that resolves spontaneously the vast majority of times. OD is due to a combination of ischemia and repetitive microtrauma to an elbow that is subjected to valgus stress, as it occurs in throwing athletes as baseball players [27]. But it can also be seen in patients with no throwing demands. Typically, patients have pain along the joint line posteriorly with symptoms consistent with locking or catching. A flexion contracture is usually present when they first visit the surgeon. Patients do not recall any significant traumatic event. In early cases of OD, posteroanterior and lateral radiographs of the elbow will show a radiolucency area in the capitellum, typically in its anterolateral aspect (Fig. 2.9). In the later stages, fragmentation, sclerosis and loose bodies may be seen (Fig. 2.10). There are several classification systems based on the integrity of the cartilage cap, presence of loose bodies and MRI appearance [28,

Table 2.1 Results after arthroscopic treatment of symptomatic synovial plica of the elbow

Author(s) (year)	Number of elbows	Procedure or approach	Mean patient age (range)	Mean follow-up (range)	Results
Kim et al. (2006) [26]	12	Arthroscopic resection	21 (71–33)	33 months (24–65)	11 patients healed 1 patient with MCL instablility
Huang et al. (2005) [23]	1	Arthroscopic resection	21	8 months	Complete relief of symptoms
Fukase et al. (2006) [7]	1	Open resection	12	12 months	Complete relief of symptoms
Aoki et al. (2003) [25]	2	Arthroscopic resection	16 (14–19)	5 months	Complete relief of symptoms
Antuña and O'Driscoll (2001) [2]	14	Arthroscopic resection	36 (27–48)	24 months (6–66)	10 patients had complete relief of symptoms 2 patients had mild pain without snapping after surgery 2 patients did not benefit: one with associated mild instability and one with recurrence of symptoms after 4 years
Akagi and Nakamura (1998) [24]	1	Combined arthroscopic-open resection	27	6 weeks	Complete relief of symptoms

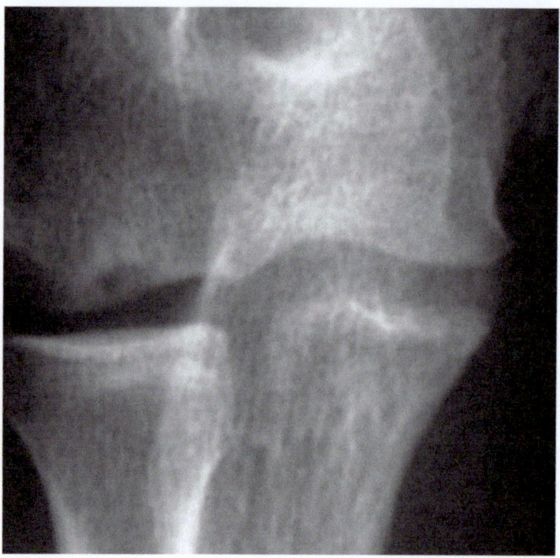

Fig. 2.9 AP radiograph of a patient with OD of the capitellum in an early stage, presenting as a radiolucent area without fragmentation

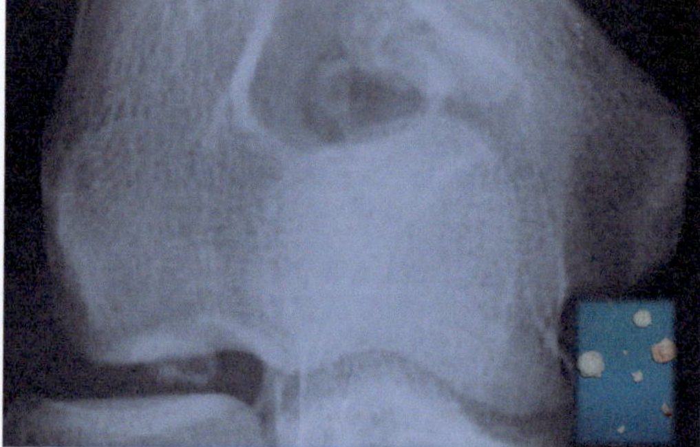

Fig. 2.10 AP radiograph of a patient with advance OD and the bony fragments which were removed arthroscopically

29]. However, Takahara has described one of the simpler classifications [30, 31] (Table 2.2). Stable lesions are those in which the patient has a full elbow range of motion and an open capitellar growth plate and localized flattening or radiolucency of the subchondral bone. These stable lesions usually heal with rest. Unstable lesions have either closed growth plates, loss of motion of more than 20° or fragmentation. Unstable lesions require surgery in order to heal. Another classification system grades lesions with intact articular cartilage as type I, lesions with cartilage fracture or displaced bone as type II and OD with completely detached fragments as type III [27]. However, there is no agreement regarding the best classification system, and no classification system has shown the ability to accurately predict healing or to direct treatment.

Surgical Technique

Patients with OD of the elbow usually come to our clinic late, when the elbow has an extension

Table 2.2 Takahara classification of OD of the capitellum

	Capitellar growth plate	Capitellar lesion	Range of motion	ICRS classification
Stable	Open	Radiolucent	Normal	I: continuous
Unstable	Closed	Fragmentation	Restricted	II: partial discontinuity
				III: complete discontinuity
				IV: dislocated or loose

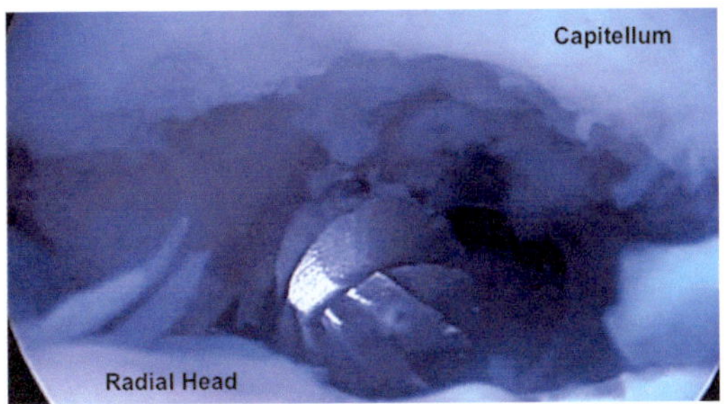

Fig. 2.11 Arthroscopic view of a remaining defect after debridement of an osteochondral defect of the capitellum

contracture and symptoms of catching and recurrent joint effusion. When an unstable, fragmented osteochondral lesion is found, the more common procedure is debridement, abrasion chondroplasty, loose body removal and microfracture (Fig. 2.11). In the very rare instance in which the patients present with an intact cartilage cap and it is considered that the injury is acute, fixation with absorbable pins can be considered. Fragment fixation is only considered for small, acute lesions. Even after successful reattachment, later collapse and joint degeneration may occur. Most studies indicate little or no clinical benefit with fragment fixation [32, 33]. When there is a big defect affecting the lateral aspect of the capitellum, compromising the tracking of the radial head, osteochondral transplantation should be considered; this procedure would be done through an open approach. Patients with stable lesions are treated conservatively, by rest, splinting and cessation of throwing activity for a minimum period of 3–6 months.

Results and Complications

Healing is achieved in 91 % of stage I lesions and 53 % of stage II lesions treated conservatively [34] (Fig. 2.12). Fragment removal alone and

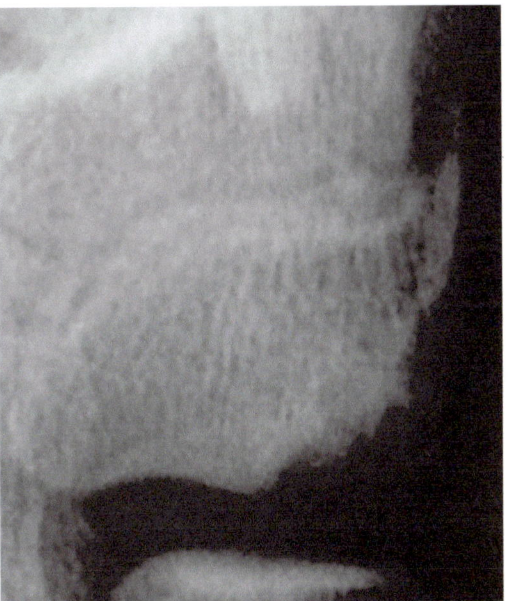

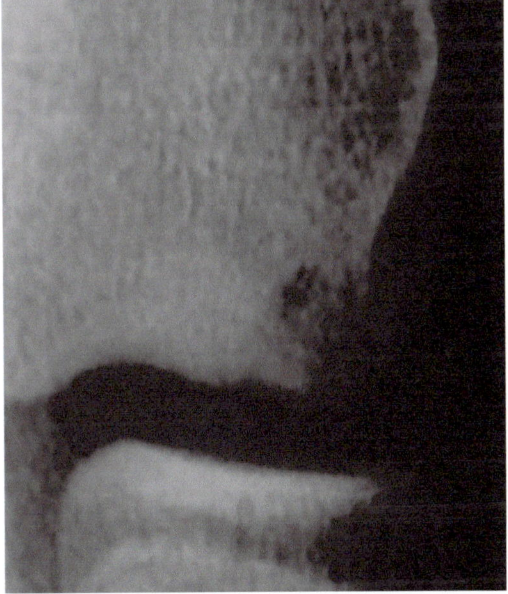

Fig. 2.12 AP radiograph of a stable OD that was treated conservatively and healed with no residual functional deficit

debridement for defects of <50 % of the capitellum results in an outcome similar to that achieved with fragment fixation or reconstruction [32, 35]. Bauer et al. presented the outcome of 31 patients with OD of the humeral capitellum treated with debridement and followed for an average of 23 years [36]. Almost half of the patients had pain, and 60 % showed radiographic progression of disease. A few series have presented the outcome of osteochondral transplantation in small group of patients with large defects and have shown very good clinical results and healing rate [37, 38].

Conclusion

Being able to make the right diagnosis in a patient with lateral elbow pain will save many unnecessary complementary studies or even unnecessary surgical procedures. The key to achieve a correct diagnosis is a detailed clinical exam. When the elbow is stiff or there is pain with resisted pronation and supination, intraarticular pathology should be suspected. LE, OD and plica may be difficult to differentiate, but in our practice very rarely coexist; therefore, every attempt should be made to locate precisely the area where pain originates. Clinical manoeuvres may help in differentiating these three entities. Many patients with lateral elbow pain will get getter with conservative treatment. If an operation is necessary, arthroscopy has become the standard approach to fully understand the pathology and correct it.

References

1. Berglund KM, Persson BH, Denison E. Prevalence of pain and dysfunction in the cervical and thoracic spine in persons with and without lateral elbow pain. Man Ther. 2008,13(4).295–9.
2. Antuña SA, O'Driscoll SW. Snapping plicae associated with radiocapitellar chondromalacia. Arthroscopy. 2001;17(5):491–5.
3. Baumgarten TE, Andrews JR, Satterwhite YE. The arthroscopic classification and treatment of osteochondritis dissecans of the capitellum. Am J Sports Med. 1998;26:520–3.
4. Naam NH, Nemani S. Radial tunnel syndrome. Orthop Clin North Am. 2012;43(4):529–36.
5. Rhyou IH, Kim KW. Is posterior synovial plica excision necessary for refractory lateral epicondylitis of the elbow? Clin Orthop Relat Res. 2013;471(1):284–90.
6. Ferdinand BD, Rosenberg ZS, Schweitzer ME, Stuchin SA, Jazrawi LM, Lenzo SR, Meislin RJ, Kiprovski K. MR imaging features of radial tunnel syndrome: initial experience. Radiology. 2006;240(1):161–8.
7. Fukase N, Kokubu T, Fujioka H, Iwama Y, Fujii M, Kurosaka M. Usefulness of MRI for diagnosis of painful snapping elbow. Skeletal Radiol. 2006;35(10):797–800.
8. Pattanittum P, Turner T, Green S, Buchbinder R. Non-steroidal anti-inflammatory drugs (NSAIDs) for treating lateral elbow pain in adults. Cochrane Database Syst Rev. 2013;5:CD003686.
9. Gosens T, Peerbooms JC, van Laar W, den Oudsten BL. Ongoing positive effect of platelet-rich plasma versus corticosteroid injection in lateral epicondylitis: a double-blind randomized controlled trial with 2-year follow-up. Am J Sports Med. 2011;39(6):1200–8.
10. Krogh TP, Bartels EM, Ellingsen T, Stengaard-Pedersen K, Buchbinder R, Fredberg U, Bliddal H, Christensen R. Comparative effectiveness of injection therapies in lateral epicondylitis: a systematic review and network meta-analysis of randomized controlled trials. Am J Sports Med. 2013;41(6):1435–46.
11. Buchbinder R, Johnston RV, Barnsley L, Assendelft WJ, Bell SN, Smidt N. Surgery for lateral elbow pain. Cochrane Database Syst Rev. 2011;3:CD003525.
12. Lo MY, Safran MR. Surgical treatment of lateral epicondylitis: a systematic review. Clin Orthop Relat Res. 2007;463:98–106. Review.
13. Wada T, Moriya T, Iba K, Ozasa Y, Sonoda T, Aoki M, Yamashita T. Functional outcomes after arthroscopic treatment of lateral epicondylitis. J Orthop Sci. 2009;14(2):167–74.
14. Nirschl RP. Elbow tendinosis/tennis elbow. Clin Sports Med. 1992;11(4):851–70.
15. Mehta JA, Bain GI. Posterolateral rotatory instability of the elbow. J Am Acad Orthop Surg. 2004;12(6):405–15. Review.
16. Sanchez-Sotelo J, Morrey BF, O'Driscoll SW. Ligamentous repair and reconstruction for posterolateral rotatory instability of the elbow. J Bone Joint Surg Br. 2005;87(1):54–61.
17. Henry M, Stutz C. A unified approach to radial tunnel syndrome and lateral tendinosis. Tech Hand Up Extrem Surg. 2006;10(4):200–5.
18. Sanders WE. Radial tunnel syndrome. An investigation of compression neuropathy as a possible cause. J Bone Joint Surg Am. 1992;74(2):309–10.
19. Lee JT, Azari K, Jones NF. Long term results of radial tunnel release–the effect of co-existing tennis elbow, multiple compression syndromes and workers' compensation. J Plast Reconstr Aesthet Surg. 2008;61(9):1095–9.
20. Jebson PJ, Engber WD. Radial tunnel syndrome: long-term results of surgical decompression. J Hand Surg Am. 1997;22(5):889–96.
21. Clarke R. Symptomatic, lateral synovial fringe (plica) of the elbow joint. Arthroscopy. 1988;4:112–6.
22. Commandre FA, Taillan B, Benezis C, Follacci FM, Hammou JC. Plica synovialis (synovial fold) of the elbow. report on one case. J Sports Med Phys Fit. 1988;28:209–10.

23. Huang GS, Lee CH, Lee HS, Chen CY. MRI, arthroscopy, and histologic observations of an annular ligament causing painful snapping of the elbow joint. AJR Am J Roentgenol. 2005;185(2):397–9.
24. Akagi M, Nakamura T. Snapping elbow caused by the synovial fold in the radiohumeral joint. J Shoulder Elbow Surg. 1998;7(4):427–9.
25. Aoki M, Okamura K, Yamashita T. Snapping annular ligament of the elbow joint in the throwing arms of young brothers. Arthroscopy. 2003;19(8):E4–7.
26. Kim DH, Gambardella RA, Elattrache NS, Yocum LA, Jobe FW. Arthroscopic treatment of posterolateral elbow impingement from lateral synovial plicae in throwing athletes and golfers. Am J Sports Med. 2006;34(3):438–44.
27. Difelice G, Meunier M, Paletta G. Elbow injury in the adolescent athlete. In: Altchek D, Andrews J, editors. The athlete's elbow. Philadelphia: Lippincott Williams & Wilkins; 2001. p. 231–48.
28. Jans LB, Ditchfield M, Anna G, Jaremko JL, Verstraete KL. MR imaging findings and MR criteria for instability in osteochondritis dissecans of the elbow in children. Eur J Radiol. 2012;81(6):1306–10.
29. Kijowski R, De Smet AA. MRI findings of osteochondritis dissecans of the capitellum with surgical correlation. AJR Am J Roentgenol. 2005;185(6):1453–9.
30. Takahara M, Mura N, Sasaki J, Harada M, Ogino T. Classification, treatment, and outcome of osteochondritis dissecans of the humeral capitellum: surgical technique. J Bone Joint Surg Am. 2008;90:47–62.
31. Takahara M, Mura N, Sasaki J, Harada M, Ogino T. Classification, treatment and outcome of osteochondritis dissecans of the humeral capitellum. J Bone Joint Surg Am. 2007;89:1205–14.
32. Baker 3rd CL, Baker Jr CL, Romeo AA. Osteochondritis dissecans of the capitellum. J Shoulder Elbow Surg. 2010;19(2 Suppl):76–82.
33. Nobuta S, Ogawa K, Sato K, Nakagawa T, Hatori M, Itoi E. Clinical outcome of fragment fixation for osteochondritis dissecans of the elbow. Ups J Med Sci. 2008;113:201–8.
34. Takahara M, et al. Conservative treatment for osteochondrosis of the humeral capitellum. Am J Sports Med. 2008;36:868–72.
35. Miyake J, Masatomi T. Arthroscopic debridement of the humeral capitellum for osteochondritis dissecans: radiographic and clinical outcomes. J Hand Surg Am. 2011;36(8):1333–8.
36. Bauer M, Jonsson K, Josefsson P, Lindén B. Osteochondritis dissecans of the elbow: a long-term follow-up study. Clin Orthop Relat Res. 1992;284:156–60.
37. Ovesen J, Olsen BS, Johannsen HV. The clinical outcomes of mosaicplasty in the treatment of osteochondritis dissecans of the distal humeral capitellum of young athletes. J Shoulder Elbow Surg. 2011;20(5):813–8.
38. Shimada K, Tanaka H, Matsumoto T, Miyake J, Higuchi H, Gamo K, Fuji T. Cylindrical costal osteochondral autograft for reconstruction of large defects of the capitellum due to osteochondritis dissecans. J Bone Joint Surg Am. 2012;94(11):992–1002.

Medial Elbow Pain

Theodore A. Blaine, Opeyemi E. Lamikanra,
Paul M. Tomaszewski, and Alem Yacob

Abstract

Pain on the medial aspect of the elbow can be a source of disability. The focus of the chapter is to provide the required knowledge to correctly diagnose patients with medial elbow pain. Since several etiologies may coexist, the emphasis on correct diagnostic strategies is provided. Ulnar collateral ligament injuries, snapping triceps, medial epicondylitis, and ulnar nerve pathology are presented with key features of clinical exam, diagnostic tests, and current aspects of treatment.

Keywords

Medial elbow pain • Diagnosis • Treatment • Epicondylitis • Pediatric • Ulnar • Throwing • Athlete

T.A. Blaine, MD, MA, AB (✉)
Department of Orthopaedics and Rehabilitation,
Yale School of Medicine,
800 Howard Avenue, New Haven, CT 06520, USA
e-mail: theodore.blaine@yale.edu

O.E. Lamikanra, MD • P.M. Tomaszewski, MD, MS
Department of Orthopaedics and Rehabilitation,
Yale University School of Medicine,
800 Howard Avenue, New Haven, CT 06519, USA
e-mail: opeyemi.lamikanra@yale.edu;
paul.tomaszewski@yale.edu

A. Yacob, MD, MSc
Department of Orthopaedics and Rehabilitation,
Yale University School of Medicine,
Yale Physicians Building, 800 Howard Avenue,
New Haven, CT 06510, USA
e-mail: alem.yacob@yale.edu

The Problem

The number of persons involved in sports with an overhead-throwing component has grown significantly over the recent years. The intensity of training and the number of games played have also steeply risen. This increase in number, time, and intensity has led to an increased incidence of injuries to the medial elbow, including tendon, ligament, and bony injuries.

When the physician faces a patient with pain in the medial aspect of the elbow, it is important to know if it is caused by repetitive throwing or not. Many patients with medial epicondylitis do not refer continuous strain on the elbow, but they may be involved in work-related movements that aggravate their symptoms. In this chapter, we will

S. Antuña, R. Barco (eds.), *Essentials in Elbow Surgery*,
DOI 10.1007/978-1-4471-4625-4_3, © Springer-Verlag London 2014

present several provocative maneuvers that have been useful in our practice to differentiate among the anatomical structure that may be causing pain: ligament, tendon, bone, or nerve. However, when managing patients with medial elbow pain, one should be aware that some of these entities might coexist at the same time.

Ulnar Collateral Ligament Injury

Functional Anatomy of the Elbow

A review of the key anatomy of the elbow is necessary to understand common injuries to the medial elbow. The osseous structures provide approximately half of the stability to varus force of the elbow in extension. The anterior capsule, the ulnar and radial collateral ligaments, and the surrounding musculature deliver the remaining stability to the elbow. The ulnar collateral ligament (UCL) is the static restraint to a valgus force, while the flexor-pronator mass is a dynamic stabilizer [1].

The UCL of the elbow is comprised of three discrete ligamentous bands: the anterior bundle, posterior bundle, and transverse bundle. The anterior bundle is the primary stabilizer during a valgus load and taut during full extension of the deceleration phase [2]. It courses from the sublime tubercle of the coronoid to the medial condyle of the humerus. It is the stiffest of all the ligaments of the elbow with an average failure load of 260 N. The posterior bundle is more fan-shaped, originates on the medial epicondyle, and inserts on the medial margin of the semilunar notch. It is taut during flexion and thus more vulnerable to injury in the overthrowers [3].

Biomechanics of Throwing

The upper extremity of an overhead-throwing athlete sees extreme force, which may result in significant morbidity and loss of playing time. The baseball throw or pitch has historically been the biomechanical model for the overhead athlete as baseball players are the most commonly affected athletes. Understanding the biomechanics of throwing is key in understanding elbow pathology in this patient population [4].

A pitch can be divided into six distinct phases. Phase one begins with the windup. Although each pitcher has a unique start, the windup begins as the elbow flexes and the forearm pronates. This phase ends with the break of the player's hands from the ball, and he then enters early cocking phase. Early cocking phase begins with activation of the deltoid and rotator cuff. The shoulder is abducted, the humerus is externally rotated, and the elbow is flexed. As the contralateral foot makes contact with the ground, the thrower begins late cocking phase. This is marked by further activation of the posterior cuff musculature resulting in full abduction, external rotation of the shoulder as well flexion of the elbow past 90°. During the transition from late cocking phase to the acceleration phase, there is a rapid change in velocity of the arm. As the arm changes direction, a large valgus force is transmitted across the medial elbow.

Increased activity of the pectoralis major, latissimus dorsi, and serratus anterior muscles marks the initiation of the acceleration phase. During this phase, there is a large forward-directed force on the upper extremity. This results in a swift valgus force, along with a forceful extension of the elbow. The kinetic energy transferred from the lower extremities and torso is primarily absorbed by the periarticular structures of the medial elbow [5].

The deceleration phase begins as the ball is released. The extreme change in velocity of the upper extremity during the deceleration phase makes it the most intense phase. The entire upper extremity musculature undergoes eccentric loads and sees extreme forces. Deceleration ends with the humerus in neutral and the elbow extended. Finally, in the follow-through phase, the body is propelled forward and toward the thrower's target. The cycle is complete when the body is at rest [3].

Mac Williams et al. describe the motion as a *kinetic chain* whose energy is generated from the lower extremities and trunk and transmitted to the upper extremity. The elbow, specifically the medial elbow, can be seen upward 65 Nm of torque generated by the humerus and 300 N of medial shear forces during each overhead pitch. It is the repetitive valgus stress that ultimately leads to injury [6].

Waris first described injury to the medial ulnar collateral ligaments in athletes in 1946 in a population of javelin throwers [7]. However, it was not until the 1980s when Los Angeles Dodgers star pitcher, Tommy John, underwent ulnar collateral ligament reconstruction on his pitching arm by Dr. Frank Jobe that surgeons started to truly believe valgus instability was of clinical importance. Since that time, the surgery, which now bears John's name, has garnished significant notoriety as many major league baseball pitchers have had Tommy John surgery [8]. The spectrum of injuries involved with the UCL is broad but can all be related back to either two broad categories: (1) overuse injury to the UCL and (2) catastrophic failure.

Valgus instability stems from thousands of pitches below the intrinsic tensile failure strength of the collagen bands of the UCL (Fig. 3.1). This repetitive loading leads to micro tears and ultimately ligamentous laxity, instability, and in some cases catastrophic failure. Patients at risk include those with poor pitching mechanics, decreased flexibility, and improper conditioning.

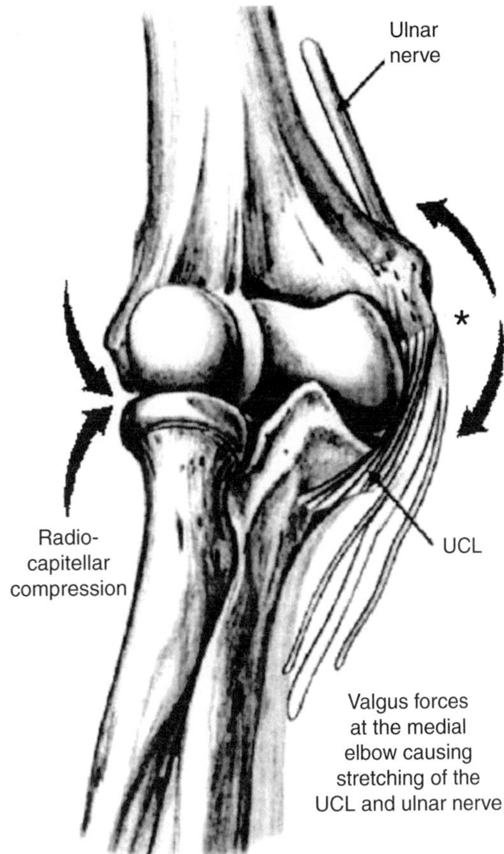

Fig. 3.1 Drawing showing the valgus forces at the elbow leading to ulnar collateral ligament deficiency (From Safran [9], figure 2, page 17)

Patient Workup

A thorough but focused history and physical exam can help to elucidate a patient's presenting diagnosis. In the overhead-throwing athlete, it is very important to understand the timing, location, and duration of the injury and what the patient's normal athletic activities consisted of prior to injury [10], for example, the point in throwing cycle when pain occurs, the initial onset of pain, whether velocity is affected, and how often the patient was pitching prior to the injury. All of these can help narrow down a diagnosis [11].

The thrower will report insidious onset of medial elbow pain during the late cocking or acceleration phase of throwing with minimal effort. They will also report a recent large volume of innings pitched. Or conversely, the patient may feel a sudden pop or inability to throw with one full force pitch. Either of these is suggestive of UCL instability. Additionally, the players may report ulnar nerve symptoms, secondary to the inflammation surrounding the cubital tunnel [12].

On physical exam, the player may have point tenderness over the medial elbow, but more importantly will have instability to valgus stress. To elicit instability on exam, there are two maneuvers that can help the clinician make the diagnosis. The first is the moving valgus stress test, which isolates the anterior band of the medical collateral ligament (Fig. 3.2). The examiner must stabilize the hand and forearm of the affected extremity. Then after unlocking the olecranon from the olecranon fossa, progressive flexion of the elbow is performed with a constant valgus

Fig. 3.2 The valgus stress test for ulnar collateral ligament deficiency

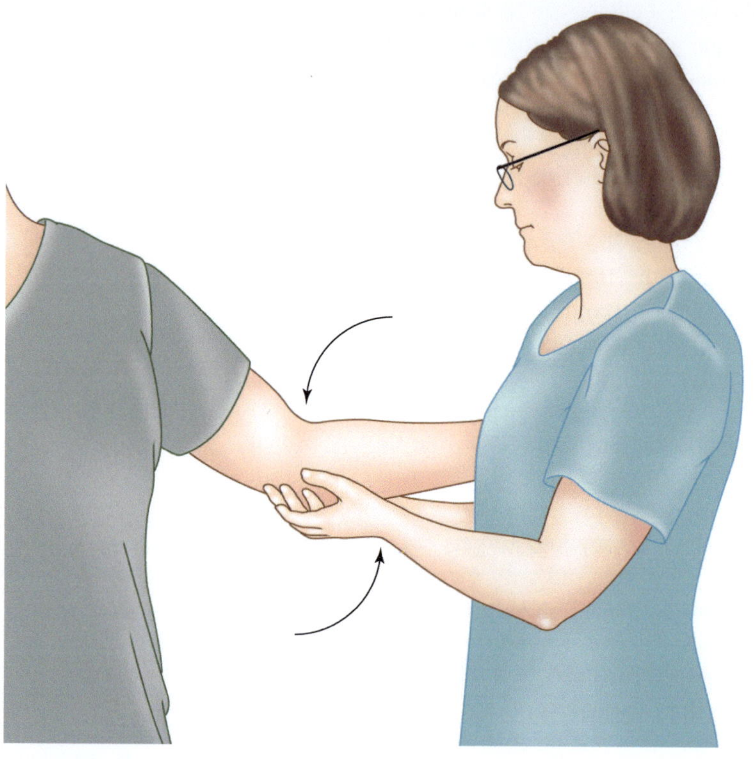

force. Pain along the medial collateral ligament, a feeling of apprehension or medial joint space widening (compared to other side), and frank loss of an end point are all signs of ligamentous injury.

The milking maneuver is similar; however, the elbow is not ranged, but rather, the elbow remains static at greater than 90 degrees of flexion. This maneuver simulates the pitching motion as the arm is fully abducted and externally rotated. Additionally, the forearm must be in full supination. The clinician then pulls on the patient's thumb placing a valgus-directed force on the medial elbow. Like the moving valgus stress test, any signs of pain during the maneuver are suggestive of valgus instability.

Imaging

Plain radiographs are static images of the osseous structures of the elbow and therefore are inherently poor at diagnosing ligamentous injury

(Fig. 3.3). However, there are some views and clues that can help in the diagnosis of valgus instability. Most radiographs reveal heterotopic ossification within the UCL; Mulligan et al. report this to be as high as 75 % [13]. If this finding is not evident, one may use a gravity view or a valgus stress view to evaluate the competence of the UCL (Fig. 3.4). Greater than 3 mm of medial joint line opening or a difference of 0.5 mm compared to the nonstress views is suggestive of UCL incompetence [14].

In addition to plain radiographs, dynamic ultrasound can be a valuable tool in the diagnostic algorithm of valgus instability. Although user dependent, ultrasound can give a real-time dynamic evaluation of the stability of the elbow. Ultrasound is a valid option that minimizes radiation and is a fraction of the cost of magnetic resonance imaging. Using the above physical exam maneuvers along with the addition of ultrasound helps to make the diagnosis of valgus instability.

MRI and MR arthrogram remain the gold standard, with a sensitivity of 86 % and

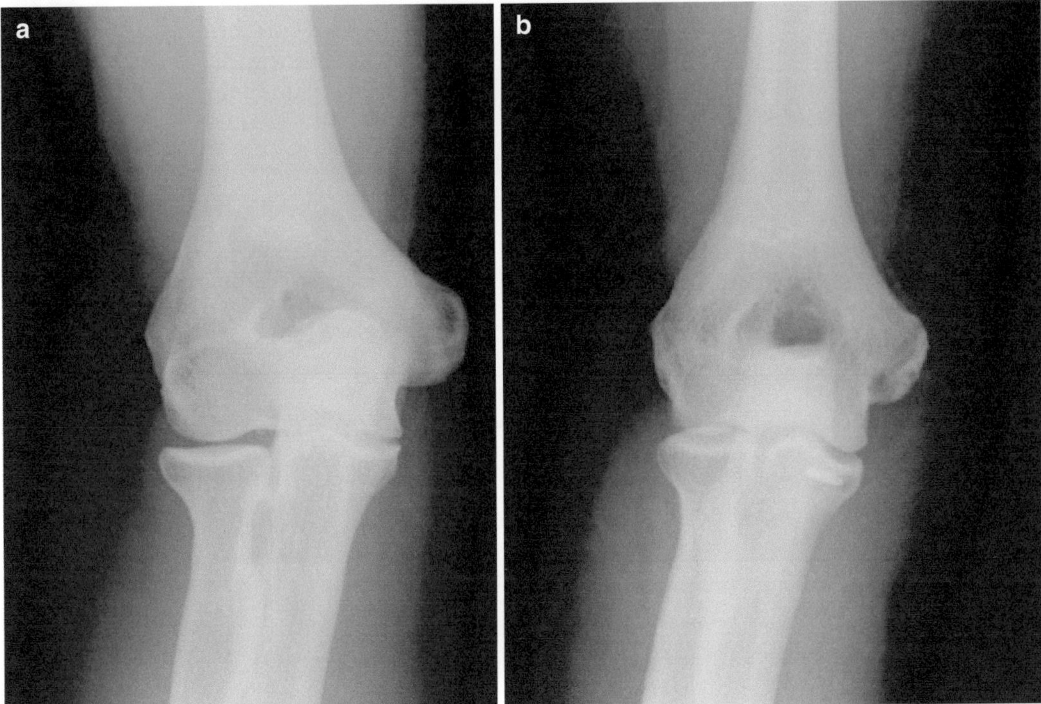

Fig. 3.3 Preoperative (**a**) and postoperative (**b**) AP radiographs in a patient with ulnar collateral ligament reconstruction using the docking technique

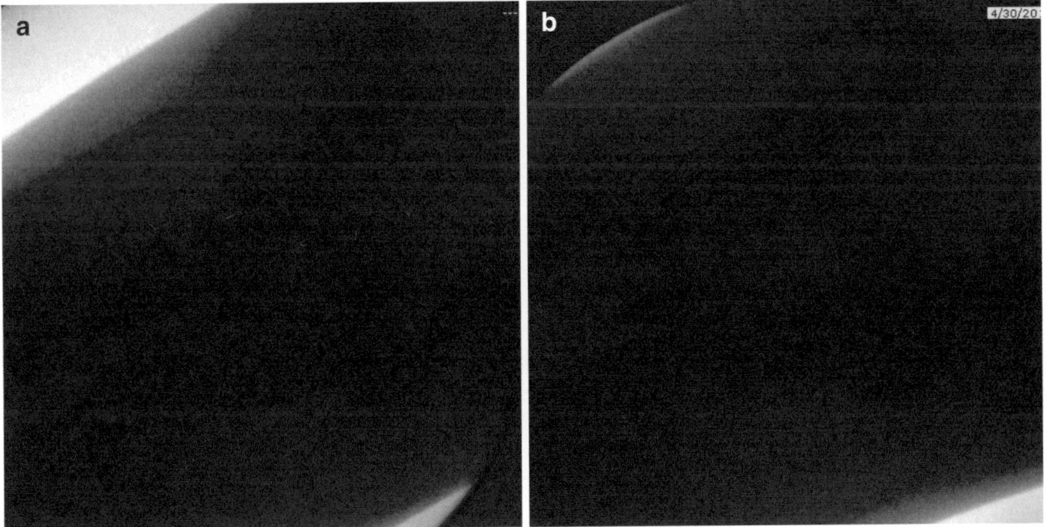

Fig. 3.4 Intraoperative fluoroscopy images of the right elbow. (**a**) Valgus stress films (**b**) show increased opening (>1 mm) of the medial ulnohumeral joint indicating ulnar collateral ligament deficiency

specificity of 100 %, according to Schwartz et al. [15]. Extravasation of contrast out of the joint represents a full-thickness tear, while the T-sign identifies a partial-thickness undersurface tear. If a patient is unable to have an MRI, a CT arthrogram remains a useful tool.

Treatment

Individualized treatment for patients with UCL injuries is based upon the goals of the athlete. Nonoperative treatment is preferred for those athletes who can avoid overhead throwing for a period of time. The program includes a brief period of rest; nonsteroidal anti-inflammatories drugs [NSAIDs], followed by focused physical therapy on flexor-pronator mass strengthening; and a change in pitching mechanics of the athlete, followed by a slow progressive throwing regimen. However, those athletes who fail nonoperative management for 6–12 months or those patients who have a catastrophic failure of the UCL and are high-demand athletes are deemed surgical candidates.

There are several different procedures that are well described for the surgical reconstruction of the ulnar collateral ligament, including the modified Jobe technique, the docking technique, and a hybrid interference screw technique.

The *Jobe technique* was first developed in the 1980s (Fig. 3.5). It was a direct medial approach to the ulnar collateral ligament, centered over the medial epicondyle, taking down the flexor-pronator mass and transposing the ulnar nerve anteriorly in the process. This was later modified to decrease morbidity on the flexor mass by taking a muscle-splitting approach. Specifically, the flexor carpi ulnaris is split to reveal the distal aspect of the ulnar collateral ligament [16]. After thorough inspection of the ligament under a valgus stress, bone tunnels are created in the ulna and humerus. A transverse tunnel is made at the insertion of the UCL at the level of the coronoid, just proximal to the insertion of the brachialis, and a longitudinal Y-shaped tunnel is made at its origin on the humerus. Care not to breach the posterior cortex and injure the ulnar nerve must be taken throughout the procedure. With the arm at 45° and using either a palmaris longus autograft, harvested from the ipsilateral arm, or an allograft, in a figure-of-eight fashion, the reconstruction is completed after tensioning the graft and suturing it securely down. The palmaris longus tendon has two potential advantages: first is the ease of harvest and second the fact that

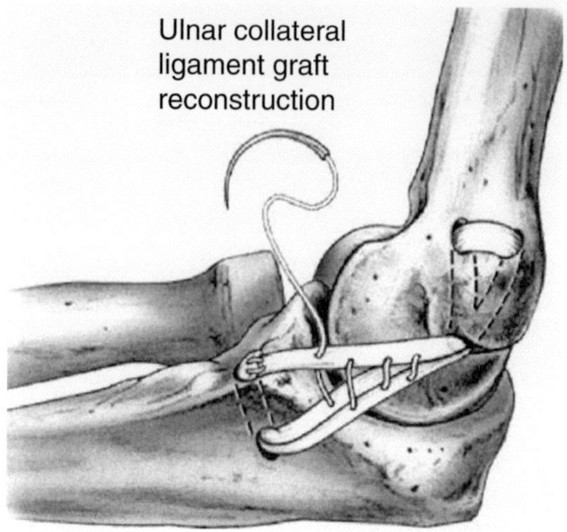

Fig. 3.5 Drawing showing the Jobe technique for ulnar collateral ligament reconstruction (From Safran [9], figure 8, page 21)

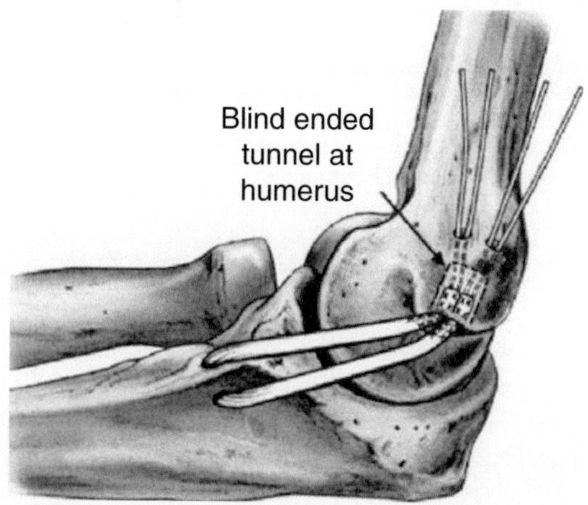

Fig. 3.6 Drawing showing the docking technique for ulnar collateral ligament reconstruction (From Safran [9], figure 9, page 22)

it has a similar tensile strength (357 N) as the native ligament. The modified Jobe technique is considered to be the gold standard for operative intervention of ulnar collateral ligament reconstruction. Ahmad et al. report that there is 93 % success rate in returning the high-performance athlete to competition after a successful modified Jobe procedure [17].

The *docking technique* is a variation on the modified Jobe technique, with a simplification of the humeral bone tunnels and graft tensioning (Fig. 3.6). Two small exit tunnels,

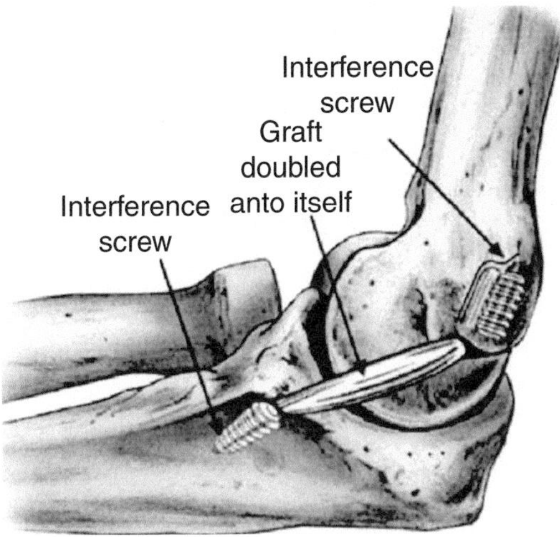

Fig. 3.7 Drawing showing the interference screw technique for ulnar collateral ligament reconstruction (From Safran [9], figure 10, page 22)

just large enough for a suture, i.e., a number one Ethibond, are used as the limbs of the Y instead of the two larger tunnels of the modified Jobe technique. Decreasing the number of drill holes on the humeral side from three to one lowers the likelihood of cortical breach [18]. Additionally, because the surgeon is not tensioning the graft through a tunnel, but instead using the suture as an anchor, it makes for graft balancing easier. Rohrbough et al. reported that 92 % of athletes, of all levels, returned to or exceeded their previous level of competition for at least 1 year [18].

Hybrid screw technique incorporates the docking techniques on the humeral fixation side while utilizing a single bone tunnel and an interference screw on the ulnar side [19] (Fig. 3.7). Advantages to this technique include easier bone tunnels and decreased morbidity of periarticular soft tissues, including the ulnar nerve. However, due to the small size of the medial ulna and medial epicondyle of the humerus, concerns exist over possible fracture with interference screw fixation.

Rehabilitation following UCL reconstruction, regardless of technique, typically takes 1 year. Care must be taken to follow specific postoperative protocols in order to obtain an optimal outcome.

Valgus Extension Overload Syndrome (VEO)

Patient Workup

Valgus instability of the elbow, which may result from UCL injury or laxity, is an entity that causes significant morbidity to the soft tissues surrounding the elbow. If medial ligamentous laxity is left untreated, repetitive impaction of olecranon into the medial olecranon fossa occurs [20]. The shear forces cause chondrosis of the olecranon fossa, posterior osteophyte formation, as well as loose bodies. Patients present with posterior medial elbow pain, especially during deceleration phase of throwing, as it is during this phase that forceful extension occurs. On exam, patients may exhibit loss of extension and/or crepitus [21]. A specific test for VEO is performed with the elbow at 20–30 degrees of flexion, as this is the angle at which stress is placed on the UCL. The elbow is then forced into terminal extension while a valgus force is applied. This test is positive if it reproduces the pain that is consistent with the patient's primary complaint [22].

Imaging

Plain radiographs may reveal olecranon osteophytes, but computed tomography, specifically the three-dimensional reconstructions, gives the most detailed view of damage to the olecranon and olecranon fossa. MR will show the ligamentous instability as well as bone marrow edema; however, CT remains the optimal imaging for this syndrome [23].

Treatment

Treatment includes all of the modalities implemented for valgus instability, such as activity modifications, corticosteroid injections, NSAID, and alterations in pitching techniques. When nonoperative treatment fails, elbow arthroscopy is indicated to perform removal of osteophytes, loose bodies, and debridement. One must remain

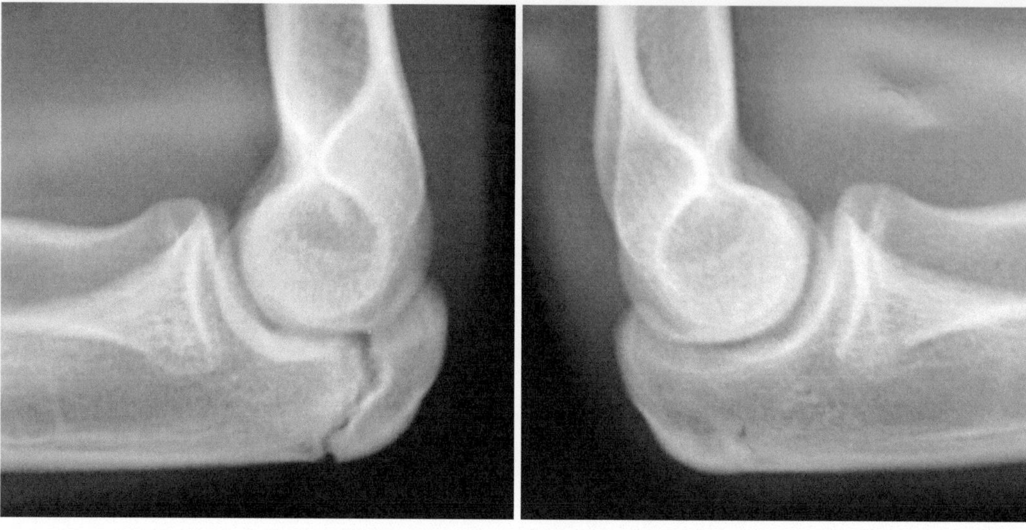

Fig. 3.8 Lateral radiographs in a patient with olecranon apophyseal fracture (**a**) and normal comparison view (**b**)

vigilant in the amount of bone removed, since excessive removal will result in increased instability and further impingement. Additionally, care must be taken to respect the close proximity of the ulnar nerve to the medial olecranon to avoid ulnar nerve injury.

Olecranon Stress Fracture

Olecranon stress fracture is a rare diagnosis usually found in overhead-throwing athletes. In an analysis of over 14,000 athletes, olecranon stress fractures were found to occur in 8.7 % of patients and most commonly in baseball players [24]. These fractures have also been described in athletes who participate in weight lifting, gymnastics, and javelin throwing [25].

There are two main categories of olecranon stress fractures, which are presumed to arise from two different mechanisms. The repetitive pull of the triceps can cause a transverse olecranon fracture or, in the case of an adolescent, a stress fracture through the olecranon physis [26, 27] (Fig. 3.8). A second mechanism of fracture involves valgus extension overload in the acceleration phase that causes the coronoid process to impinge on the intercondylar notch, causing an oblique-type fracture [28].

Patient Workup

These patients describe elbow pain that occurs during or after an overhead-throwing motion. This pain is located over the olecranon and can also include medial elbow pain. Upon physical exam, they have pain with palpation that is noted to be more distal and lateral on the olecranon than that seen in VEO. Additionally, forced extension of the elbow may reproduce pain [22].

Imaging

Diagnosis should begin with plain radiographs (AP, lateral, and oblique), which may identify the stress fracture. More sensitive imaging such as CT, MRI, or bone scan may be needed for diagnosis or characterization of the fracture.

Treatment

Athletes who are diagnosed with an olecranon stress fracture should be instructed to take a period of active rest from overhead throwing or any other activities that may trigger symptoms. The athlete's symptoms and bony healing on x-ray determine the length of this period. Active rest is followed by a gradual return to throwing activity with an emphasis on technique and subsequent return to play. If bony union is not achieved after a period of rest, determined by the patient and surgeon, surgical intervention is considered.

The standard surgical treatment for an isolated olecranon stress fracture includes single-screw fixation across the fracture site, and the obliquity of the fracture determines the trajectory of the fixation. This screw is placed through a single posterior stab incision that splits the triceps. Transverse fractures are compressed with a perpendicular screw, while mid-proximal oblique fractures are stabilized with an antegrade medullary screw. Paci and coauthors found that single cannulated screw fixation of refractory olecranon fractures led to a high rate of union with timely return to sports at or above the level of play established preoperatively. Upon long-term follow-up, the majority of these patients required additional surgeries, including hardware removal, UCL reconstruction, and/or removal of loose bodies [25]. Patients are immobilized in 90 degrees of flexion postoperatively for approximately 7–10 days to allow for wound healing. Range-of-motion exercises may begin after this period, but active flexion past 90° is avoided for 6 weeks. The patient may then slowly return to throwing activities through a strengthening and technique program.

Medial Epicondylitis

Medial epicondylitis, or "golfer's elbow," is much less common than the well-known tennis elbow or lateral epicondylitis. In fact, it has a reported prevalence of less than 1 % in the general population. However, in certain populations, such as those who see repetitive flexion of the wrist and pronation of the forearm, it is as high as 6 %. The patients at risk include the middle aged (male=female), laborers, smokers, and the overweight patient. It occurs 75 % of the time in the dominant arm. In addition to plumbers and carpenters, the overhead athlete makes up a large percentage of the patients [29].

Repetitive overhead activities place large torque and shear forces across the medial elbow. During the acceleration phase, the valgus stresses described above place significant strain on the common flexor-pronator mass, in particular the pronator teres and the flexor carpi radialis. After thousands of repetitions, the tendons may undergo metaplasia in response to the increased stimuli, and the tendons histologically show signs of angiofibroblastic hyperplasia.

Patient Workup

Patients will present with a history of insidious onset of medial elbow pain in the setting of repetitive gripping, flexion, and pronation activities. A systematic review by Van Rijn showed that patients who are involved in activities in which objects greater than 5 kg are handled for greater than 2 h per day or objects greater than 10 kg are handled more than ten times per day are at high risk for golfer's elbow [30].

On physical exam, there is pain with resisted forearm pronation and wrist flexion. Patients are tender to palpation at and just distal to the insertion of the flexor-pronator mass on the medial epicondyle, and a flexion contracture may be present. Careful neurologic exam is necessary as ulnar neuritis is common in these patients; some report as high as 50 % [31]. It is thought that patients with a concomitant cubital tunnel syndrome have worse outcomes than those with golfer's elbow alone.

Imaging

Imaging modalities may be helpful in the diagnoses of medial epicondylitis. Radiographs for the most part are normal, except for when the duration of the microtrauma is significant as calcifications or traction osteophytes may be seen within the flexor tendon mass. MRI is the imaging modality of choice (Fig. 3.9).

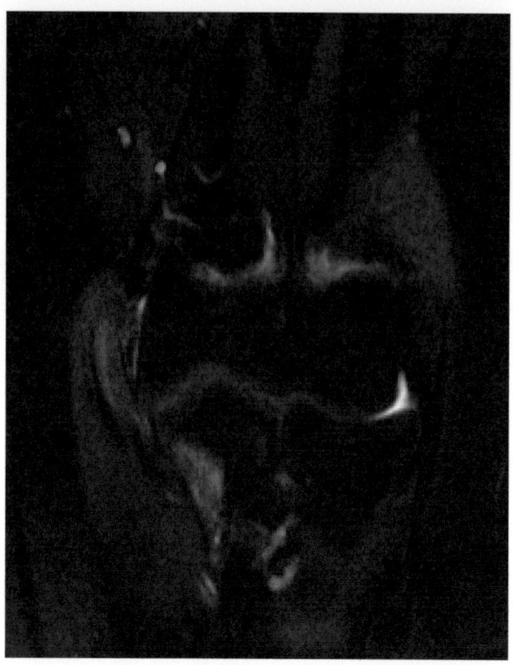

Fig. 3.9 Coronal view MRI scan of the right elbow showing increased signal in the common flexor origin at the medial epicondyle consistent with medial epicondylitis

Treatment

Like most overuse injuries, nonoperative management is the preferred initial treatment. NSAIDs, activity modification, rest, counterforce bracing, corticosteroid injections, physical therapy, and equipment modifications are all tools that the treating physician may initiate before considering operative intervention. However, if the patient has failed nonoperative treatment for 6–12 consecutive months and the pain limits his/her function, then surgery is warranted. Although arthroscopy is this author's preferred technique for lateral epicondylitis, open debridement is still favored in medial epicondylitis with an 80–85 % success rate [32].

Open treatment includes debridement of the tendinosis of pronator teres and flexor carpi radialis and, when necessary, resection of pathologic tendon with reattachment to the medial epicondyle. This can be performed through an oblique incision anterior to the medial epicondyle. Dissection is carried down to the flexor-pronator origin with care to preserve the medial antebrachial cutaneous nerve. Pathologic tissue is excised down to the level of the UCL. After debridement, decortication of the medical epicondyle is often done to enhance healing of the tendon, which is reattached with suture [33].

Arthroscopic treatment has traditionally been thought to be unsafe due to the danger of ulnar nerve injury or injury to the UCL complex, but Zonno recently described effective arthroscopic debridement in a cadaveric study. The flexor-pronator origin is visualized after a partial capsulectomy is made on the anteromedial aspect of the humerus, and the fibers of the flexor-pronator origin are debrided until the fibers of the UCL are visualized. This debridement was performed without injury to the medial epicondyle, ulnar nerve, or UCL complex [34].

Postoperatively, the patient may be placed in a long arm posterior splint for a short, 10–14-day period of immobilization, after which the patient is started on a range-of-motion program. However, volar flexion of the wrist is avoided until soft tissue inflammation subsides. Complications include damage or inflammation to the medial antebrachial cutaneous nerve.

Adolescent Medial Elbow Pain

The pediatric population presents a unique set of diagnoses and symptoms due to their open physes. Awareness of these differences allows for better evaluation of the pediatric patient. Ossification of the elbow continues through early adolescence, allowing for age-related injuries. After primary ossification, secondary ossification centers include the capitellum, radial head, medial epicondyle, trochlea, olecranon, and lateral epicondyle, which ossify in that order. Ossification of the capitellum begins by approximately age 2 and the subsequent centers ossify every 2 years until the lateral epicondyle ossification occurs at 10 years old in girls and 12 years old in males [35].

Elbow injuries in the immature athlete population are more common than shoulder injuries. Approximately 50–75 % of all baseball players report elbow pain at some time point. Many of these injuries are chronic in nature; however, there are those who suffer acute elbow injuries [36].

Little Leaguer's Elbow

Little Leaguer's elbow is defined as any injury to the elbow with associated medial elbow or forearm pain. In 1960, this clinical condition was first described in the pitching arm of two Little League pitchers by Brogdon and Crow [37]. Like valgus instability in the adult, this syndrome stems from excessive valgus hyperextension overload during throwing, and repetitive microtrauma leads to inflammation and apophysitis. Repetitive trauma can be seen from throws of excessive speed, especially noted in pitchers. The UCL, most specifically the anterior bundle, absorbs the majority of the valgus stress during a throw [38]. Speeds greater than 80 mph cause injury to the UCL; however, children with open physes are more likely to have apophysitis [39].

Patient Workup

On history and physical exam, the patient will display medial elbow pain, even at rest. Additionally, they report a loss of throwing distance, decreased accuracy, and a loss in velocity and may even present with a flexion contracture of the elbow [40]. Physical exam reveals increased carrying angle, point tenderness over medial epicondyle and/or flexor mass, and positive valgus stress test.

Imaging

AP, lateral, and oblique elbow radiographs of the affected extremity are usually non-revealing by themselves. However, when compared to the unaffected arm, many of these patients have hypertrophy of the medial epicondylar apophysis or the medial humeral cortex, separation of the medial epicondyle, and/or fragmentation of the medial epicondyle apophysis [40]. Valgus stress radiographs in older children may reveal joint widening greater than 2 mm when compared to the unaffected side, which may indicate a UCL injury. MRI studies may show edema at the apophysis and/or UCL and can be very useful in diagnosing a ligamentous tear [39].

Treatment

Initial management of Little Leaguer's elbow includes a rest from activity for 4–6 weeks along with ice and NSAIDs. An extension brace may also be used for those patients who present with a flexion contracture. Following this period of rest, the patient can be instructed to begin a noncompetitive, gradual throwing program with an emphasis on technique and strength. The average return to playtime is approximately 12 weeks. If the patient has any complaints of medial elbow pain during recovery, they should repeat a period of rest for at least 2–3 days [39]. Young patients who return to pitching should be counseled about the fact that the number of pitches in a single game should be limited to 75 to diminish the chances of elbow pain and that throwing more than 600 pitches in a single season is also a risk factor for elbow pain [41].

Medial Epicondylar Avulsion Fractures

Medial epicondyle fractures are usually caused by a distinct traumatic event in adolescents between the ages of 9 and 14. The patient may report feeling a "pop" or "giving way" [36]. Many different mechanisms of fracture have been proposed. A strong contraction of the flexor mass leading to an avulsion can occur during activities such as arm wrestling or overhead throwing [35]. A second mechanism involves the child falling onto a hyperextended elbow, causing a valgus force and a pull of the flexor mass on the medial epicondyle [42]. Lastly, these fractures can occur in association with an elbow dislocation in which case the ulnar collateral ligament traction on the epicondyle leads to fracture [35].

Imaging

Most medial epicondyle avulsion fractures can be identified on plain radiographs, and the degree of displacement guides treatment. Younger children tend to have larger fracture fragments that may involve the entire epicondyle, while older patients have small fragments once physeal fusion has occurred [36]. Particular attention must be paid to ensure that no osseous fragments are incarcerated within the joint.

Treatment

Minimally displaced, stable fractures are treated with 2–3 weeks of immobilization. Operative

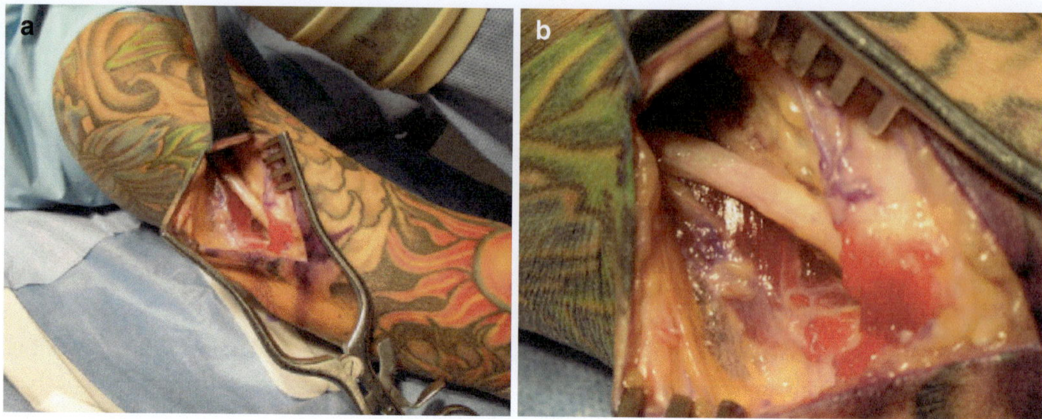

Fig. 3.10 Intraoperative photographs of a patient with ulnar nerve compression. (**a**) The nerve passes behind an expansion of anconeus (anconeus epitrochlearis) attached to the medial epicondyle (**b**)

intervention is indicated for any fracture with an incarcerated fragment or clinical valgus instability. However, controversy exists regarding fractures displaced >5 mm as studies have shown good to excellent results with both operative and nonoperative treatment [43, 44].

Ulnar Nerve Entrapment

Ulnar nerve compression at the elbow can present with symptoms of medial elbow pain. Cubital tunnel syndrome is the second most common peripheral neuropathy of the upper extremity after carpal tunnel syndrome.

The ulnar nerve is formed from the C8 and T1 nerve roots and continues from the medial cord of the brachial plexus [45, 46]. As it travels distally, it can be compressed by either intrinsic or extrinsic forces [45]. Intrinsic causes include medial elbow ganglia which are rare but can be a cause of cubital tunnel syndrome [47]. Extrinsic lesions include tendon, muscle, and vascular lesions [45].

The radial and median nerves also cross the elbow joint, but their pathology does not usually cause medial elbow pain. The radial nerve tends to cause symptoms that affect the lateral elbow [48]. Though the median nerve can become entrapped near the elbow, it tends to present as forearm and wrist pain.

Compression of the Ulnar Nerve

Ulnar nerve entrapment can occur at several sites around the elbow. Approximately 10 cm from the elbow, the ulnar nerve pierces the medial intermuscular septum and travels with the medial head of the triceps muscle [45, 46] (Fig. 3.10). Proximal to the elbow joint, this compression can occur at the medial intermuscular septum and at the medial epicondyle [46]. The cubital tunnel, located distal to the elbow, is another possible source of compression [46] (Fig. 3.11). Further distal to the elbow, and unlikely to cause medial elbow pain, the ulnar nerve can be compressed as the nerve exits from flexor carpi ulnaris [46]. Compression sites can be found 10 cm proximal to the elbow and as far as 5 cm distal to the elbow [46].

The arcade of Struthers is a musculofascial band. The proximal border was noted to be located an average of 8 cm from the medial epicondyle [49] and the distal end of the arcade was approximately 6 cm from the medial epicondyle [2]. The average length of the arcade was noted to be 4 cm [2]. It has been noted to be found in anywhere from 70 to 85 % of anatomical dissections [45, 50]. It has variously been described as a "thickening of the deep investing fascia of the distal arm" and as "a thickening of the brachial fascia" (type 1), due to "the internal brachial ligament" (type 2) and due to a thickening of the medial intermuscular septum (type 3) [45, 50].

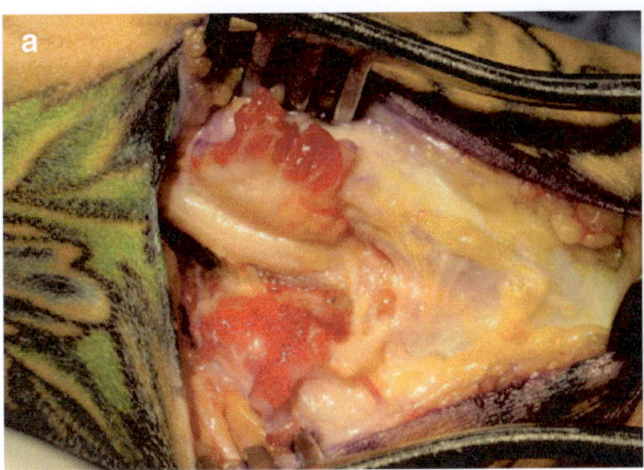
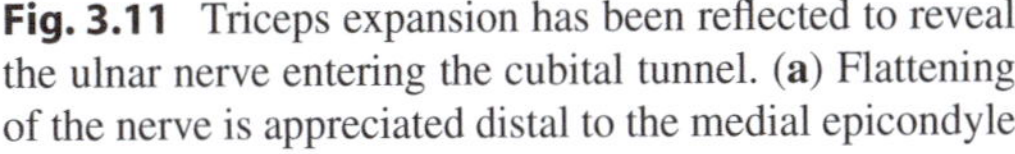
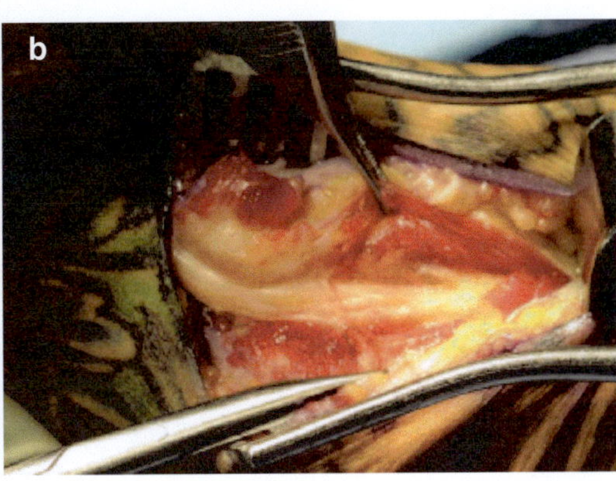

Fig. 3.11 Triceps expansion has been reflected to reveal the ulnar nerve entering the cubital tunnel. (**a**) Flattening of the nerve is appreciated distal to the medial epicondyle at the cubital tunnel retinaculum (ligament of Osborne). Ligament has been divided (**b**) to expose the flattened ulnar nerve

As the ulnar nerve approaches the elbow, it continues between the medial epicondyle and the olecranon. Here, it enters a groove located on the medial epicondyle. Just prior to entering this fibro-osseous groove, the nerve is exposed to potential compression from a valgus deformity at the elbow [46]. This deformity could be a result of malunion secondary to an old fracture. The lateral border of the groove is the olecranon, the medial border is a fibroaponeurotic band, and the anterior border is the medial epicondyle [46, 51]. As the nerve passes through the groove, it runs with the anastomotic arterial system composed of the superior and inferior ulnar collateral arteries from above and the posterior ulnar recurrent artery from below [46]. Causes of compression in the groove can be secondary to post-traumatic injury, inflammatory pathology, tumors, and vascular injury or pathologic growth. It is also here that the ulnar nerve can be described to be dynamically subluxating or dislocating out of the groove and into a position that causes compression [46] (Fig. 3.12). In this situation, the nerve tends to subluxate out of the groove with elbow flexion and reduce into the groove with elbow extension [46]. As the ulnar nerve exits the groove, it is exposed and susceptible to extrinsic compression from resting of the medial elbow on hard objects [46].

After leaving the ulnar groove, the ulnar nerve traverses the joint and continues toward the ulnar part of the forearm. The nerve enters what has been called "the cubital tunnel," a term that was first coined in 1958 by Feindel and Stratford [52]. The pathway of the tunnel is between the ulnar and humeral heads of the flexor carpi ulnaris (FCU), which is innervated by the ulnar nerve [53]. The humeral head of the FCU originates at the medial epicondyle and the ulnar head of the FCU originates at the olecranon and the posterior border of the ulna [53]. The roof of the cubital tunnel is formed by the cubital tunnel retinaculum, which is a fibrous band that attaches between the medial epicondyle and the tip of the olecranon [54]. The roof is thought to be a continuation of the fibroaponeurotic covering of the epicondylar groove [46]. This fibrous band has been variously called "Osborne's ligament, the triangular ligament, the arcuate ligament, and the humeroulnar arch" [46]. The floor of the cubital tunnel is formed by the capsule of the elbow and the posterior transverse parts of the medial collateral ligament of the elbow [46, 54]. As the elbow flexes, Osborne's ligament becomes taut, the medial collateral ligament relaxes, and the canal shape flattens or narrows [46]. The change in the canal increases the pressure on the nerve and can cause mechanical deformation of the nerve [46].

Patient Workup

As with other areas of the body, the physician's exam should include inspection, palpation, and

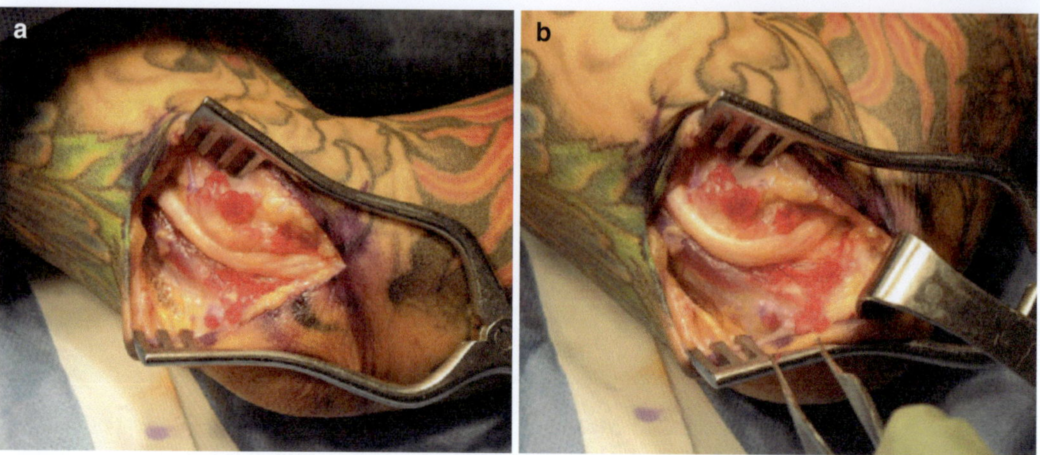

Fig. 3.12 Ulnar nerve in extension (**a**) and flexion (**b**) demonstrating subluxation out of its groove over the medial epicondyle

percussion. Inspection should assess the elbow and arm for signs of trauma, healing bony or soft tissue injuries, and masses. Physical exam focused on medial elbow pain should include a neurologic exam of the upper extremity. This exam should also rule out radiculopathy that could be emanating from the cervical spine [45]. The ulnar nerve should also be examined for potential sites of compression. This includes sites proximal and distal to the elbow. Focused exam of the ulnar nerve should include palpation of the nerve along its course from the axilla to the hand [45]. A positive Tinel's sign, distal tingling on percussion, supports a diagnosis of nerve compression proximal to the area of tingling [55]. This sign was originally described to assess the degree of regeneration after a wartime injury to a peripheral nerve [55]. Palpation and inspection should also inform the examiner of the patient's carrying angle and allow appreciation of ulnar nerve subluxation with elbow range of motion [45]. Vascular exam should assess for pulsating masses and symmetric perfusion of the hand distally. Sensory testing should isolate the nerve in question based on a thorough understanding of upper extremity anatomy. Testing can utilize gross touch, 2-point discrimination, vibration testing, and the Semmes-Weinstein monofilament testing. The Semmes-Weinstein monofilament test is considered the most sensitive at detecting early nerve compression [56].

Motor testing should focus on the muscles innervated by the ulnar nerve. In the forearm, this includes the flexor carpi ulnaris and flexor digitorum profundus. In the hand, the hypothenar muscles are the opponens digiti minimi, abductor digiti minimi, and flexor digiti minimi. The remaining hand muscles include the palmaris brevis, dorsal interossei, palmar interossei, lumbricals (3rd and 4th), adductor pollicis, and deep part of the flexor pollicis brevis [53]. Motor weakness is usually not associated with nerve compression [45]. Testing of the intrinsic muscles of the hand includes the crossover sign (crossing the index and middle finger test to evaluate the function of the 1st palmar and 2nd dorsal interossei [45]). Other exam findings include Froment's sign (thumb flexion during pinching) indicating weakness of the 1st dorsal interossei, 2nd palmar interosseous, or adductor pollicis muscles. Flexion at the IP joint during lateral pinch occurs due to weakness of the adductor pollicis and it is being overpowered by the flexor pollicis longus [45]. The Wartenberg sign is abduction of the little finger when the patient attempts to extend all the fingers. This is caused by unopposed ulnar insertion of extensor digiti quinti [45].

Imaging

Imaging should start with radiographs to rule out causes of compression secondary to bony

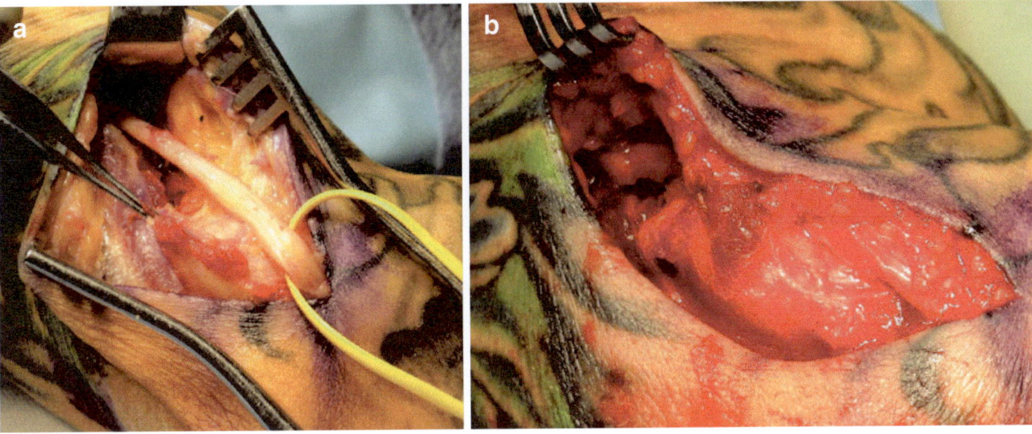

Fig. 3.13 Ulnar nerve is mobilized from the ligament of Struthers to the ligament of Osborne and transposed anterior to the medial epicondyle (**a**). A subcutaneous transposition is performed (**b**)

compression or fracture malunion. Ultrasound can be helpful if there is concern for a soft tissue mass and ultrasound is readily available in the office. One study showed that ultrasound measurement of the ratio of the ulnar nerve to the cross-sectional area of the cubital tunnel seems to most closely correlate with electrodiagnostic studies [57]. Providing more detail yet is an MRI of the elbow though this is not considered absolutely necessary for a diagnosis of ulnar nerve compression. In pathologic cases, MRI may show high signal intensity of T1-weighted images in the muscles surrounding the ulnar nerve. For example, in cubital tunnel syndrome, the FCU and FDP may show increased signal intensity of T1-weighted images and the ulnar nerve may show increased signal on T2-weighted images suggestive of neuritis [58]. Further, muscles innervated by the ulnar nerve may show signs of atrophy or fatty degeneration in chronic cases of compression [58].

Electrodiagnostic studies include electromyography (EMG) and nerve conduction studies (NCS) of both motor and sensory nerves. Motor nerve conduction studies are notably reduced in amplitude and speed in the setting of compression [59]. Testing is done in progressive segments along the arm looking for the maximal change or drop in speed and amplitude of the signal which identifies the area of maximal compression [59].

Treatment

Nonsurgical management is the initial treatment for ulnar nerve compression syndrome. Activity modification and splinting along with anti-inflammatory medications can be useful for the majority of patients who present with mild forms of ulnar compression [60]. Since the cubital tunnel is narrowest in flexion, braces that limit elbow flexion and encourage patients to resist prolonged periods of resting their arms with their elbows flexed have shown benefit [60]. Patients who were treated closest to the onset of symptoms also fared better than those with long-standing symptoms [60].

Surgically, the intervention options vary from in situ decompression of the cubital tunnel or other site of compression to a medial elbow epicondylectomy to transposition of the ulnar nerve. Zlowodzki and coauthors concluded in their meta-analysis of 4 studies, 261 patients and 21 months of average follow-up, that there was no difference between motor nerve conduction velocity or clinical outcome scores between simple decompression and either type of ulnar nerve transposition (two studies used a subcutaneous transposition and two studies used a submuscular transposition) in patients with no history of prior trauma [61] (Fig. 3.13). Macadam and coauthors in their meta-analysis found that there was no statistically significant difference in clinical outcomes between decompression and transposition but did suggest that there was a trend toward better outcomes with transposition [62]. Of note, Bartels and coauthors found that there was a significantly lower complication rate, 9.6 % vs 31.1 % (risk ratio 0.32), in the simple decompression arm of their prospective randomized controlled study compared to the anterior subcutaneous transposition group [63].

Snapping Medial Triceps Tendon

A potential reason for failure of ulnar nerve transposition is a missed diagnosis of snapping medial triceps tendon. This condition usually occurs in association with a dislocating ulnar nerve and is a result of the medial triceps (muscle belly, tendon, or fascia) catching on the medial epicondyle, leading to medial elbow pain. Patients are more commonly male and in adolescence or early adulthood. If an associated subluxing ulnar nerve is present, these patients may have ulnar neuritis in addition to medial elbow pain.

Patient Workup

Detailed physical exam can demonstrate two snaps while taking the elbow through a range of motion. During passive elbow flexion, the ulnar nerve dislocates at 70–90° and the triceps at approximately 115° [64]. The elbow should also be taken through active and passive motion against resistance to check for subluxation.

Imaging

Further diagnosis can be confirmed with dynamic ultrasound [65]. CT or MRI in multiple degrees of flexion may demonstrate the subluxing of the medial triceps and/or ulnar nerve [66].

Treatment

Surgical intervention may be considered if the patient fails 3–6 months of conservative treatment

and involves either resection or transposition of the affected triceps in addition to treatment of the subluxating ulnar nerve. If an underlying deformity is present, this should also be addressed. Following a brief period of immobilization, patients return to range-of-motion exercises and are expected to have excellent results [67].

Conclusion

Medial elbow pain is a common source of elbow pathology that may occur in all age groups. It is particularly common in overhead-throwing athletes; ulnar collateral ligament injuries and valgus extension overload syndrome may occur in throwers due to excessive valgus forces at the elbow. Multiple techniques for ligament reconstruction have been described based on the original "Tommy John" operation, with successful results in returning pitchers to throwing. Golfer's elbow (medial epicondylitis) is another common source of elbow pain that is typically treated by nonoperative means. Pediatric patients have a unique set of pathologies that must be considered due to open physes, and these may include olecranon apophysitis and Little Leaguer's elbow. These conditions may often be treated nonoperatively. Finally, ulnar nerve compression is a common cause of medial elbow pain. When nonoperative treatment is unsuccessful, surgical decompression and/or transposition can lead to successful results in these patients.

References

1. Park MC, Ahmad CS. Dynamic contributions of the flexor-pronator mass to elbow valgus stability. J Bone Joint Surg Am. 2004;86-A(10):2268–74. Epub 2004/10/07.
2. Regan WD, Korinek SL, Morrey BF, An KN. Biomechanical study of ligaments around the elbow joint. Clin Orthop Relat Res. 1991;271:170–9. Epub 1991/10/01.
3. Callaway GH, Field LD, Deng XH, Torzilli PA, O'Brien SJ, Altchek DW, et al. Biomechanical evaluation of the medial collateral ligament of the elbow. J Bone Joint Surg Am. 1997;79(8):1223–31. Epub 1997/08/01.

4. Miller CD, Savoie 3rd FH. Valgus extension injuries of the elbow in the throwing athlete. J Am Acad Orthop Surg. 1994;2(5):261–9. Epub 1994/10/01.

5. Fleisig GS, Andrews JR, Dillman CJ, Escamilla RF. Kinetics of baseball pitching with implications about injury mechanisms. Am J Sports Med. 1995; 23(2):233–9. Epub 1995/03/01.

6. MacWilliams BA, Choi T, Perezous MK, Chao EY, McFarland EG. Characteristic ground-reaction forces in baseball pitching. Am J Sports Med. 1998;26(1):66–71. Epub 1998/02/25.

7. Waris W. Elbow injuries of javelin-throwers. Acta Chir Scand. 1946;93(6):563–75. Epub 1946/01/01.

8. Jobe FW, Stark H, Lombardo SJ. Reconstruction of the ulnar collateral ligament in athletes. J Bone Joint Surg Am. 1986;68(8):1158–63. Epub 1986/10/01.

9. Safran MR. Injury to the ulnar collateral ligament: diagnosis and treatment. Sports Med Arthrosc. 2003; 11:15–24.

10. Cain Jr EL, Dugas JR, Wolf RS, Andrews JR. Elbow injuries in throwing athletes: a current concepts review. Am J Sports Med. 2003;31(4):621–35. Epub 2003/07/16.

11. Chen FS, Rokito AS, Jobe FW. Medial elbow problems in the overhead-throwing athlete. J Am Acad Orthop Surg. 2001;9(2):99–113. Epub 2001/04/03.

12. Jobe FW, Kvitne RS. Elbow instability in the athlete. Instr Course Lect. 1991;40:17–23.

13. Mulligan SA, Schwartz ML, Broussard MF, Andrews JR. Heterotopic calcification and tears of the ulnar collateral ligament: radiographic and MR imaging findings. AJR Am J Roentgenol. 2000;175(4):1099–102. Epub 2000/09/23.

14. Rijke AM, Goitz HT, McCue FC, Andrews JR, Berr SS. Stress radiography of the medial elbow ligaments. Radiology. 1994;191(1):213–6. Epub 1994/04/01.

15. Schwartz ML, al-Zahrani S, Morwessel RM, Andrews JR. Ulnar collateral ligament injury in the throwing athlete: evaluation with saline-enhanced MR arthrography. Radiology. 1995;197(1):297–9. Epub 1995/10/01.

16. Thompson WH, Jobe FW, Yocum LA, Pink MM. Ulnar collateral ligament reconstruction in athletes: muscle-splitting approach without transposition of the ulnar nerve. J Shoulder Elbow Surg. 2001;10(2):152–7. Epub 2001/04/18.

17. Ahmad CS, ElAttrache NS. Elbow valgus instability in the throwing athlete. J Am Acad Orthop Surg. 2006;14(12):693–700. Epub 2006/11/02.

18. Rohrbough JT, Altchek DW, Hyman J, Williams 3rd RJ, Botts JD. Medial collateral ligament reconstruction of the elbow using the docking technique. Am J Sports Med. 2002;30(4):541–8. Epub 2002/07/20.

19. Ahmad CS, Lee TQ, ElAttrache NS. Biomechanical evaluation of a new ulnar collateral ligament reconstruction technique with interference screw fixation. Am J Sports Med. 2003;31(3):332–7. Epub 2003/05/17.

20. Ahmad CS, Park MC, Elattrache NS. Elbow medial ulnar collateral ligament insufficiency alters posteromedial olecranon contact. Am J Sports Med. 2004;32(7):1607–12. Epub 2004/10/21.

21. Wilson FD, Andrews JR, Blackburn TA, McCluskey G. Valgus extension overload in the pitching elbow. Am J Sports Med. 1983;11(2):83–8. Epub 1983/03/01.

22. Dugas JR. Valgus extension overload: diagnosis and treatment. Clin Sports Med. 2010;29(4):645–54. Epub 2010/10/05.

23. Conway JE, Jobe FW, Glousman RE, Pink M. Medial instability of the elbow in throwing athletes. Treatment by repair or reconstruction of the ulnar collateral ligament. J Bone Joint Surg Am. 1992;74(1):67–83. Epub 1992/01/01.

24. Iwamoto J, Sato Y, Takeda T, Matsumoto H. Analysis of stress fractures in athletes based on our clinical experience. World J Orthop. 2011;2(1):7–12. Epub 2011/01/18.

25. Paci JM, Dugas JR, Guy JA, Cain Jr EL, Fleisig GS, Hurst C, et al. Cannulated screw fixation of refractory olecranon stress fractures with and without associated injuries allows a return to baseball. Am J Sports Med. 2013;41(2):306–12. Epub 2012/12/12.

26. Suzuki K, Minami A, Suenaga N, Kondoh M. Oblique stress fracture of the olecranon in baseball pitchers. J Shoulder Elbow Surg. 1997;6(5):491–4. Epub 1997/11/14.

27. Rettig AC, Wurth TR, Mieling P. Nonunion of olecranon stress fractures in adolescent baseball pitchers: a case series of 5 athletes. Am J Sports Med. 2006;34(4):653–6. Epub 2006/03/25.

28. Kvidera DJ, Pedegana LR. Stress fracture of the olecranon. Orthop Rev. 1983;12:113–6.

29. Taylor SA, Hannafin JA. Evaluation and management of elbow tendinopathy. Sports Health. 2012;4(5):384–93. Epub 2012/09/28.

30. van Rijn RM, Huisstede BM, Koes BW, Burdorf A. Associations between work-related factors and specific disorders at the elbow: a systematic literature review. Rheumatology (Oxford). 2009;48(5):528–36. Epub 2009/02/20.

31. Gabel GT, Morrey BF. Operative treatment of medical epicondylitis. Influence of concomitant ulnar neuropathy at the elbow. J Bone Joint Surg Am. 1995;77(7):1065–9. Epub 1995/07/01.

32. Vangsness Jr CT, Jobe FW. Surgical treatment of medial epicondylitis. Results in 35 elbows. J Bone Joint Surg Br. 1991;73(3):409–11.

33. Ciccotti MG, Ramani MN. Medial epicondylitis. Tech Hand Up Extrem Surg. 2003;7(4):190–6. Epub 2006/03/07.

34. Zonno A, Manuel J, Merrell G, Ramos P, Akelman E, DaSilva MF. Arthroscopic technique for medial epicondylitis: technique and safety analysis. Arthroscopy. 2010;26(5):610–6. Epub 2010/05/04.

35. Rockwood CA, Beaty JH, Kasser JR. Rockwood and Wilkins' fractures in children. 7th ed. Philadelphia: Wolters Kluwer/Lippincott Williams & Wilkins; 2010. xiii, 1076 p.

36. Chen FS, Diaz VA, Loebenberg M, Rosen JE. Shoulder and elbow injuries in the skeletally immature athlete.

J Am Acad Orthop Surg. 2005;13(3):172–85. Epub 2005/06/09.

37. Brogdon BG, Crow NE. Little leaguer's elbow. Am J Roentgenol Radium Ther Nucl Med. 1960;83:671–5. Epub 1960/04/01.

38. Morrey BF, An KN. Articular and ligamentous contributions to the stability of the elbow joint. Am J Sports Med. 1983;11(5):315–9. Epub 1983/09/01.

39. Benjamin HJ, Briner Jr WW. Little league elbow. Clin J Sport Med. 2005;15(1):37–40. Epub 2005/01/18.

40. Hang DW, Chao CM, Hang YS. A clinical and roentgenographic study of Little League elbow. Am J Sports Med. 2004;32(1):79–84. Epub 2004/02/03.

41. Lyman S, Fleisig GS, Waterbor JW, Funkhouser EM, Pulley L, Andrews JR, et al. Longitudinal study of elbow and shoulder pain in youth baseball pitchers. Med Sci Sports Exerc. 2001;33(11):1803–10. Epub 2001/11/02.

42. Smith FM. Medial epicondyle injuries. JAMA. 1950;142(6):396–402, illust. Epub 1950/02/11.

43. Hines RF, Herndon WA, Evans JP. Operative treatment of medial epicondyle fractures in children. Clin Orthop Relat Res. 1987;223:170–4. Epub 1987/10/01.

44. Josefsson PO, Danielsson LG. Epicondylar elbow fracture in children. 35-year follow-up of 56 unreduced cases. Acta Orthop Scand. 1986;57(4):313–5.

45. Elhassan B, Steinmann SP. Entrapment neuropathy of the ulnar nerve. J Am Acad Orthop Surg. 2007;15(11):672–81. Epub 2007/11/09.

46. Posner MA. Compressive ulnar neuropathies at the elbow: I. Etiology and diagnosis. J Am Acad Orthop Surg. 1998;6(5):282–8. Epub 1998/10/01.

47. Kato H, Hirayama T, Minami A, Iwasaki N, Hirachi K. Cubital tunnel syndrome associated with medial elbow Ganglia and osteoarthritis of the elbow. J Bone Joint Surg Am. 2002;84-A(8):1413–9. Epub 2002/08/15.

48. Tsai P, Steinberg DR. Median and radial nerve compression about the elbow. Instr Course Lect. 2008;57:177–85. Epub 2008/04/11.

49. Tiyaworanan P, Jianmongkol S, Thammaroj T. Anatomical study of arcade of Struthers. Hand Surg. 2010;15(3):157–9. Epub 2010/11/23.

50. Tubbs RS, Deep A, Shoja MM, Mortazavi MM, Loukas M, Cohen-Gadol AA. The arcade of Struthers: an anatomical study with potential neurosurgical significance. Surg Neurol Int. 2011;2:184. Epub 2012/01/26.

51. Hansen JT, Netter FH. Netter's clinical anatomy. Philadelphia: Saunders/Elsevier; 2010. Available from: http://www.mdconsult.com/public/book/view?title=Hansen:+Netter's+Clinical+Anatomy.

52. Feindel W, Stratford J. Cubital tunnel compression in tardy ulnar palsy. Can Med Assoc J. 1958;78(5):351–3. Epub 1958/03/01.

53. Hansen JT, Frank H, Netter MD. (1906-1991): the artist and his legacy. Clin Anat. 2006;19(6):481–6. Epub 2006/05/10.

54. O'Driscoll SW, Horii E, Carmichael SW, Morrey BF. The cubital tunnel and ulnar neuropathy. J Bone Joint Surg Br. 1991;73(4):613–7. Epub 1991/07/01.

55. Bower JO, Hawkins IL. TInel's sign, formication or distal tingling on percussion and deep pressure sensation. Arch Neurol Psychiatry. 1920;4(6):17.

56. Gelberman RH, Szabo RM, Williamson RV, Dimick MP. Sensibility testing in peripheral-nerve compression syndromes. An experimental study in humans. J Bone Joint Surg Am. 1983;65(5):632–8. Epub 1983/06/01.

57. Yoon JS, Kim BJ, Kim SJ, Kim JM, Sim KH, Hong SJ, et al. Ultrasonographic measurements in cubital tunnel syndrome. Muscle Nerve. 2007;36(6):853–5. Epub 2007/09/20.

58. Andreisek G, Crook DW, Burg D, Marincek B, Weishaupt D. Peripheral neuropathies of the median, radial, and ulnar nerves: MR imaging features. Radiographics. 2006;26(5):1267–87. Epub 2006/09/16.

59. Miller RG. The cubital tunnel syndrome: diagnosis and precise localization. Ann Neurol. 1979;6(1):56–9. Epub 1979/07/01.

60. Szabo RM, Kwak C. Natural history and conservative management of cubital tunnel syndrome. Hand Clin. 2007;23(3):311.

61. Zlowodzki M, Chan S, Bhandari M, Kalliainen L, Schubert W. Anterior transposition compared with simple decompression for treatment of cubital tunnel syndrome. A meta-analysis of randomized, controlled trials. J Bone Joint Surg Am. 2007;89(12):2591–8. Epub 2007/12/07.

62. Macadam SA, Gandhi R, Bezuhly M, Lefaivre KA. Simple decompression versus anterior subcutaneous and submuscular transposition of the ulnar nerve for cubital tunnel syndrome: a meta-analysis. J Hand Surg. 2008;33(8):1314.e1–12. Epub 2008/10/22.

63. Bartels RH, Verhagen WI, van der Wilt GJ, Meulstee J, van Rossum LG, Grotenhuis JA. Prospective randomized controlled study comparing simple decompression versus anterior subcutaneous transposition for idiopathic neuropathy of the ulnar nerve at the elbow: part 1. Neurosurgery. 2005;56(3):522–30; discussion -30. Epub 2005/02/26.

64. Spinner RJ, Goldner RD. Snapping of the medial head of the triceps: diagnosis and treatment. Tech Hand Up Extrem Surg. 2002;6(2):91–7. Epub 2006/03/08.

65. Jacobson JA, Jebson PJ, Jeffers AW, Fessell DP, Hayes CW. Ulnar nerve dislocation and snapping triceps syndrome: diagnosis with dynamic sonography – report of three cases. Radiology. 2001;220(3):601–5. Epub 2001/08/30.

66. Spinner RJ, Hayden Jr FR, Hipps CT, Goldner RD. Imaging the snapping triceps. AJR Am J Roentgenol. 1996;167(6):1550–1. Epub 1996/12/01.

67. Spinner RJ, Goldner RD. Snapping of the medial head of the triceps and recurrent dislocation of the ulnar nerve. Anatomical and dynamic factors. J Bone Joint Surg Am Vol. 1998;80(2):239–47. Epub 1998/03/05.

Distal Humerus Fractures

4

Joaquin Sanchez-Sotelo

Abstract

Distal humerus fractures can be very challenging injuries. Patient's age, activity requirements, the presence of comminution, and the level of the fracture may increase their complexity. This chapter includes specific information on the epidemiology, the specific challenges these fractures pose, and the favored surgical plan to manage complex articular fractures. Details on exposure, internal fixation techniques, and arthroplasty are provided along with information on postoperative measures and expected outcomes.

Keywords

Distal humeral fractures • Supracondylar • Surgical treatment

Distal humerus fractures are among the most challenging elbow injuries to manage. The outcome of these injuries has been greatly improved by (1) better understanding of these injuries, facilitated by more widespread use of computed tomography with tridimensional reconstructions; (2) improved internal fixation implants and techniques; and (3) selected use of elbow arthroplasty [1].

J. Sanchez-Sotelo, MD, PhD
Department of Orthopedic Surgery, Mayo Clinic, 200 First Street SW, Rochester, MN 55905, USA
e-mail: sanchezsotelo.joaquin@mayo.edu

Epidemiology

The rate of distal humerus fractures in the United States has been estimated to be 43 for every 100,000 people, which translates in approximately 130,000 distal humerus fractures every year [2]. The incidence of these injuries is expected to increase over time, especially as the number of elderly individuals continues to grow.

Fractures of the distal humerus have a trimodal epidemiology distribution. In the pediatric age, children tend to sustain supracondylar fractures or partial articular physeal injuries; these injuries fall out of the scope of this book chapter. Most high-energy distal humerus fractures are seen in active middle-age adults as a result of motor vehicle accidents, falls from a height, or – rarely – sport-related

S. Antuña, R. Barco (eds.), *Essentials in Elbow Surgery*,
DOI 10.1007/978-1-4471-4625-4_4, © Springer-Verlag London 2014

injuries. Elderly patients with underlying osteopenia may sustain low transcondylar fractures or comminuted fractures of the articular surface and/or columns with falls from a standing height.

Classification and Characterization of the Injury

Various classification schemes have been proposed for fractures affecting the distal end of the humerus. Some of these classifications may be of interest mostly for research purposes. The most commonly used classification is the AO/ASIF/OTA, with three broad categories: A (partial articular), B (extra-articular), and C (intra-articular) [3]. From a practical clinical perspective, four major fracture patterns should be distinguished (Fig. 4.1):

1. *Supraintercondylar/column fractures.* This type represents the classic distal humerus fractures most of us think about when we hear such term. The entire distal humerus is fractured through the columns and the articular surface. There may be comminution at either the articular level, the supracondylar level, or both. Anatomic reduction of the articular surface is pursued in order to decrease the risk of post-traumatic arthritis and stiffness. Stable fixation of the whole distal humerus is pursued to avoid nonunion and stiffness.
2. *Articular fractures.* These fractures shear the articular surface of the humerus, but do not extend into the columns [4]. Fractures of the capitellum represent the classic example. More complex fractures of the articular surface of the distal humerus extend into the lateral epicondylar region or the trochlear portion of the distal humerus and have only been fully recognized recently.
3. *Low transcondylar fractures.* A single extra-articular fracture line consistently exits just proximal to the medial epicondyle and through the mid-portion of the lateral epicondyle. This

fracture is relatively more common in the elderly patient.

4. *Partial articular fractures.* A large portion of the articular segment and adjacent column is fractured off as a single piece. This fracture pattern is uncommon, tends to affect children or younger adults with good bone strength, and most times is easier to treat with internal fixation.

Interestingly, the decision to proceed with internal fixation or arthroplasty is based mostly on the age of the patient, preexisting articular pathology, bone quality, comminution, and surgeon experience [1]. Partial articular fractures are almost always best treated with internal fixation. Internal fixation or arthroplasty may be considered for the other three types. When internal fixation is attempted, each fracture type presents some unique features:

- Supraintercondylar column fractures usually require exposure through an olecranon osteotomy or its alternatives, anatomic restoration of the articular surface, and plate fixation of each column.
- Selected fractures of the capitellum with no or limited extension to the trochlea can be approached laterally, whereas fractures with more medial extension may require exposure through an olecranon osteotomy or its alternatives. Multiple screw and/or wire fixation may be adequate for most fractures, but some may require plate fixation. Fixation of small articular fragments may require neutralization with an external fixator with or without distraction.
- Low transcondylar fractures may be fixed with plates on each column applied by working on both sides of the triceps. Their main challenge is to obtain adequate plate anchorage in the very small distal fragment.
- Partial articular fractures in individuals with adequate bone strength may be fixed with a single plate along the affected column, but augmentation of the fixation with screws from the opposite side without a plate will increase the stability of the construct if needed.

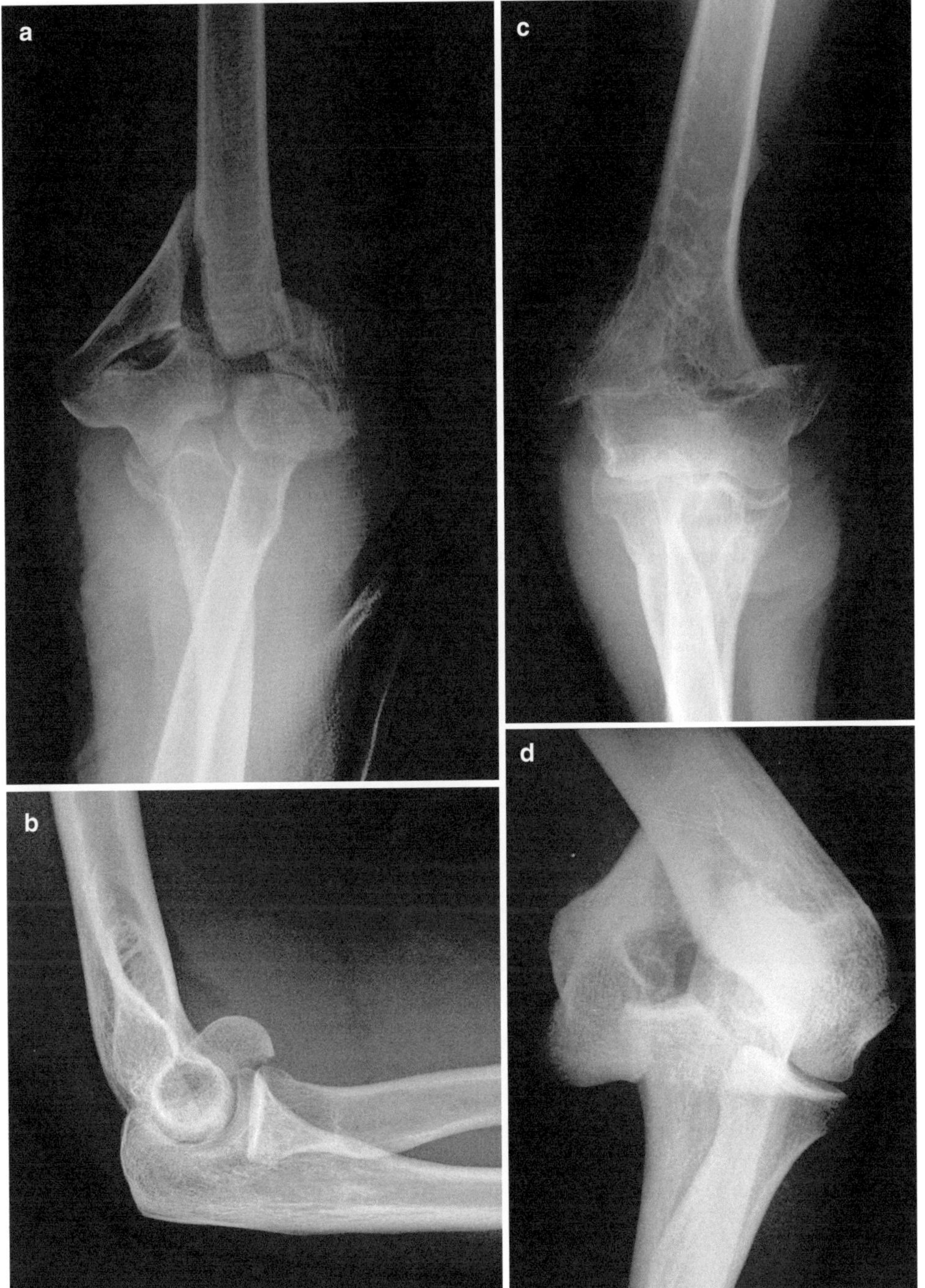

Fig. 4.1 Four major patterns for distal humerus fractures. (**a**) Supraintercondylar column fractures. (**b**) Articular fractures (fracture of the capitellum). (**c**) Low transcondylar fractures. (**d**) Partial articular fractures

Patient Workup

The patient's history and physical examination should concentrate on identification of preexisting elbow pathology (i.e., inflammatory arthritis, previous injuries) that may lead toward arthroplasty, assessment of the soft-tissue envelope (open fractures, frail skin), identification of associated fractures (both in the same upper extremity and other locations), and careful assessment and documentation of the integrity or dysfunction of the median, radial, and ulnar nerves [1].

Plain anteroposterior and lateral radiographs may be sufficient for the more simple fracture patterns (low supracondylar, partial articular, fractures of the capitellum). We have a low threshold to obtain a CT scan with three-dimensional reconstruction (Fig. 4.2) when the morphology of the fracture is difficult to understand on plain radiographs (supraintercondylar column fractures, more complex articular fractures), unless it has already been decided to proceed with elbow arthroplasty, in which case a CT scan provides little help intraoperatively. Traction

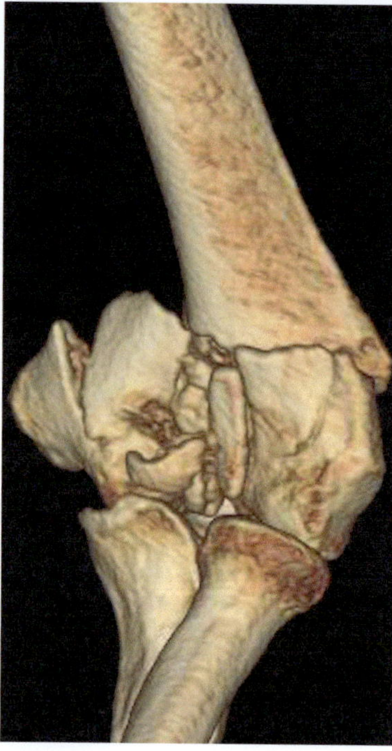

Fig. 4.2 Computed tomography with three-dimensional reconstruction facilitates fracture visualization and preoperative planning

radiographs obtained with the patient under anesthesia prior to surgery may add useful information to plan the internal fixation strategy.

Articular Fractures

Selection of Surgical Treatment

Internal fixation is selected for most patients with articular fractures of the distal humerus. Arthroplasty is considered for the elderly patient (over 65 years old) with poor bone quality, comminution, and/or preexisting pathology.

Internal Fixation

Fractures of the capitellum with minimal or no extension to the trochlea are exposed laterally through the anterior interval of the so-called lateral column procedure (Fig. 4.3a). The common extensor group is split in line with Lister's tubercle anterior to the location of the lateral collateral ligament complex; the exposure is continued proximally by elevating the muscle origins off the lateral column of the humerus. The detached muscle group is retracted anteriorly. The fracture is anatomically reduced under direct vision. We favor the use of cannulated headless compression screws from anterior to posterior and from lateral to medial (Fig. 4.3b). Very small fragments may require use of wires, absorbable pins, or even suture fixation.

Surgeons with extensive experience in elbow arthroscopy may be able to perform arthroscopically assisted reduction and fixation of fractures of the capitellum [5]. Arthroscopy is associated with less morbidity and allows accurate assessment of the quality of the reduction on the articular side. Percutaneous fixation may then be performed using cannulated screws, usually inserted from posterior to anterior.

Fractures with more extensive medial extension oftentimes require exposure through the extensor mechanism (Fig. 4.4). We favor an olecranon osteotomy (see below). The fractured fragments are reduced anatomically and fixed with multiple cannulated headless screws, wires, or pins. In cases of severe comminution of the

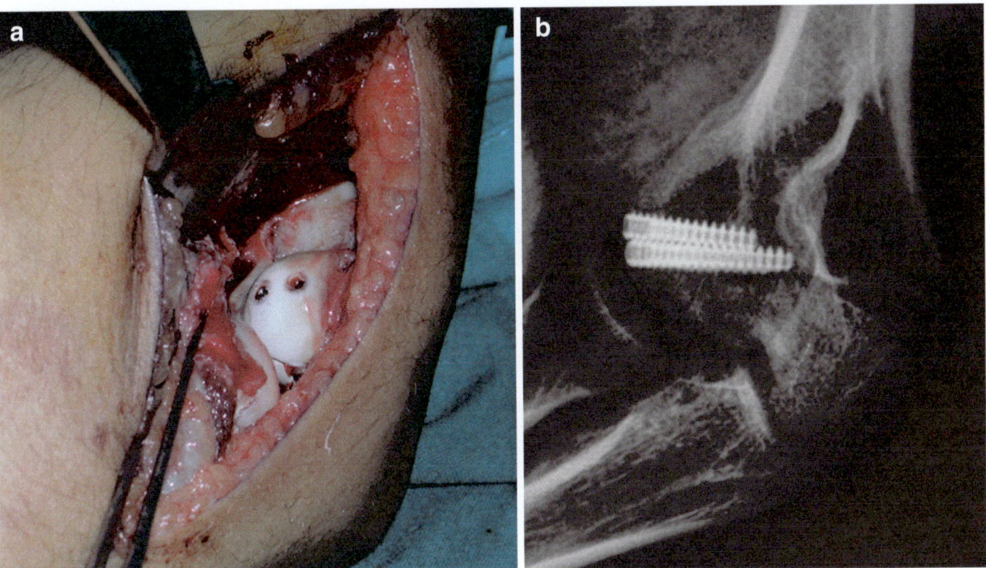

Fig. 4.3 (**a**) Articular fractures of the lateral aspect of the distal humerus are adequately exposed through the anterior interval of the lateral column procedure. (**b**) Most are fixed with headless compression screws

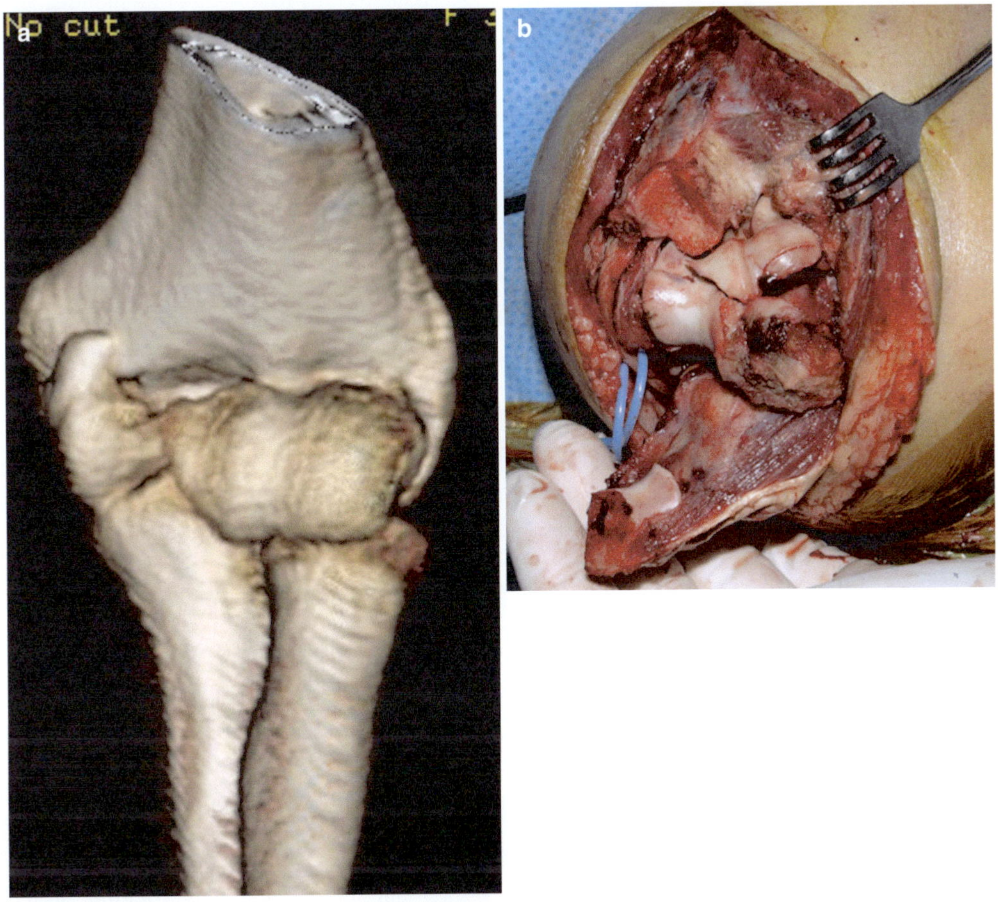

Fig. 4.4 Complex articular fractures with substantial medial extension require more ample exposure, such as an olecranon osteotomy. (**a**) Preoperative computed tomography. (**b**) Intraoperative findings

lateral and/or medial epicondyles, plates may be required to achieve stable fixation.

When the size and bone quality of the fragments lead to tenuous fixation, postoperative range of motion may lead to fracture displacement secondary to shear forces created by the proximal ulna and radius. In these circumstances, consideration should be given to the temporary use of an external fixator. We favor the use of a dynamic external fixator. Some distraction may be applied to minimize intra-articular shear forces. The fixator is typically removed after 3–6 weeks.

Arthroplasty

When arthroplasty is selected for true articular distal humerus fractures, distal humerus hemiarthroplasty represents an attractive alternative, since the origins of the medial and lateral collateral ligament complexes are mostly intact [6, 7]. In these circumstances, implantation of the humeral component without taking down the extensor mechanism is possible but difficult. Exposure for arthroplasty may be obtained through Kocher's approach (detaching and repairing the lateral collateral ligament complex), through an osteotomy of the lateral epicondyle, or through an olecranon osteotomy.

A linked total elbow arthroplasty may be the best treatment option for the elderly patient with a comminuted articular fracture. Exposure may be obtained though the extensor mechanism (triceps reflection, triceps split, or triceps tongue) or by resecting part of the intact non-fractured columns, leaving the triceps on. Additional details about the technique for elbow arthroplasty in fractures are detailed below.

Outcome

Several authors have reported the outcome of internal fixation for articular fractures of the distal humerus. There are no publications focused on the outcome of total elbow arthroplasty specifically for articular fractures of the distal humerus, although the expected results could be extrapolated from publications on arthroplasty for all causes (see below).

Ring et al. reported on 21 elbows followed for an average of 3.3 years [4]. The mean arc of motion was from 27 degrees of extension to 123 degrees of flexion, and the overall results were considered satisfactory in 76 %. Reoperations included contracture release (six elbows), ulnar nerve decompression (two elbows), early loss of fixation (one elbow), and need for hardware removal (one elbow).

Dubberley et al. reported on 28 elbows followed for a mean of 4.6 years [8]. Average extension and flexion ranged from 29° to 138°, with an 89 % rate of satisfactory results. Reoperations included contracture release (seven elbows), revision internal fixation (two elbows), salvage with an elbow arthroplasty (two elbows), and hardware removal from the olecranon (seven elbows).

Mighell et al. reported on a selected group of 18 elbows with large coronal shear fractures of the capitellum and lateral aspect of the trochlea [9]. At an average follow-up of 26 months, all but one patient had good or excellent results; three showed evidence of osteonecrosis on radiographs, with limited clinical importance.

Supraintercondylar Column Fractures

Selection of Surgical Treatment

Internal fixation is the treatment of choice for most supraintercondylar column fractures. However, better outcomes and a faster recovery may be obtained with arthroplasty in the elderly patient with an unfixable fracture.

Internal Fixation

Controversy remains regarding the ideal technique for internal fixation of supraintercondylar column fractures. Use of a plate on each column has become the standard of care; luckily, internal fixation techniques using only wires, screws, or one plate have been largely abandoned. For the more simple fractures with no comminution, orthogonal and parallel dual plating probably provide equivalent results. However, for the

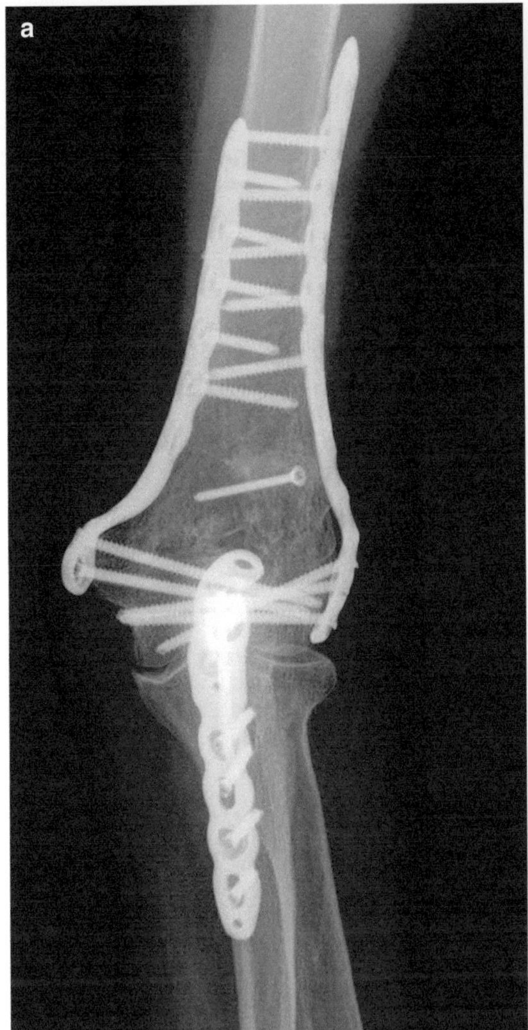
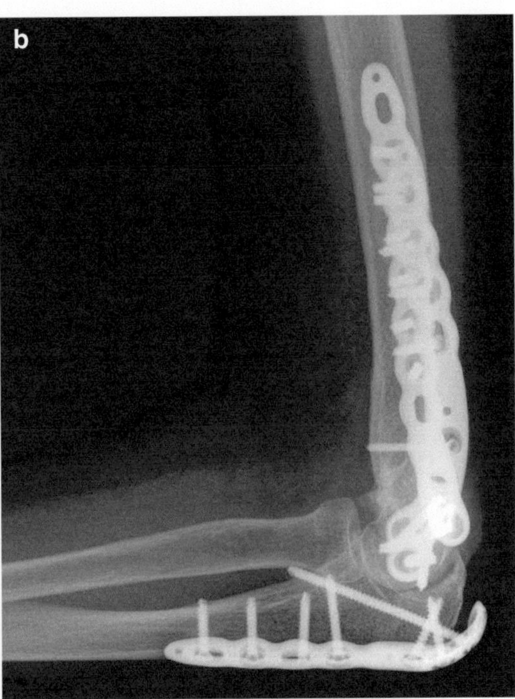

Fig. 4.5 Postoperative anteroposterior (**a**) and lateral (**b**) radiographs after open reduction and internal fixation using parallel-plating technique

complex distal humerus fracture, parallel plating is superior [10]. Since many surgeons do not have the opportunity of treating many of these fractures each year, it does not make sense to master two techniques. For those reasons, we would recommend to master the parallel-plating technique (Fig. 4.5) [11, 12].

Exposure and the Ulnar Nerve

We favor exposure of these fractures through an olecranon osteotomy. The shape of the osteotomy probably is not critical; a chevron osteotomy provides a larger bone surface for healing and more intrinsic stability. Fractures with a single intra-articular fracture line may be approached by experienced surgeons working on both sides of the triceps. Once distal humerus fracture fixation is complete, the olecranon osteotomy may be fixed with a plate, tension-band wiring, an intramedullary screw with or without a tension band, or an intramedullary nail. Plate fixation probably is the most stable, but we have noticed a larger rate of soft-tissue complications (wound dehiscence, infection) when plates are used. We favor tension-band wiring or intramedullary nails for most patients.

The ulnar nerve needs to be formally identified and decompressed; oftentimes, it needs to be mobilized for adequate fracture reduction and fixation. Traditionally, the ulnar nerve is transposed in an anterior subcutaneous pocket; more recently, some surgeons favor relocating the nerve in its anatomic position at the end of the case. The rate of postoperative ulnar nerve symptoms is probably underreported. Currently, the available literature does not allow determining whether the ulnar nerve should be transposed or left in situ [13, 14].

Osteosynthesis

Parallel plating has been well described in the literature [11, 12]. The articular surface should be anatomically reduced and provisionally fixed with fine wires close to the articular cartilage. Medial and lateral plates are applied according to the Mayo Clinic principles, so that (1) every distal screw contributes not only to fixation of the articular fragments but also to anchorage of the plates on the distal fragments and (2) true compression at the supracondylar level is achieved.

Provisional placement of each plate through a Steinmann pin distally and a screw in an oblong hole proximally allows fine-tuning of plate positioning. Distal fixation is achieved next by placing multiple distal long screws across the distal fragments from side to side. The distal Steinmann pins may be exchanged for screws without drilling to avoid breaking the drill bit. Compression at the supracondylar level may be achieved with a large reduction clamp and maintained or increased by application of proximal screws in the compression mode.

Management of bone loss is often times challenging. For moderate bone loss at the supracondylar level secondary to comminution, *metaphyseal shortening* is extremely useful [15]. The concept underneath metaphyseal shortening is to accept a nonanatomic reduction at the supracondylar level by shortening or shifting the distal segment in reference to the shaft in order to maximize contact in compression. The space to receive the coronoid and radial head in flexion in the anterior compartment of the elbow may be recreated by translating the distal segment anteriorly. The space to receive the olecranon posteriorly may be recreated by burring away bone from the distal aspect of the diaphysis to develop a new olecranon fossa.

Comminution of the central portion of the trochlea may be managed with an *intercalary graft* to avoid narrowing of the distal humerus with mediolateral compression. The graft does not need to articulate with the proximal ulna and can be recessed from the articular surface. Very large areas of bone loss involving a substantial portion of the distal humerus may require structural bone graft with or without cartilage, but the outcome of such reconstructions is largely unknown.

Postoperative Care

The nature of these injuries and the additional morbidity associated with internal fixation lead to a very substantial inflammatory response in the soft tissues around the elbow. Edema control is the mainstay of early postoperative care: the elbow is lightly wrapped in a compressive dressing, an anterior plaster splint is applied to keep the elbow in extension, the elbow is elevated for one or more days, and ice may be applied.

Elbow range of motion exercises are initiated as soon as the soft-tissue response seems to be reasonably well controlled. Active and active-assisted range of motion exercises are instructed; motion may be facilitated by the use of continuous passive motion (CPM) or static braces. CPM seems to be extremely useful to accelerate recovery and may lead to a better final motion arc. However, it is labor-intensive, expensive, and not devoid of complications, including wound problems and nerve irritation in some instances. We do recommend CPM for compliant patients and transition them to static braces between 2 and 4 weeks after surgery. Prevention of heterotopic ossification with postoperative radiation should probably be avoided due to the increased risk of nonunion [16]; the role of postoperative indomethacin in this regard is unknown.

Outcome

The outcome of internal fixation for supraintercondylar distal humerus fractures is difficult to interpret, as the severity of injuries included in different studies is difficult to compare, and there may be variations in the accuracy of elbow motion measurements. The outcome of parallel-plating fixation techniques was first reported for a group of 34 elbows with complex injuries: 45 % were open, and most were classified as AO C3 [11]. At most recent follow-up, 83 % of the patients reported no or mild pain, average motion was from 26 degrees of extension to 124 degrees of flexion, and fracture union was achieved in all but one elbow. Complications included deep infection (one elbow), heterotopic ossification (five elbows), and osteonecrosis (one elbow). Higher nonunion rates have been documented with orthogonal versus parallel plating [10].

Few studies have focused on complications following internal fixation of distal humerus fractures, but interestingly the nature of complications has shifted over time. We recently reviewed the complications experienced after internal fixation of 89 consecutive distal humerus fractures. Forty-three elbows (48 %) had at least one complication. There were five distal humerus nonunions (5.6 %), 14 wound complications or deep infection (15.7 %), persistent ulnar neuropathy in 9 %, heterotopic ossification visible on radiographs in 41.6 % (although it was surgically removed in only 6.7 %), and post-traumatic osteoarthritis or stiffness requiring release in approximately 6 % of the elbows. Wound complications were much more common when plates were used for olecranon osteotomy fixation.

Arthroplasty

Total elbow arthroplasty is recommended for selected patients with supraintercondylar fractures. In our opinion, distal humerus hemiarthroplasty makes less sense in these fractures (as opposed to the true articular fractures) due to the need to stabilize the columns and/or ligament origins in order to obtain stability.

Total elbow arthroplasty provides a number of benefits for distal humerus fractures: bone union is not required, patients recover relatively easier and return faster to independent activities of daily living, and both nonunion and post-traumatic arthritis are avoided. However, elbow arthro-plasty is associated with a certain rate of mechanical failure, patients need to accommodate to restrictions for the rest of their lives, and some complications – such as a deep periprosthetic infection – may be catastrophic [1]. In our practice, its indications are limited to elderly patients (over 70 if possible) with severely comminuted fractures, especially in the presence of previous articular pathology.

Exposure and the Ulnar Nerve

Elbow arthroplasty may be performed in this setting leaving the extensor mechanism intact, a major attractiveness in order to decrease complications related to olecranon nonunion or triceps weakness and to allow early unprotected return to activities of daily living. Removal of the fractured fragments on either side of the triceps creates enough space for canal instrumentation and implant placement. Use of a linked implant is mandatory in these circumstances (Fig. 4.6).

Much like in the case of internal fixation, the rate of postoperatively ulnar symptoms is probably higher than reported, and the management of the ulnar nerve is controversial. A recent study has reported a much higher rate of postoperative neuropathy than previously documented [17]. We continue to transpose the ulnar nerve in all elbow arthroplasties performed for distal humerus fractures.

Bone Preparation and Implant Placement

The humeral canal is easy to access by delivering it on the medial side of the triceps. Humeral instrumentation is completed with the usual instrumentation, but because of the fracture, landmarks for implant height and rotational orientation are more difficult to identify. Insertion of the humeral component parallel to the posterior cortex of the distal humerus seems to be quite reliable for rotational alignment, although some recent data seems to show a 15° internal rotation difference between the posterior cortex and the axis of flexion and extension of the elbow joint. Implant depth of insertion can be based off the roof of the olecranon fossa when intact; it should be confirmed with trial reduction of the implants to assess for adequate soft-tissue tension.

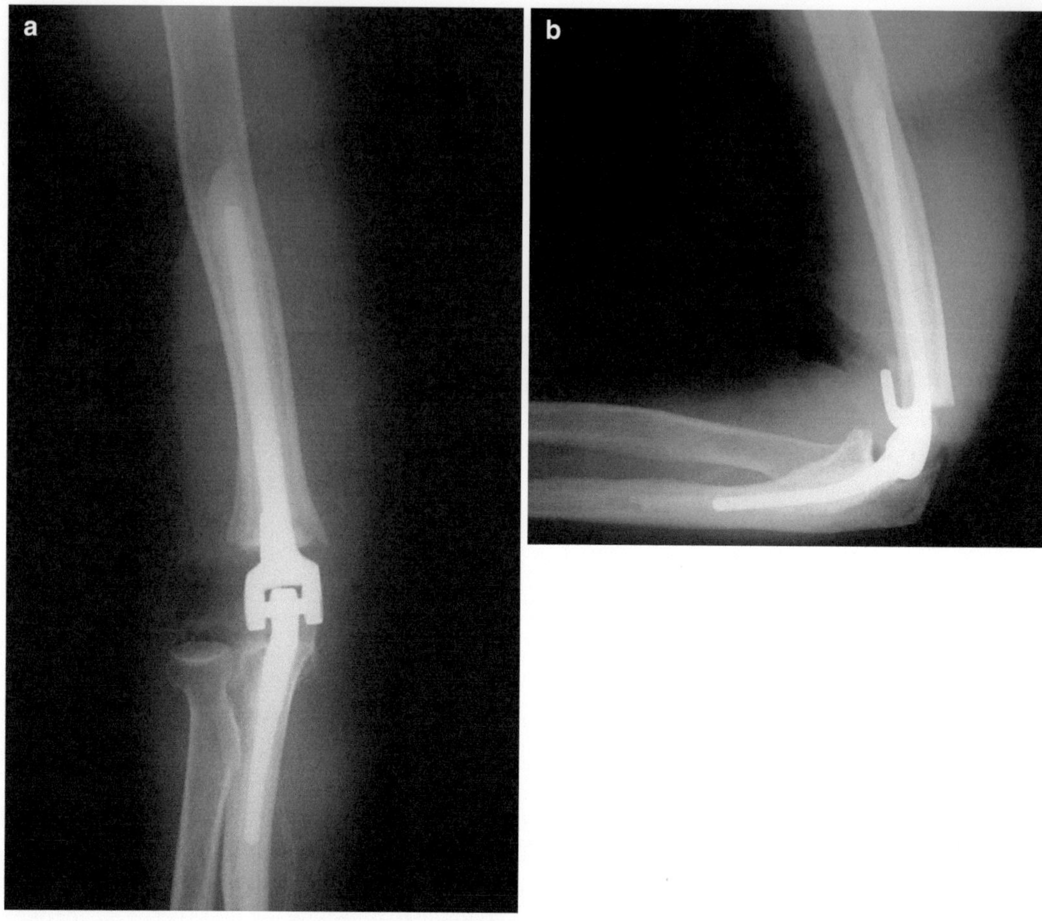

Fig. 4.6 Postoperative anteroposterior (**a**) and lateral (**b**) radiographs after elbow replacement for a distal humerus fracture. Note the absence of the resected condyles

Adequate preparation of the ulna and implantation of the ulnar component is more challenging. Subperiosteal elevation of the very medial margin of the triceps off the olecranon facilitates rotating the ulna and visualizing the center of the coronoid. Depth of insertion on the ulnar side is aimed to place the center of the articulation equidistant from the olecranon and coronoid tips. Rotationally, the implant should be parallel to the flat dorsal aspect of the olecranon.

We routinely add vancomycin and methylene blue to the bone cement used for implant fixation. Both components can be fully seated prior to linking, regardless of the system selected, since the absence of condyles facilitates linking.

Postoperative Care

As detailed above for internal fixation, edema control is pursued by keeping the elbow compressed in extension and elevated for a few days. Active-assisted and active range of motion exercises are initiated as tolerated. Interestingly, stiffness does not seem to be very common when elbow arthroplasty is performed for distal humerus fractures. Continuous passive motion is not used, and braces are rarely used unless unexpected stiffness is confirmed in the early (4 weeks) postoperative period.

Patients are recommended to avoid heavy lifting with the affected upper extremity for the rest of their lives. As a general guideline, patients are restricted from lifting over 2 to 5 kg as a single event or over 1–2 kg on a repetitive basis. Some modern implants are hoped to have better wear performance with weight lifting. Hopefully, these implants will allow heavier use of the replaced joint with a reasonable mechanical failure rate.

Outcome

The first report on total elbow arthroplasty for distal humerus fractures was published by Cobb and Morrey on a series of 21 elbows treated at the Mayo Clinic. In that study, the mean range of flexion and extension was from 25° to 130°, and the overall results were graded as excellent in 15 elbows and good in five elbows [18]. Similar reports have been reported later from other centers (Table 4.1).

The Mayo Clinic experience has been updated twice. Kamineni et al. reported on 43 elbows followed for an average of 7 years [24]. Mean range of motion was from 24° to 132°, and the mean Mayo Elbow Performance Score (MEPS) was high (93 points), but five patients required revision surgery.

Streubel et al. just updated the outcome of this procedure at the Mayo Clinic to specifically analyze those elbows followed for a minimum of 5 years (*unpublished data*). Between 1982 and 2002, 43 consecutive linked semiconstrained total elbow arthroplasties were performed for the treatment of a distal humerus fractures. In the first 5 postoperative years, 3 patients were lost to follow-up, 11 patients died with their implants in place, and 4 early failures occurred, including infection in 2 elbows, ulnar loosening in 1 elbow, and a periprosthetic ulnar fracture in 1 elbow.

For the 25 elbows followed for a minimum of 5 years (average follow-up, 9.7 years, range, 5–15 years), the mean MEPS was 79.3 points (range, 35–100 points), and results were graded as excellent or good in 85 % of the elbows. However, the complication rate was 38 % and the reoperation rate was 31 %. Complications included deep infection (4 elbows), aseptic loosening (5 elbows), and periprosthetic fractures (5 elbows). Reoperations included implant revision in 7 elbows and irrigation and debridement or resection in 4 elbows.

Two separate studies have compared internal fixation and arthroplasty for distal humerus

Table 4.1 Results of total elbow arthroplasty for selected patients with distal humerus fractures

Study	Cases	Mean age	F/U	ROM	MEPS	Comments
Short-term follow-up studies						
Cobb 1997 [18]	21	72	3.3 years	25–130°	Exc 15, good 5	Ulnar component fracture (1)
Ray 2000 [19]	7	82	3 years	20–103°	Exc 5, good 2	Superficial infection (1)
Gambirasio 2001 [20]	10	84	17.8 months	23.5–125°	94 (80–100)	No complications
Garcia 2002 [21]	16	73	3 years	24–125°	93 (80–100)	No complications
Antuna 2012 [17]	16	73	4.7 years	28–117°	73 (35–100) 31 % moderate–severe pain	Sensory ulnar neuropathy in 50 % Infection (3), humeral loosening (1)
Comparative studies						
Frankle 2003 [22]	12	72	3.75 years	15–120°	Exc 11, good 1	Disengagement (1) and superficial infection (2)
McKeee 2009 [23]	25	77	2 years	26–133°	86	Reoperations for stiffness (2) and deep infection (1)
Mid-term and long-term follow-up studies						
Kamineni 2004 [24]	43	67	7 years	24–132°	93	Revision in five cases
Streubel et al. 2012	25	67	10 years	30–133°	79.3	Revision in seven elbows Deep infection in four elbows

fractures. Frankle et al. compared 24 fractures in women older than 65 years old [22]. Arthroplasty provided better motion and overall results. McKee et al. described a prospective randomized study on patients older than 65 years old, with 20 elbows assigned to internal fixation and 20 to arthroplasty. There were five intraoperative conversions from internal fixation to arthroplasty. Elbow arthroplasty was associated with a substantial reduction in the operative time, better elbow scores, and less overall disability as measured with the Disabilities of the Arm, Shoulder, and Hand score. There was a trend to better motion and fewer reoperations in the arthroplasty group, but the differences were not statistically significant.

Low Transcondylar and Partial Articular Fractures

Low Transcondylar Fractures

Low transcondylar distal humerus fractures are quite particular and interestingly have not received detailed attention as a separate entity in the literature until recently. The injury is not common (5 % of all distal humerus fractures in our experience) and tends to affect the elderly patient with osteopenia. The fracture line is transverse and extra-articular and exits through or below the lateral epicondyle and at the level or just above the medial epicondyle.

On one hand, internal fixation is appealing due to the extra-articular nature of the fracture and the possibility to stabilize the fracture with parallel plates working on both sides of the triceps (Fig. 4.7). On the other hand, stable fixation is hard to achieve because of the very small thickness of the distal fragment, in addition to the already mentioned common osteopenia.

We recently reviewed the outcome of 14 consecutive low transcondylar fractures treated with internal fixation at the Mayo Clinic and followed for approximately 1 year (unpublished data). All but two fractures healed, but there were some additional complications, including delayed union (two elbows), deep infection (one elbow),

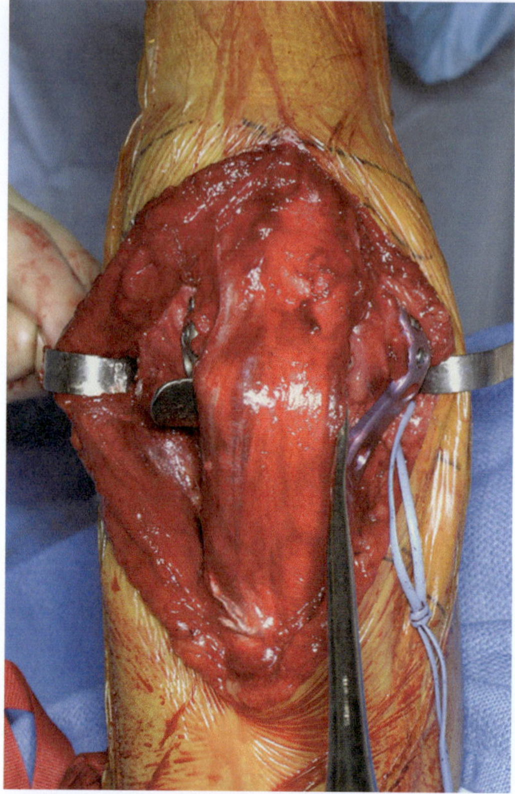

Fig. 4.7 Low transcondylar fractures can be stabilized with parallel plates applied by working on both sides of the triceps, without violating the extensor mechanism

and heterotopic ossification limiting motion (one elbow). The mean flexion-extension arc was 95°, and the mean MEPS was 85 points (satisfactory in 12 of 14 elbows).

Based on these results, we tend to favor internal fixation for the low transcondylar fracture, but do consider arthroplasty for the elderly patient with severe osteopenia, especially when compliance with postoperative care is of concern.

Partial Articular Fractures

Fractures affecting only one column of the distal humerus are also relatively uncommon, but also quite particular. They typically affect the younger patient and are almost universally treated with internal fixation.

In the absence of articular comminution, these fractures may be properly exposed leaving the extensor mechanism undisturbed. In patients with very good bone quality, a single plate applied on the fractured column will provide sufficient stability. When suboptimal stability is achieved with a single plate, insertion of additional screws from the opposite column without the need for a plate provides improved stability. The overall morbidity of the surgical exposure may be decreased by using a direct medial or direct lateral skin incision – as opposed to a posterior midline skin incision – provided the need for an olecranon osteotomy is not anticipated.

Conclusion

Distal humerus fractures may lead to a devastating outcome when treated poorly. When complications occur, salvage options are commonly suboptimal and oftentimes lead to an unsatisfactory result. Widespread use of computed tomography with three-dimensional reconstruction has improved the management of the more complex fractures. Internal fixation remains the mainstay of treatment. Parallel plating using precontoured periarticular plates is our fixation technique of choice. However, internal fixation should not be pursued at all costs, and many elderly patients with comminuted injuries are much better off with elbow arthroplasty. Articular fractures, low transcondylar fractures, and partial articular fractures are specific subtypes with their own nuances.

Advances still need to be made in order to improve the overall outcome of these injuries. Hardware failure and nonunion have decreased over the last decade, thanks to the selective use of elbow arthroplasty for elderly patients with osteopenia and the use of precontoured periarticular parallel plates when fixation is attempted. However, we have made little progress in developing less invasive exposures, preventing wound complications, infection, and heterotopic ossification, or improving the management of the ulnar nerve. These may be the areas of research that will lead to even better management of distal humerus fractures in the near future.

References

1. Sanchez-Sotelo J. Distal humeral fractures: role of internal fixation and elbow arthroplasty. J Bone Joint Surg Am. 2012;94(6):555–68.
2. Kim SH, Szabo RM, Marder RA. Epidemiology of humerus fractures in the United States: nationwide emergency department sample, 2008. Arthritis Care Res (Hoboken). 2012;64(3):407–14.
3. Marsh JL, et al. Fracture and dislocation classification compendium – 2007: Orthopaedic Trauma Association classification, database and outcomes committee. J Orthop Trauma. 2007;21(10 Suppl):S1–133.
4. Ring D, Jupiter JB, Gulotta L. Articular fractures of the distal part of the humerus. J Bone Joint Surg Am. 2003;85-A(2):232–8.
5. Kuriyama K, Kawanishi Y, Yamamoto K. Arthroscopic-assisted reduction and percutaneous fixation for coronal shear fractures of the distal humerus: report of two cases. J Hand Surg Am. 2010; 35(9):1506–9.
6. Adolfsson L, Nestorson J. The Kudo humeral component as primary hemiarthroplasty in distal humeral fractures. J Shoulder Elbow Surg. 2012;21(4):451–5.
7. Burkhart KJ, et al. Distal humerus hemiarthroplasty of the elbow for comminuted distal humeral fractures in the elderly patient. J Trauma. 2011;71(3):635–42.
8. Dubberley JH, et al. Outcome after open reduction and internal fixation of capitellar and trochlear fractures. J Bone Joint Surg Am. 2006;88(1):46–54.
9. Mighell M, et al. Large coronal shear fractures of the capitellum and trochlea treated with headless compression screws. J Shoulder Elbow Surg. 2010;19(1): 38–45.
10. Shin SJ, Sohn HS, Do NH. A clinical comparison of two different double plating methods for intraarticular distal humerus fractures. J Shoulder Elbow Surg. 2010;19(1):2–9.
11. Sanchez-Sotelo J, Torchia ME, O'Driscoll SW. Complex distal humeral fractures: internal fixation with a principle-based parallel-plate technique. J Bone Joint Surg Am. 2007;89(5):961–9.
12. Sanchez-Sotelo J, Torchia ME, O'Driscoll SW. Complex distal humeral fractures: internal fixation with a principle-based parallel-plate technique. Surgical technique. J Bone Joint Surg Am. 2008;90(Suppl 2 Pt 1):31–46.
13. Vazquez O, et al. Fate of the ulnar nerve after operative fixation of distal humerus fractures. J Orthop Trauma. 2010;24(7):395–9.
14. Chen RC, et al. Is ulnar nerve transposition beneficial during open reduction internal fixation of distal humerus fractures? J Orthop Trauma. 2010;24(7):391–4.
15. O'Driscoll SW, Sanchez-Sotelo J, Torchia ME. Management of the smashed distal humerus. Orthop Clin North Am. 2002;33(1):19–33, vii.
16. Hamid N, et al. Radiation therapy for heterotopic ossification prophylaxis acutely after elbow trauma: a prospective randomized study. J Bone Joint Surg Am. 2010;92(11):2032–8.

17. Antuna SA, et al. Linked total elbow arthroplasty as treatment of distal humerus fractures. Acta Orthop Belg. 2012;78(4):465–72.
18. Cobb TK, Morrey BF. Total elbow arthroplasty as primary treatment for distal humeral fractures in elderly patients. J Bone Joint Surg Am. 1997;79(6):826–32.
19. Ray PS, et al. Total elbow arthroplasty as primary treatment for distal humeral fractures in elderly patients. Injury. 2000;31(9):687–92.
20. Gambirasio R, et al. Total elbow replacement for complex fractures of the distal humerus: an option for the elderly patient. J Bone Joint Surg Br. 2001;83: 974–8.
21. Garcia JA, Mykula R, Stanley D. Complex fractures of the distal humerus in the elderly: the role of total elbow replacement as primary treatment. J Bone Joint Surg Br. 2002;84:812–6.
22. Frankle MA, et al. A comparison of open reduction and internal fixation and primary total elbow arthroplasty in the treatment of intraarticular distal humerus fractures in women older than age 65. J Orthop Trauma. 2003;17(7):473–80.
23. McKee MD, et al. A multicenter, prospective, randomized, controlled trial of open reduction–internal fixation versus total elbow arthroplasty for displaced intra-articular distal humeral fractures in elderly patients. J Shoulder Elbow Surg. 2009;18(1):3–12.
24. Kamineni S, Morrey BF. Distal humeral fractures treated with noncustom total elbow replacement. J Bone Joint Surg Am. 2004;86-A(5):940–7.

Fractures and Dislocations of the Proximal Ulna and Radial Head

5

Parham Daneshvar, J. Whitcomb Pollock, and George S. Athwal

Abstract

This chapter presents a comprehensive review of isolated fractures of the proximal ulna and radial head, along with the most complex patterns of injury, including fracture-dislocations of the elbow. The epidemiology, pathomechanics, and diagnostic plan are exposed along with modern strategies for elbow reconstruction. Tips and tricks for radial head reconstruction or arthroplasty, coronoid fixation, and ligament repair are described. A standardized protocol for dealing with the most complex elbow fracture-dislocations and an algorithm to understand the most appropriate treatment for these patients are provided.

Keywords

Radial head • Coronoid • Ligament • Elbow dislocation

P. Daneshvar, MD (✉)
Department of Orthopedic Surgery,
University of British Columbia/
Providence Health Care, 1081 Burrard Street,
Vancouver, BC V6Z 1Y6, Canada
e-mail: pdane050@uottawa.ca

J.W. Pollock, MD, MSc, FRCSC
Department of Surgery, The Ottawa Hospital,
The University of Ottawa, Ottawa,
ON K1H 8L6, Canada
e-mail: jwpollock@gmail.com

G.S. Athwal, MD, FRCSC
HULC, St. Joseph's Health Care,
268 Grosvenor street,
London ON N6A 4L6, Canada
e-mail: gathwal@uwo.ca

Epidemiology

Radial head fractures make up about one-third of all elbow fractures and 1.7–5.4 % of all fractures in adults [1]. Eighty five percent of radial head fractures occur in patients who are between 20 and 60 years old. These fractures are more common in females with a male to female ratio of 2:3 [2, 3].

In conjunction with a radial head fracture, 10–23 % of patients sustain other upper extremity fractures; most common of which is a coronoid fracture (4–16 %) [2, 3]. Other ligamentous and soft tissue injuries are also common. These associated injuries are crucial to identify based on the history, physical exam, and appropriate imaging studies.

Fractures of the coronoid process almost always occur in conjunction with other elbow

S. Antuña, R. Barco (eds.), *Essentials in Elbow Surgery*,
DOI 10.1007/978-1-4471-4625-4_5, © Springer-Verlag London 2014

injuries. These fractures occur in 10 % of elbow dislocations [4]. The pattern of injury plays a key role in the location of the coronoid fracture and the type of instability to suspect.

Olecranon fractures comprise 10 % of all elbow fractures [5] and are more common in the elderly population [6]. With higher-energy trauma, olecranon fractures are associated with other fractures around the elbow.

Classification and Characterization of the Injury

Radial Head Fractures

Fractures of the radial head were initially classified by Mason et al. in 1954 into three types [7]. This was modified by Johnston in 1962 to include type IV, which was described as a radial head fracture in association with an elbow dislocation [8]. In 1987 Broberg and Morrey modified the Mason classification by quantifying the amount of displacement and size of radial head fragment [9, 10]:

- Type I<2 mm displacement
- Type II>2–3 mm displacement and >30 % head involvement
- Type III comminuted fracture
- Type IV radial head fracture associated with an elbow dislocation

Coronoid Fractures

Coronoid fractures can be classified based on the size and location of the fragment(s). Regan and Morrey classified coronoid fractures into three types based on size of the fragment on a lateral radiograph and identified them as tip fracture (<10 %), ≤50 % coronoid height, and >50 % coronoid height [4]. O'Driscoll et al. classified coronoid fractures into three main types and seven subtypes (Fig. 5.1) based on the location of the fracture [11]. This classification is useful in identifying the type of instability, guiding management decisions, and selecting the surgical approach.

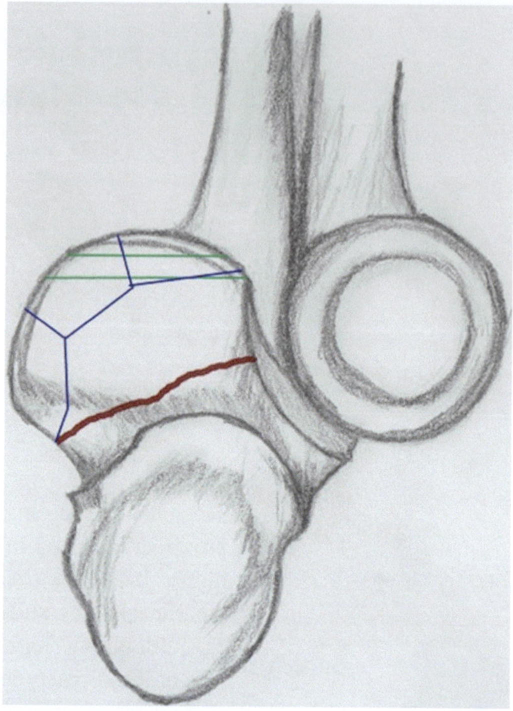

Fig. 5.1 O'Driscoll classification of coronoid fractures. Tip subtype fractures are represented in green. Anteromedial subtype which includes the tip, anteromedial rim, and sublime tubercle is represented in blue, and base fracture subtype is represented in brown

Olecranon Fractures

Fractures of the olecranon process occur as a result of direct or indirect trauma. Direct trauma is often caused by a fall onto the elbow which is flexed at about 90° [6]. Indirect fractures may occur as a result of eccentric triceps contraction leading to avulsion of the olecranon tip.

Olecranon fractures are all intra-articular fractures. There are multiple classification systems described for these fractures. We prefer the Mayo classification, which describes olecranon fractures based on their stability, displacement, and comminution [1]. Type I fractures are undisplaced and stable. Type II fractures are displaced fractures with a stable ulnohumeral joint as the collateral ligaments are intact. Type III fractures are displaced and unstable. Any type of fracture can then be classified as comminuted (A) or non-comminuted (B).

Patient Workup

History and Clinical Examination

As with any trauma, the history can provide important details about the mechanism of injury and raise suspicion about possible associated injuries. Identifying the force involved (high energy versus low energy) and the position of the body and the arm (elbow extension or flexion, forearm supinated or pronated) is helpful in determining the pattern of injury. It is also important to note the patient demographics, comorbidities, and history of previous injuries and surgeries.

After a complete history, a thorough examination is conducted. Inspection of the elbow and wrist will identify areas of bruising, inflammation, and deformity. Palpating ligamentous attachment sites will help identify associated injuries. Point tenderness over the lateral epicondyle or region of the supinator crest may indicate a lateral ulnar collateral ligament injury. Tenderness at anteroinferior aspect of the medial epicondyle or on the sublime tubercle suggests a medial collateral ligament injury.

Generally, it is difficult to conduct conclusive instability tests acutely as the patient's elbow is swollen, stiff, and painful. Nevertheless, a gentle assessment of ligamentous stability should be done. This should include assessment of valgus and varus instability as well as posterolateral rotatory instability (PLRI) and posteromedial instability (PMRI).

In the case of radial head fractures, it is important to identify an associated MCL injury as well as any blocks to elbow and forearm motion. Assessment of the forearm, wrist, and specifically the distal radioulnar joint (DRUJ) is essential in ruling out interosseous membrane involvement and DRUJ instability. Tenderness at the DRUJ or instability should raise suspicion of an Essex-Lopresti-type injury [12].

A thorough neurovascular assessment should be performed following any injuries around the elbow. Although neurologic injuries are rare with elbow dislocations, up to 20 % of patients can develop ulnar neuropathy within 2 years of the injury [13]. Hence, a baseline exam is important.

Imaging

Imaging of the injured elbow should start with orthogonal and oblique plain radiographs. The oblique radiographs are helpful in identifying associated injuries such as small bony avulsions involving the ligaments. The plain radiographs should be meticulously assessed for any abnormalities of the bony anatomy and the alignment and congruity of the ulnohumeral and radiocapitellar joints.

In patients with associated wrist symptoms, appropriate radiographic views of the wrist and the DRUJ are required. Contralateral limb comparisons may be necessary in selected cases.

Once a fracture has been diagnosed, computed tomography can be helpful to further characterize the fracture providing valuable information for preoperative planning, surgical approach, and type of fixation. Subtle incongruences of the joints will assist with diagnosis of ligamentous injuries and instability patterns.

Magnetic resonance imaging is rarely indicated, although can be helpful in identifying associated soft tissue injuries and assessment of chondral injuries and loose bodies as well as any bone bruising.

Simple Elbow Dislocations

Simple elbow dislocations refer to dislocations without associated fractures. The annual incidence of elbow dislocations is 6 per 100,000 population. This is only second to shoulder dislocations [14]. Most elbow dislocations are posterolateral or direct posterior. It is critical to reduce these in a timely manner and to mobilize the patient early within 2 weeks to avoid contractures and poorer outcomes [15].

Once the elbow is reduced, it should be examined for stability. This is done by gradually extending the elbow from a fully flexed and reduced position. As the elbow is being extended, the examiner determines the flexion angle when the elbow becomes unstable. This should be done in pronation, neutral, and supination to assess rotational effects on stability. If the elbow is completely stable after reduction, a short period of rest (approximately a week) is followed by early range of motion.

If the elbow is stable up to 30–45° of extension, the forearm is placed in the position of most stability, which is generally in pronation and about 90° of elbow flexion. In these patients, range of motion is started 7–10 days post injury; however, the amount of extension allowed is limited to the zone of stability. The extension limit is progressively increased 10–15° per week under the supervision of a therapist. Forearm rotation exercises are only performed with the elbow in flexion for the first 6 weeks.

In unstable simple elbow dislocations, which are defined as those dislocating at >30–45° of flexion, surgery is recommended. The surgical approach typically involves open repair of the LCL and the extensor mass. Stability is then reassessed intraoperatively. If still unstable, the MCL and the flexor-pronator mass are repaired. In the rare case of persistent instability, a temporary static or dynamic external fixator is recommended for 3–4 weeks. Postoperatively, early active range of motion within the safe zone of stability is recommended. The extension limit is progressively increased at 10–15° per week. Forearm rotation is only permitted with the elbow in greater than 90° of flexion for the first 6 weeks.

Isolated Radial Head Fractures

Indications for Treatment

The decision to operate on radial head fractures is dependent on several factors, including how much of the head is involved, the displacement, and whether there is a block to motion. With Mason type I fractures, there is generally no block to motion. These fractures are treated nonoperatively, with early range of motion.

For Mason II fractures, the treatment decision is based on whether there is a block to motion, the size of the fragment, and the magnitude of displacement. If the patient has a block to elbow or forearm motion, surgery is recommended. In displaced partial articular fractures of the radial

head (Mason type II) with no block to motion, our treatment of choice is nonoperative. Presently, there are no randomized controlled studies comparing surgery to nonoperative management. If nonoperative management is selected, early range of motion is initiated. If there is any uncertainty about a block to motion, a CT scan of the elbow with the arm in maximal supination and pronation can be utilized to identify a mechanical block.

Mason type III radial head fractures are typically managed with surgery. The decision is between ORIF, excision, and arthroplasty. In our practice, if fracture fixation is not feasible, then radial head arthroplasty is preferred over excision. In general, fractures with more than three articular fragments have better outcome with arthroplasty [16].

Excision of the radial head is an option in isolated comminuted radial head fractures. Radial head resection is associated with high prevalence of radiographic arthritis but with variable symptomatology [17–20]. Most displaced comminuted radial head fractures are not isolated, and excision is contraindicated [2].

Fracture fragment excision is only performed if the fragment is small and not amendable to fixation, and the remaining defect on the radial head does not engage with the PRUJ resulting in a block to forearm rotation. Figure 5.2 outlines our treatment algorithm for RH fractures.

Preferred Surgical Approach

The surgical approach is based on the fracture location, and whether the LCL is intact. The patient is placed supine with a bolster placed under the ipsilateral scapula and the arm across the chest. A sterile tourniquet is used to allow appropriate draping and sterility of the upper arm. Before the skin is incised, an examination under anesthesia is conducted to assess elbow instability and collateral ligament injuries. For isolated radial head fractures, a lateral skin incision is sufficient. However, the authors typically prefer a posterior incision as it allows access to both sides of the elbow joint. The posterior incision has

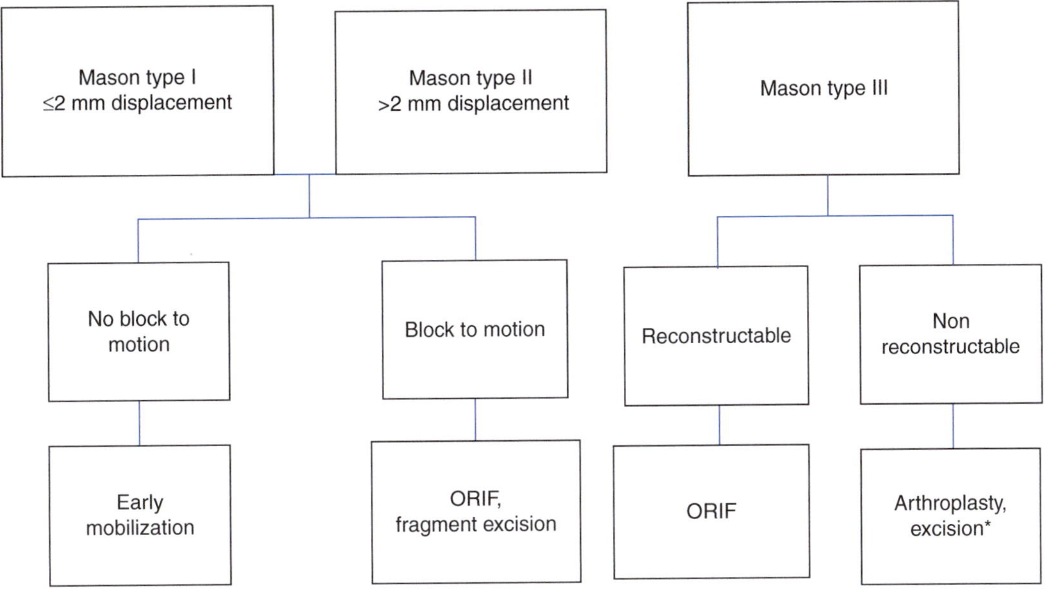

Fig. 5.2 Treatment algorithm for radial head fractures

been shown to best preserve cutaneous nerves about the elbow [21].

Partial articular fractures most often involve the anterolateral portion of the radial head. In the presence of an intact LCL and a typical antero-lateral fragment, an anterolateral approach such as the EDC split is preferred. This approach allows optimal visualization of the fracture for manipulation and fixation while being anterior to the origin of the LCL. If a LCL injury is suspected during the intraoperative examination, the Kocher approach is used because it allows excellent visualization of the radial head as well as optimal exposure for LCL repair.

Surgical Technique

With improvements in fixation and radial head arthroplasty, we rarely perform a radial head excision. At the time of surgery, all radial head fractures should be assessed for ORIF. If deemed irreparable, then consideration should be given for replacement or excision. The fixation implants that are generally used are headless compression screws or low-profile small-diameter (1.5–2.4 mm) screws, allowing the head of the screw to be countersunk beneath the cartilage surface. Fractures with substantial radial neck involvement or comminution may benefit from plate fixation (Fig. 5.3). For such fractures, the radial head plate must be placed in the "safe zone," as described by Smith and Hotchkiss [22], in order to minimize interference with rotational range of motion. This nonarticular region of the radial head typically has thinner and greyish appearing cartilage. The safe zone is described as 110° of nonarticular zone which includes 65° anterior and 45° posterior to a mark placed on lateral aspect of the RH with the arm in neutral rotation (Fig. 5.4).

In cases where excision of the radial head is being considered, it is critical to ensure that there is no longitudinal forearm instability and that the medial collateral ligament is intact. The radius pull test, described by Smith et al., is used to examine for longitudinal instability [23]. This is an intraoperative test and requires direct visualization of the proximal radial shaft. With the shoulder in 90° of abduction and full internal rotation and elbow flexed at 90° and in neutral rotation, a bone reduction clamp is applied to the

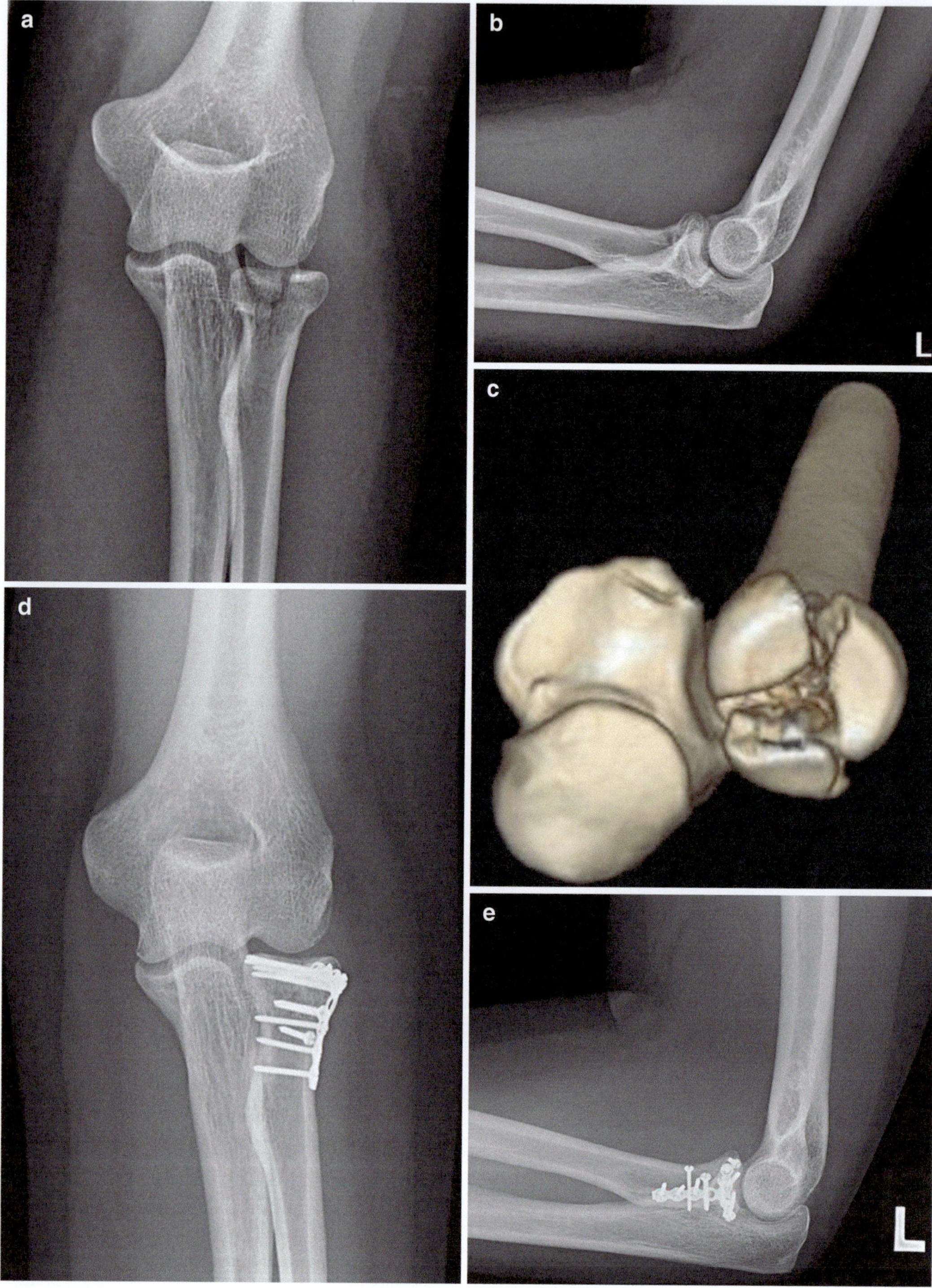

Fig. 5.3 Comminuted left radial head fracture, with three large fragments as demonstrated on the 3-dimentional CT reconstructions (**a–c**). After reduction and lag fixation of the radial neck fracture extension, the radial head fracture was treated with a low-profile plate placed in the "safe zone" (**d–e**)

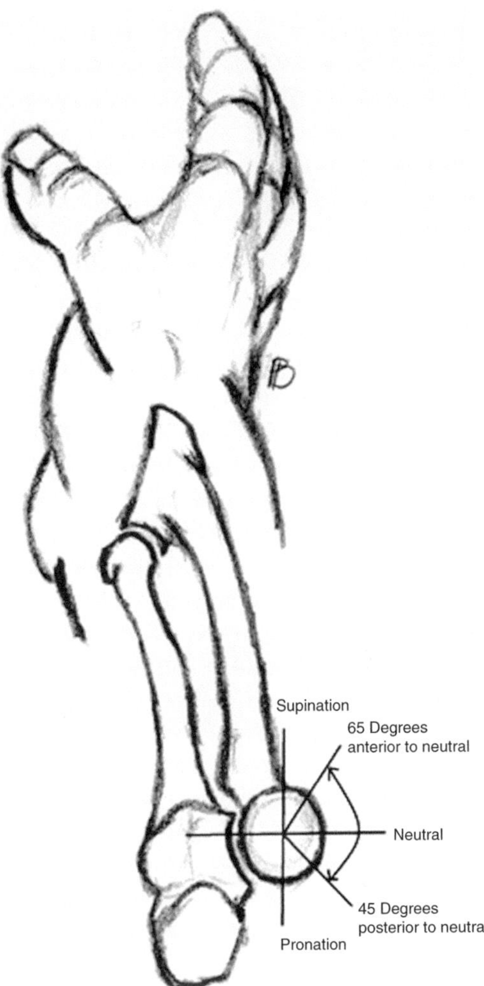

Fig. 5.4 "Safe zone" is described as the region of the radial head which does not articulate with the lesser sigmoid notch throughout forearm rotation. Smith and Hotchkiss describe placing a mark on the lateral aspect of the radial head with the arm in neutral rotation, full supination, and full pronation. The zone of safety is about 65° anterior to the neutral mark and 45° posterior to the neutral mark. This should always be individualized as total arc of motion is different for each patient. It is important to assess your rotation after the fixation is placed to ensure no blocks to motion exist despite being in the boundaries of the safe zone

proximal radial shaft and pulled longitudinally with approximately 20 lb of force. Fluoroscopic images of the wrist are taken before, during, and after the force is applied. With ≥3 mm of proximal migration of the radius or increased ulnar variance, the diagnosis of interosseous membrane disruption is made.

In cases of severe radial head comminution with poor bone quality, radial head arthroplasty should be considered. Ring et al. have described poorer outcomes of radial head ORIF if there are greater than three fragments. This number of fragments can be used as a guideline to assist with decision making for radial head arthroplasty; however, each fracture must be assessed independently and the patient's age and activity level should be considered [16].

When the decision is made to replace the radial head, it is critical to select an appropriate-sized radial head implant. The major fracture fragments should be assembled and used as a template to assess the diameter and height of the radial head (Fig. 5.5) [24]. It is critical to determine the correct height of the radial head. The height of the radial head can be measured from the articular surface to the fracture line. If the radial head is overlengthened or undersized, there is increased risk of early degenerative wear and instability, respectively [25]. To ensure appropriate height of the radial head implant, certain reference points can be utilized. The two main reference points we use to determine the correct length/height are the lesser sigmoid notch and the lateral coronoid edge [26, 27]. These reference points are important in helping to choose the appropriate implant height, especially if the radial head is highly fragmented and can't be used to accurately estimate height. It is important to assess the radial head and neck sizes independently and utilize a modular radial head replacement system which allows this accommodation.

Using the proximal aspect of the lesser sigmoid notch as the proximal level of the radial head implant and the length of the lesser sigmoid notch as the height of the radial head is a useful intraoperative landmark [26]. Additionally, direct visualization of the opening of the lateral ulnohumeral joint indicates overlengthening of the radius or overstuffing of the joint [28].

Radiographs may also be useful in the determination of radial head overlengthening. Typically, the medial ulnohumeral joint space should be parallel, and radiographic widening of this joint space is a sign of significant radial implant overlengthening. Radiographic lateral ulnohumeral

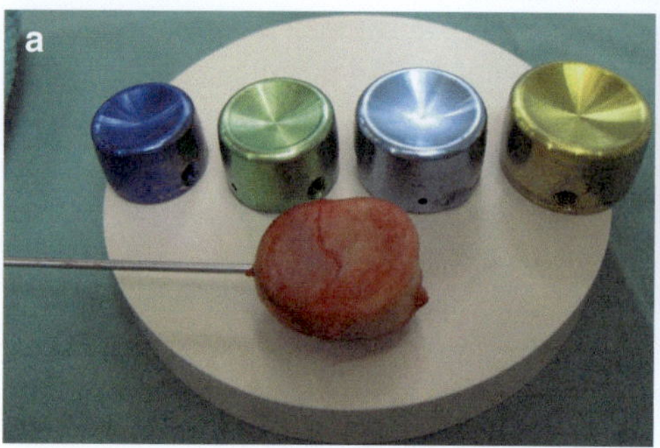

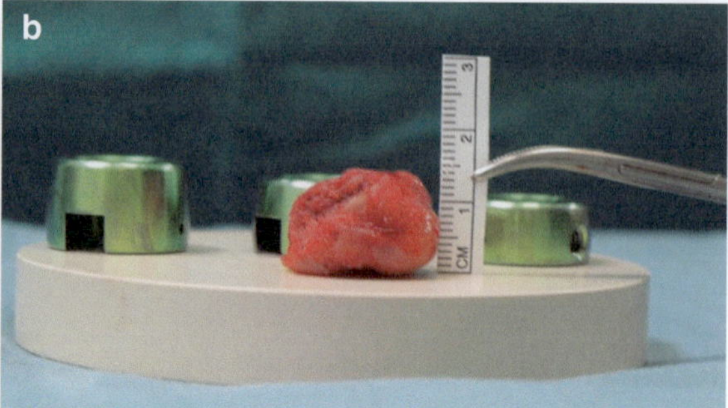

Fig. 5.5 Radial head fragments should be utilized to determine the appropriate diameter (**a**) and height (**b**) of the prosthesis

joint space widening should not be used as an indicator for overlengthening as the articular cartilage thickness has been shown to be variable [29]. Finally, an anteroposterior radiograph of the contralateral elbow can be a helpful guide to assess for joint subluxation and incongruity due to an incorrectly sized radial head implant.

Results and Complications

The pattern of injury, associated injuries, type of head fracture, surgical treatment received, and postoperative care all contribute to the clinical outcome. In general, more simple fractures, such as Mason type I or marginal type II fractures without associated ligamentous injuries do best. To achieve successful outcomes it is critical that patients are seen early and mobilization is started as soon as possible.

Complications associated with radial head fractures include stiffness, post-traumatic arthritis, nonunion, osteonecrosis, heterotopic ossification, and instability. Additional risks associated with surgical treatment of radial head fractures include infection, PIN palsy, implant complications, and an increased risk of heterotopic bone formation.

Radial head excision has been shown to adversely affect elbow kinematics [30]. If there is an associated MCL injury, excision is contraindicated. However, with radial head excision and an intact MCL, Antuna and colleagues have demonstrated good long-term function and pain relief in younger patients, despite uniform long-term arthritic changes [31]. Long-term results of ORIF

have demonstrated better functional and radiographic outcomes compared to radial head excision [32]. Ring et al. demonstrated better functional outcome in arthroplasty versus ORIF of radial head fractures with greater than three fragments [16].

Isolated Olecranon Fractures

Indications for Treatment

Most displaced olecranon fractures are treated surgically as they are intra-articular and separate the extensor mechanism of the elbow from the ulna. Nonsurgical management is indicated when fractures are undisplaced or patients are critically ill.

Tension band fixation is now less commonly used with the availability of the pre-contoured, low-profile plates. However, for proximal transverse non-comminuted fracture patterns, tension band fixation is a suitable option and much less expensive than plate fixation, although with increased hardware irritation and removal rates [33]. On the other hand, open reduction and internal fixation with plates is recommended in the treatment of oblique, comminuted, and osteoporotic olecranon fractures. Pre-contoured locking compression plates, although expensive, can be useful in osteoporotic bone.

Preferred Surgical Approach

Olecranon fractures are approached with a posterior incision over the olecranon and proximal

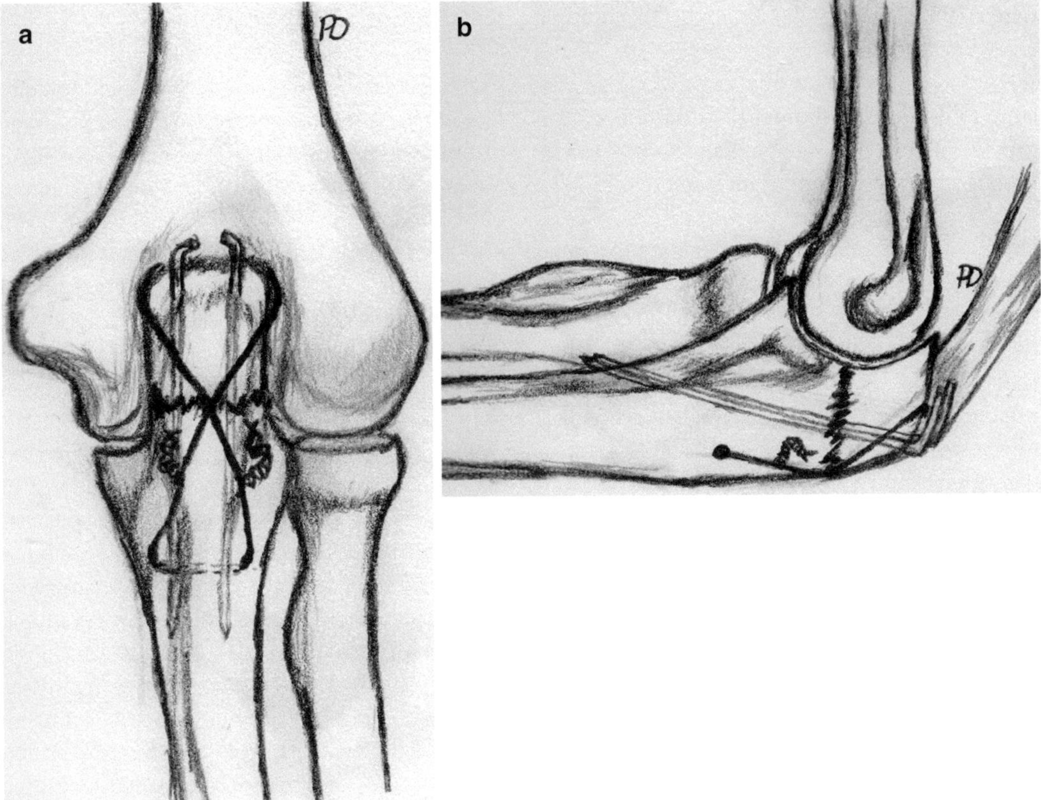

Fig. 5.6 Tension band construct demonstrating appropriate placement of the K-wires with anterior cortex purchase (**b**). Note the crossing of the tensioning wire at the fracture site and tightening of the wire on both sides of the construct (**a**)

ulna. The ulnar nerve must be protected. We routinely do not mobilize or transpose the ulnar nerve during this procedure. However, to achieve adequate exposure for complex multi-fragmented fractures involving the medial ulna or anteromedial coronoid, ulnar nerve release and mobilization are often necessary.

Surgical Technique

When tension band fixation is chosen, two 0.0625-in. K-wires are used in a parallel fashion starting dorsal proximal and aiming for the anterior cortex. The tension band wire is inserted through a drill hole in the dorsal aspect of the proximal ulna. This distance between the fracture and drill hole should equal the distance between the fracture and the olecranon tip. The wire is crossed at the fracture site in a figure of eight fashion. Both

sides of the band should be tensioned equally and simultaneously to allow balanced compression at the fracture site. The K-wires are pulled back slightly, bent, cut, and tapped back beneath the triceps tendon and through the anterior cortex (Fig. 5.6).

When using plate fixation, locking options are useful in osteoporotic bone but not required in younger healthy bone. Our preferred technique for non-comminuted fractures is to obtain reduction and temporary fixation with K-wires. The plate is carefully contoured to match the olecranon as closely as possible, including special care to recreate the proximal ulnar dorsal angulation [34]. A full-thickness split in the triceps is required to position the plate directly onto the olecranon and minimize plate prominence. The plate is first secured distally and compression holes can be used to advance the plate closer to the olecranon tip. At this point the proximal fragment is fixated with multiple screws without crossing the fracture site. These screws should be unicortical but as long as possible to optimize proximal fixation. Once fixation is obtained proximally, distal screws can be used to compress appropriate fractures. Finally, the most proximal axial screw(s) can be inserted from the olecranon tip into the anterior ulnar diaphysis crossing the fracture site. At conclusion of the case, the elbow is taken through gentle range of motion to ensure that no grinding is felt due to proud screws in the ulnohumeral joint and that rotation is not blocked secondary to screws into the proximal radioulnar joint or the radial shaft. Imaging is critical to demonstrate appropriate screw placement. Due to the complex shape of the articular surface, oblique images and live fluoroscopy are necessary to ensure that all screws are the appropriate length and extra-articular.

In the case of comminuted fractures, bridge plating is performed instead of compression plating to maintain articular congruity. Small threaded K-wires can be used to secure small articular fragments, not amendable to screw purchase (Fig. 5.7). In the case of osteoporotic bone or when it is felt that there is insufficient fixation in the proximal olecranon fragment, a triceps off-loading suture can be used to fixate the triceps tendon to the plate thereby decreasing tension on the proximal olecranon fragment [35].

If the fracture is too comminuted for any fixation, excision of comminution and advancement of the triceps insertion are performed. This is a viable option in the elderly, low-demand patient with a comminuted fracture which is deemed unreconstructable [36]. Good to excellent results have been demonstrated with this treatment in the appropriate patient [37, 38]. This procedure is contraindicated in the patient with ligamentous injury and instability. Biomechanical studies have demonstrated increasing angular and rotational instability with sequential excision of the olecranon. Therefore, the amount excised should be kept to a minimum [39].

Results and Complications

The functional outcome of olecranon fracture fixation is good to excellent independent of type of fixation [40]. Plate fixation of displaced olecranon fractures has demonstrated good functional outcomes with low rates of complications [41]. The degree of articular integrity and accuracy of the articular reduction plays an important role in decreasing the rate of early arthritic changes [42].

The main complication associated with ORIF of the olecranon is symptomatic internal fixation [43]. This often requires removal of the hardware after fracture union. Infection and wound dehiscence are always a concern especially in the elderly patient with little subcutaneous tissue and friable skin. Elbow stiffness is another complication of this injury and is associated with prolonged immobilization. However, with simple olecranon fractures, the loss of range of motion is often minimal. Iatrogenic anterior interosseous nerve injury has been described when using tension band wires, related to over penetration of the K-wires through the anterior cortex of the ulna [44]. Nonunion of olecranon fractures is 1–5 % [45]. In the case of a nonunion, preoperative modification of risk factors, such as smoking cessation, blood glucose control, and appropriate diet, is recommended [46]. Several factors that predispose the olecranon fracture to nonunion include lack of compression at the fracture site, infection, bone loss, inadequate fixation, and overaggressive elbow range of motion.

Fracture-Dislocations

Terrible Triad

Indications for Treatment

The "terrible triad" was termed by Hotchkiss due to poor prognosis associated with the injury. This injury involves an elbow dislocation in association with radial head and coronoid fractures. Most terrible triad injuries occur as a result of indirect forces on the elbow resulting in a posterolateral dislocation. The most common mechanism of

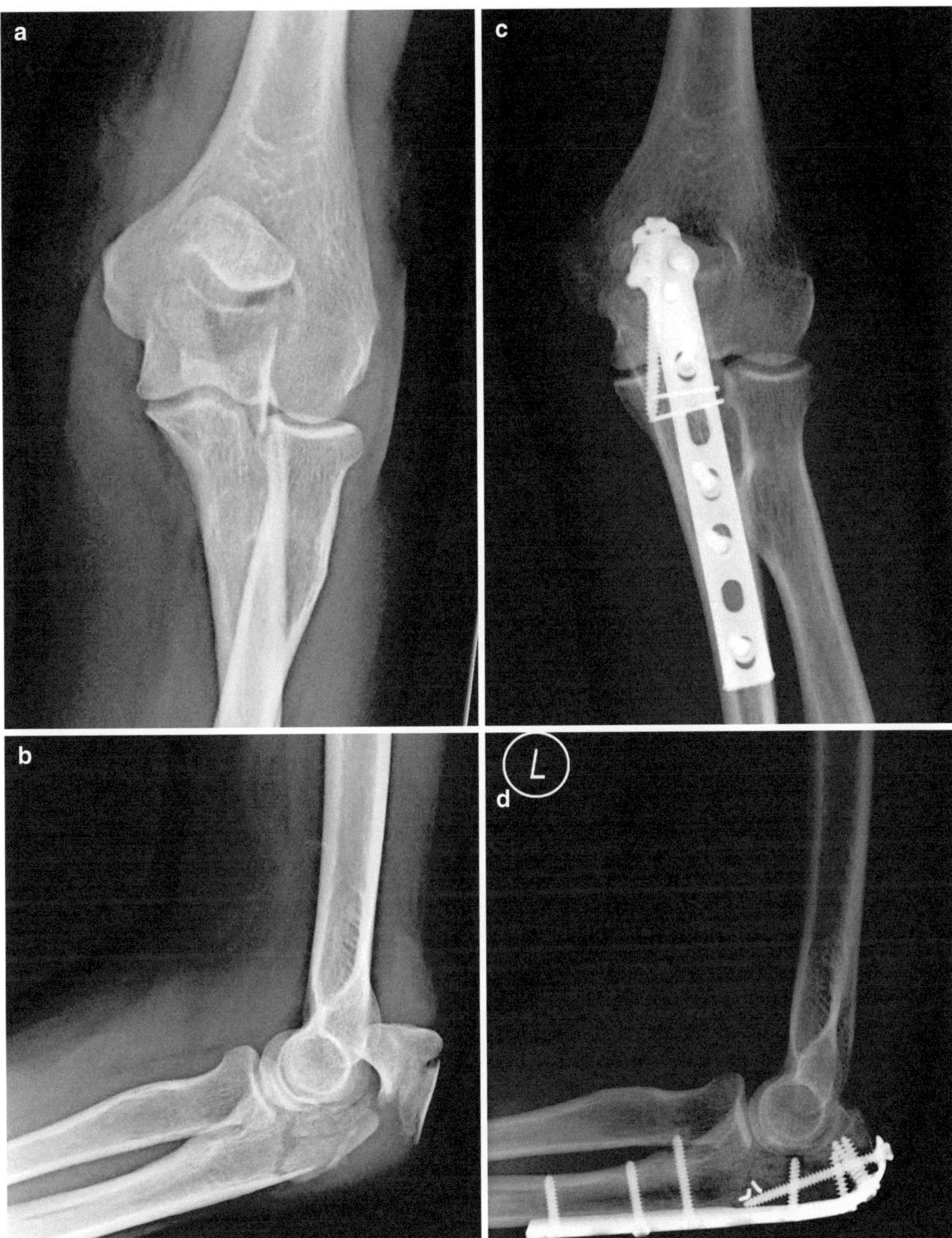

Fig. 5.7 Comminuted olecranon fracture requiring plate fixation (**a–b**). A low-profile olecranon plate was used to bridge the fracture (**c–d**). Note the use of threaded K-wires to secure small intercalary fragments which were too small to capture with the plate and screws. Alternatively, a secondary plate could have been applied orthogonally along the medial or lateral cortices

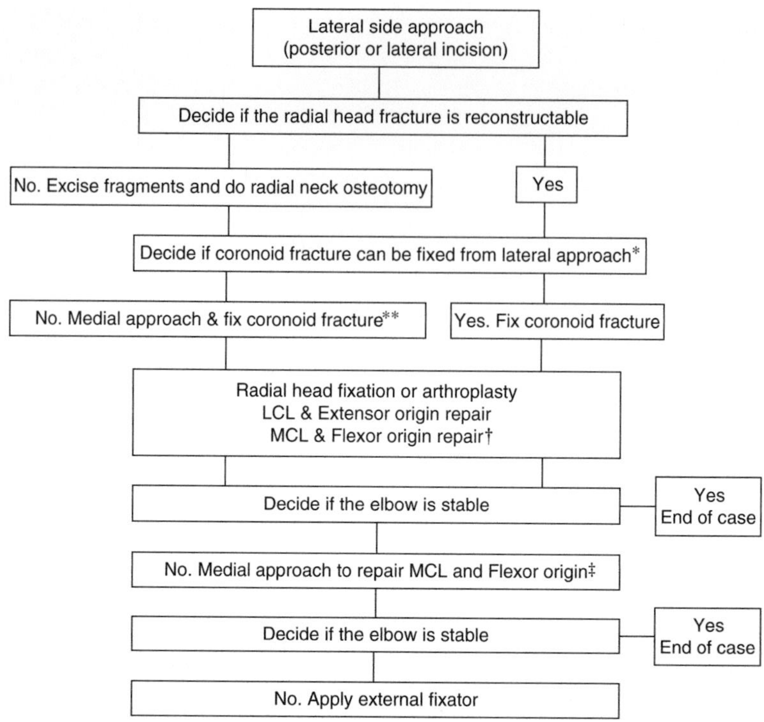

Fig. 5.8 Terrible triad algorithm

∗ Small tip coronoid fractures do not require fixation

∗∗ Can use same posterior incision or if a lateral incision used, make a new medial incision

† Only if you have done a medial approach to fix the coronoid fracture

‡ This step is already completed if a medial approach was used to fix the coronoid fracture

a terrible triad injury is a valgus axial load on a supinated forearm [47, 48]. It is crucial to obtain a good history in order to understand the mechanism of injury and help guide appropriate investigations. A preoperative CT scan can help determine the surgical approach and type of fixation.

Most terrible triad injuries require an operation. Radial head fractures which are small and undisplaced (unusual in the setting of a terrible triad injury) can be treated nonsurgically. With a terrible triad injury, radiocapitellar contact must be restored in order to assist with elbow stability and protect ligament repairs. In these injuries, radial head excision is contraindicated as there are significant ligamentous and soft tissue injuries.

Small coronoid tip fractures may be treated nonoperatively; otherwise surgery is indicated.

After the radial head and coronoid have been addressed, the lateral ulnar collateral ligament and extensor muscle origin are repaired. Most elbows will be stable at this point. However, if instability persists, the medial side of the elbow is approached and the MCL and flexor-pronator origin are repaired. In the rare case of continued instability, a static or dynamic external fixator is recommended. The surgical algorithm for a terrible triad injury is outlined in Fig. 5.8.

Preferred Surgical Approach

Our preferred incision is a universal posterior incision. The lateral side of the elbow is approached first for a terrible triad injury. The lateral collateral ligament is usually avulsed from its origin along with the extensor mechanism. It

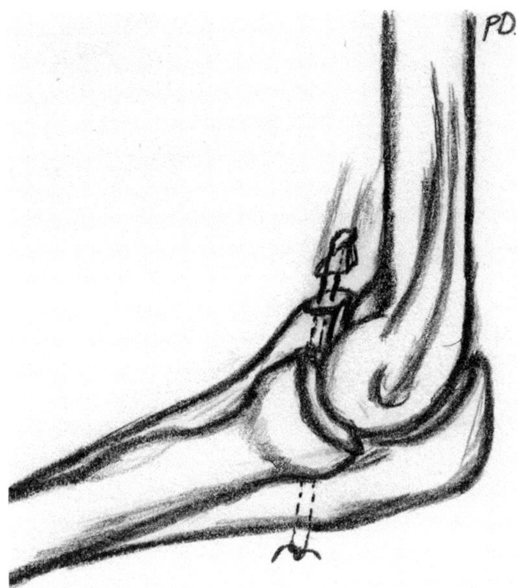

Fig. 5.9 Trans-osseous suture technique allows fixation of small coronoid tip fracture/comminution by grasping the fragment with part of the attached anterior capsule to assist in reduction

is important to recognize the six different patterns of LCL injuries as described by McKee and colleagues [49], with the most common involving avulsion of the ligament from its proximal origin. If the decision is made to perform a radial head arthroplasty, the radial neck osteotomy is performed to improve access to the coronoid fracture from the lateral side. The coronoid can usually be fixed through the radial fracture or osteotomy if arthroplasty is indicated. Exposure to the coronoid can be improved by hinging the elbow open through the LCL injury. However, in rare cases, to adequately visualize or fixate the coronoid fracture, a separate medial approach is required. If the fracture involves the anteromedial facet or sublime tubercle, a separate medial approach is preferred.

Surgical Technique

In general, coronoid fractures that require fixation (fractures involving >10 % of the coronoid) in the terrible triad elbow injury are reduced and stabilized with a trans-osseous suture technique or retrograde screws. For smaller tip fractures, a strong suture can be used though trans-osseous tunnels to capture and reduce the fragment from the subcutaneous border of the ulna (Fig. 5.9). For larger coronoid fractures, the fragment is reduced and stabilized with a targeted guide wire which is then exchanged for a cannulated screw from the subcutaneous border of the ulna. In certain cases a buttress plate is necessary to help reduce and maintain reduction of the coronoid fracture.

After addressing the coronoid and radial head fractures, attention is directed towards the LCL. The LCL is repaired back to the isometric point of origin with strong nonabsorbable sutures via a trans-osseous technique or with a suture anchor. When utilizing the trans-osseous technique, the sutures can be tied over a small plate to prevent cut out through bone. Care should be taken to avoid over tensioning the LCL repair, particularly in the setting of an MCL injury [50]. The final step on the lateral side is to repair the extensor mechanism to the supracondylar ridge (Fig. 5.10).

After repairing the coronoid, radial head, and the LCL, the stability of the elbow is examined under fluoroscopy with arm in neutral, pronation, and supination. If the elbow is stable up to 30° of flexion, MCL repair is not required. Otherwise a trans-osseous repair of the MCL is performed at its origin at the anteroinferior base of the medial epicondyle. The ulnar nerve must be identified and protected during this procedure, while transposition of the nerve is rarely required. It is quite rare for the elbow to continue to be unstable after both sides have been addressed. If this is the case, an external fixator is used.

Results and Complications

Despite earlier reports of the poor prognosis associated with terrible triad injuries, with appropriate treatment, the outcomes have been more favorable [13, 51–53]. In a multicenter series of 36 patients treated for terrible triad injuries, at a mean follow-up of 34 months, it was found that the flexion-extension arc averaged 112° ± 11° and forearm rotation 136° ± 16°. Based on the Mayo Elbow Performance Score, 15 patients were reported as excellent, 13 as good, seven as fair, and one as poor. Eight patients (22 %) required revision surgeries (2 synostosis, 1 recurrent instability, 4 contracture release and implant removal, and 1 wound infection) [53].

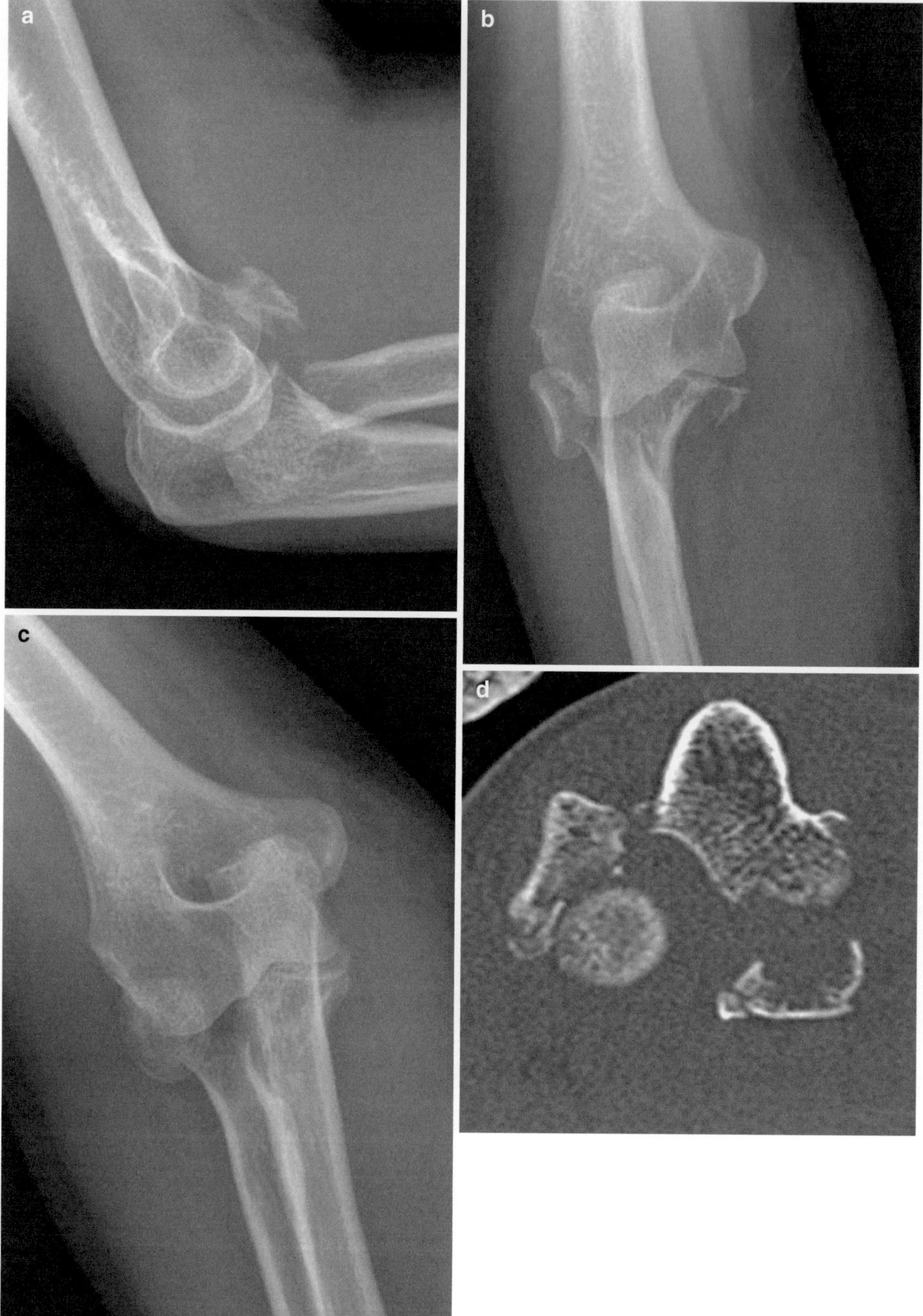

Fig. 5.10 Radiograph and computed tomography with 3-dimentional reconstruction of patient sustaining a terrible triad injury. Note the radial head is extruded laterally, and the coronoid fracture involves the tip and the antero-medial rim (**a–h**). She required a radial head arthroplasty. The coronoid fracture was fixated with retrograde screws, and the LCL repaired using trans-osseous tunnels, with sutures tied over a small plate (**i–j**). Following appropriate postoperative rehabilitation, the patient gained excellent range of motion and function (**k–n**)

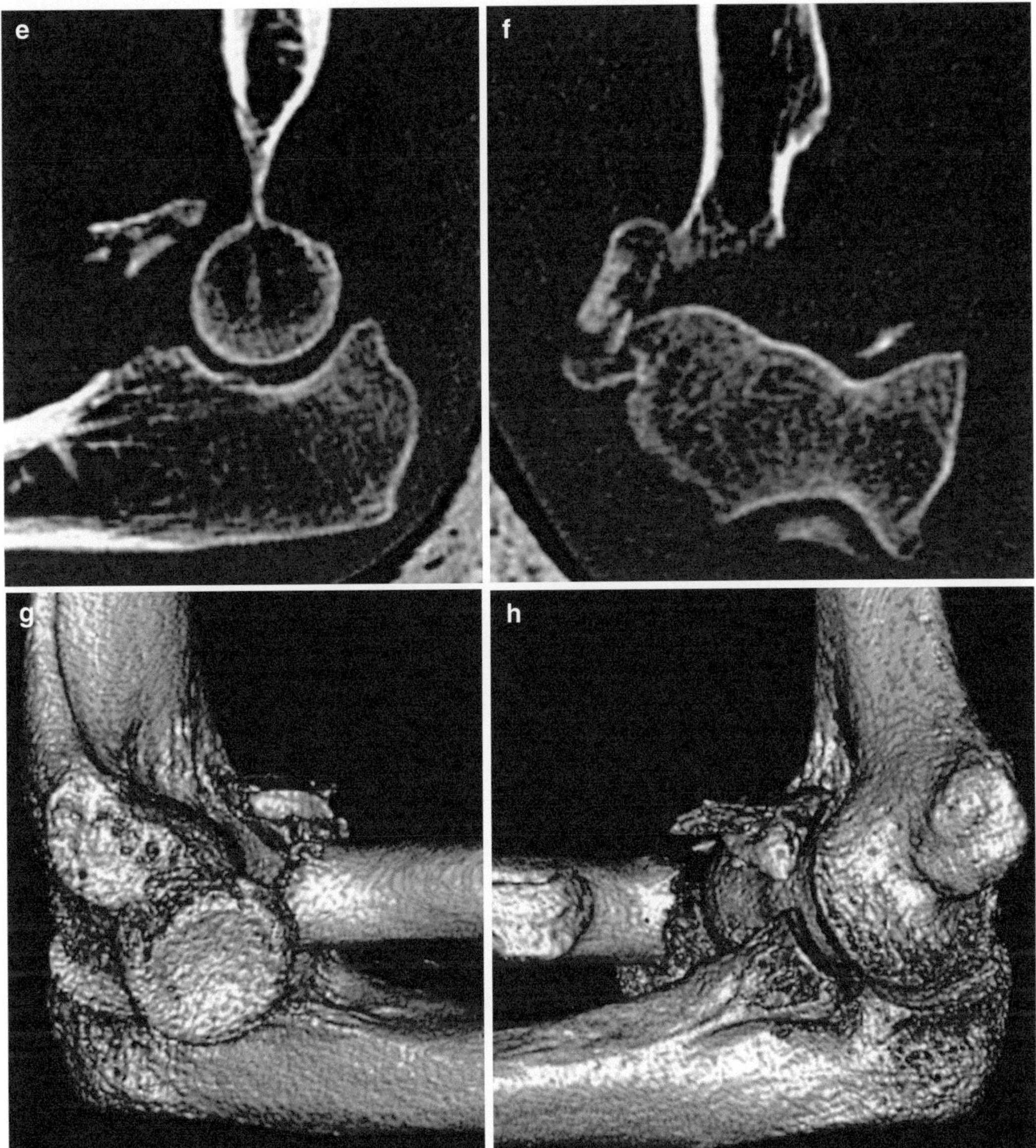

Fig. 5.10 (continued)

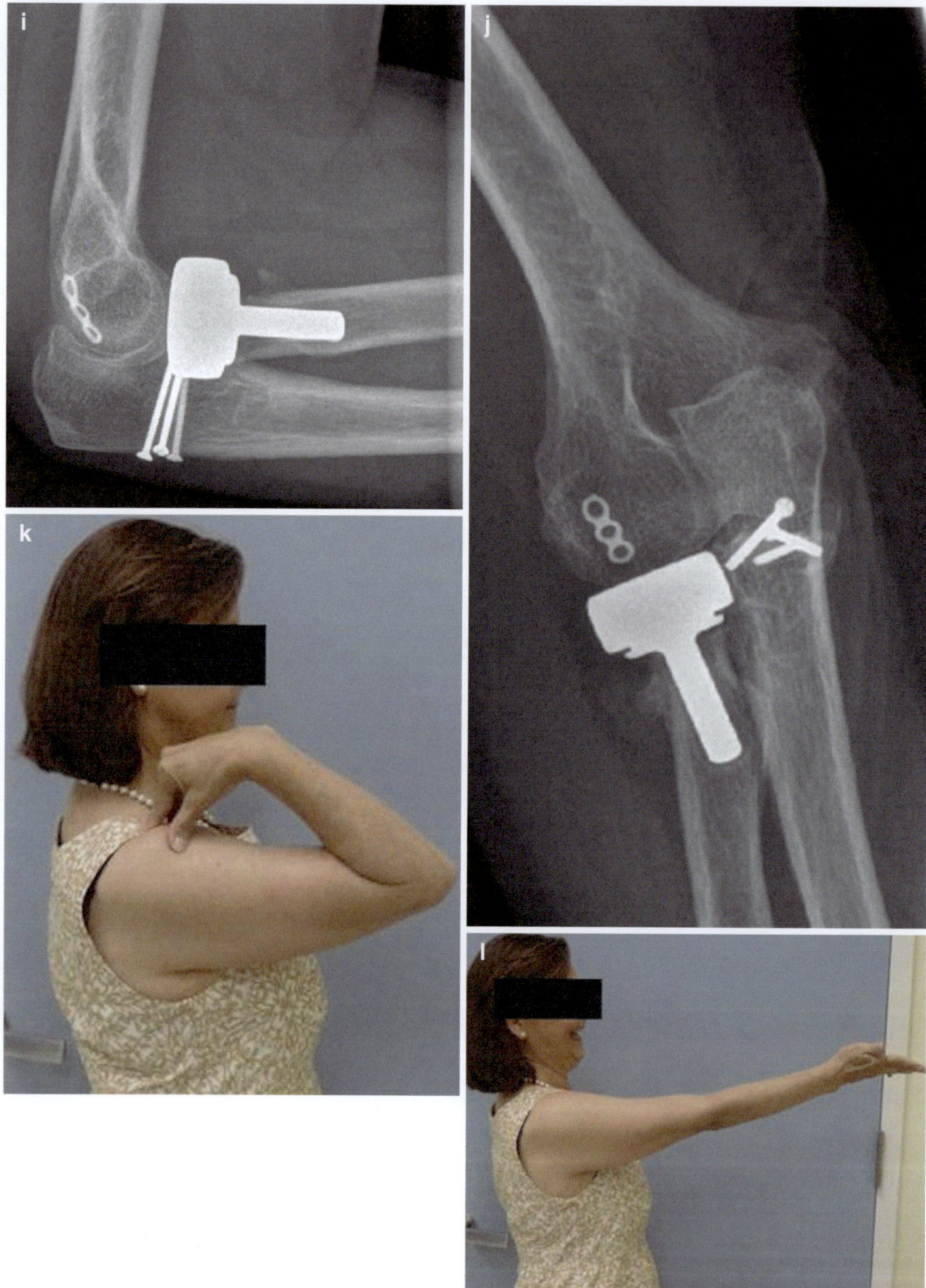

Fig. 5.10 (continued)

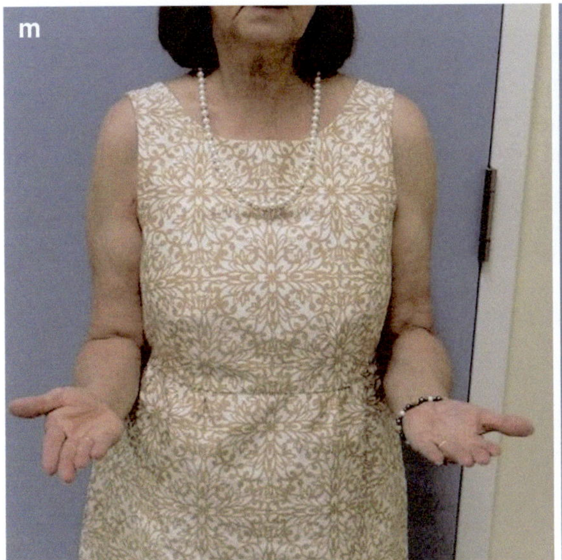
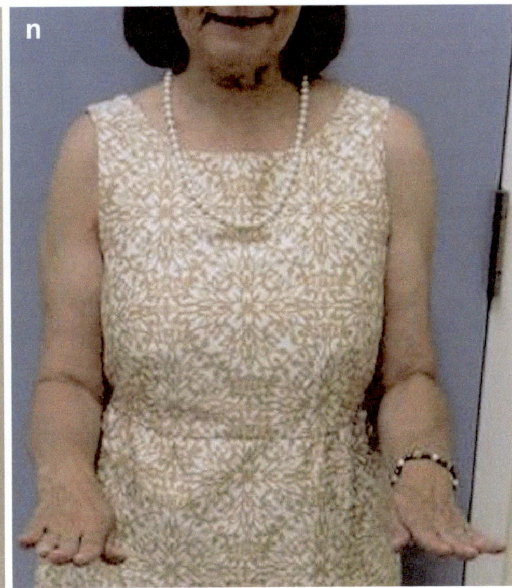

Fig. 5.10 (continued)

Similarly, Pugh and McKee demonstrated an arc of motion in flexion-extension of 115° and 135° in rotation. They demonstrated that delay in treatment and requirement for revision surgery were associated with approximately 20 % less arc of motion. Revision surgery was required in about 15–25 % of patients [52].

Common complications requiring revision surgery include instability, malunion, nonunion, infection, hardware problems, contractures, wound dehiscence, heterotopic ossification, and ulnar neuropathy [13, 52–54].

Anteromedial Coronoid Fracture-Dislocation

Indications for Treatment

Biomechanical studies have demonstrated the importance of the anteromedial coronoid facet in providing varus and posteromedial stability to the elbow [55]. This facet is prone to injury as about 58 % of it is not supported by the proximal ulnar metaphysis [56]. Anteromedial facet injuries are easy to overlook as the fracture can be small and superimposed by other structures on plain radiography. The double crescent sign on lateral radiograph is suspicious for an anterome-

dial facet fracture [57, 58]. If a coronoid fracture is suspected on radiographs, a CT scan should be obtained to better evaluate the injury.

The anteromedial facet fracture is associated with injuries to the posterior bundle of the MCL, LCL, and other lateral soft tissue stabilizers. These injuries result in posteromedial rotatory instability and varus subluxation of the ulnohumeral joint, leading to abnormal biomechanics and rapid degenerative changes of the ulnohumeral joint [59].

Several case series have demonstrated the benefits of early recognition and surgical treatment of anteromedial coronoid facet fractures [59–61]. In our practice these fractures are usually fixed surgically, and if the LCL is torn as is often the case, it should be repaired. Early protected range of motion is preferred, but not always possible. If the coronoid fracture is too comminuted for fixation, the elbow should be reduced, the LCL repaired, and consideration should be given to application of an external fixator (hinged or non-hinged).

Preferred Surgical Approach

A posterior incision is generally utilized to decrease injury to superficial nerves [21]. Both the medial and lateral sides of the elbow are approached through this incision. However, dual incisions can also be performed.

Surgical Technique

Using a posterior incision, the medial side and coronoid fracture is approached first. A full-thickness medial fasciocutaneous flap is raised. The ulnar nerve is released and gently mobilized. The coronoid is then approached through the floor of the ulnar nerve. This approach allows adequate visualization of the anteromedial coronoid and the sublime tubercle. The flexor-pronator mass is partially released from the medial epicondyle to improve visualization.

Once the coronoid is exposed, the fracture is reduced and stabilized with a reduction clamp and small K-wires. A buttress plate is used to stabilize the coronoid fragment(s). Pre-contoured or malleable plates (1.5–2.0 mm) can be used for the anteromedial facet fixation (Fig. 5.11).

After the coronoid fracture is stabilized, the lateral side is addressed. A full-thickness fasciocutaneous flap is raised laterally. A Kocher approach is used to repair the LCL. If present, extensor muscle origin injuries are also repaired. In rare circumstances, when solid fixation of the coronoid has been obtained, the LCL injury can be managed nonoperatively.

If the coronoid fracture is too comminuted for screw fixation, small threaded K-wires can be used to stabilize the fragments. In these cases of tenuous coronoid fixation, we recommend the use of an external fixator to maintain joint stability and allow healing of the LCL and the fracture fragments.

Results and Complications

Anteromedial coronoid fracture-dislocations can result in posteromedial rotatory instability. Without early recognition and appropriate management of anteromedial coronoid fractures, the elbow may become unstable and early arthritis can develop. There are very few reports of outcomes of nonoperative and surgical management of such injuries. Doornberg and Ring reported on 18 patients treated for anteromedial facet fractures, nine with plate fixation, one with screw fixation, one with suture fixation, and seven nonoperatively. These patients were followed for an average of 26 months. Six of the eighteen patients healed with malalignment of the fracture and varus displacement of the ulnohumeral joint, with eventual arthrosis and poor outcomes. Of these six patients, four were from the nonoperative group, and two had lost reduction of their fractured anteromedial facet. The remaining patients had good to excellent outcomes. This study highlights the importance of the anteromedial facet for elbow function and stability and supports surgical treatment of these fracture patterns [59].

Monteggia

Indications for Treatment

Monteggia fractures were originally termed to describe an anterior dislocation of the radial head in conjunction with a fracture of the proximal ulna. Bado classified the Monteggia lesions into four types based on the direction of the radial head dislocation [62]. Jupiter and colleagues further classified the posterior Monteggia lesion into types A to D depending on the location of the ulnar fracture: type A involving the coronoid and distal olecranon, type B being more distal at the junction of the metaphysis and diaphysis, type C involving the diaphysis, and type D extending along the entire proximal third to half of the ulna [63].

Incomplete Monteggia fractures or plastic deformations seen in children can be successfully treated with closed reduction and immobilization. However, these types of injuries do not occur in adults, and any Monteggia variant will have complete cortical disruption. Such injuries are better treated with surgical intervention.

In general, once the ulnar fracture is anatomically reduced, the radial head will reduce. If after fracture reduction, the radial head is still dislocated, the surgeon should assess the accuracy of the ulnar reduction. After the ulnar fracture is anatomically reduced and stabilized, the stability of the elbow is assessed. If the elbow continues to be unstable with hypersupination or varus stress, the LCL and annular ligament should be repaired. Postoperatively, active range of motion of the elbow is performed with the forearm in pronation to protect the lateral sided repair. For the first 6 weeks, forearm rotation is only allowed at flexion angles greater than 90°.

Preferred Surgical Approach

The key to a successful reduction of the radial head is anatomic reduction and stable fixation of the ulnar fracture. This fracture is

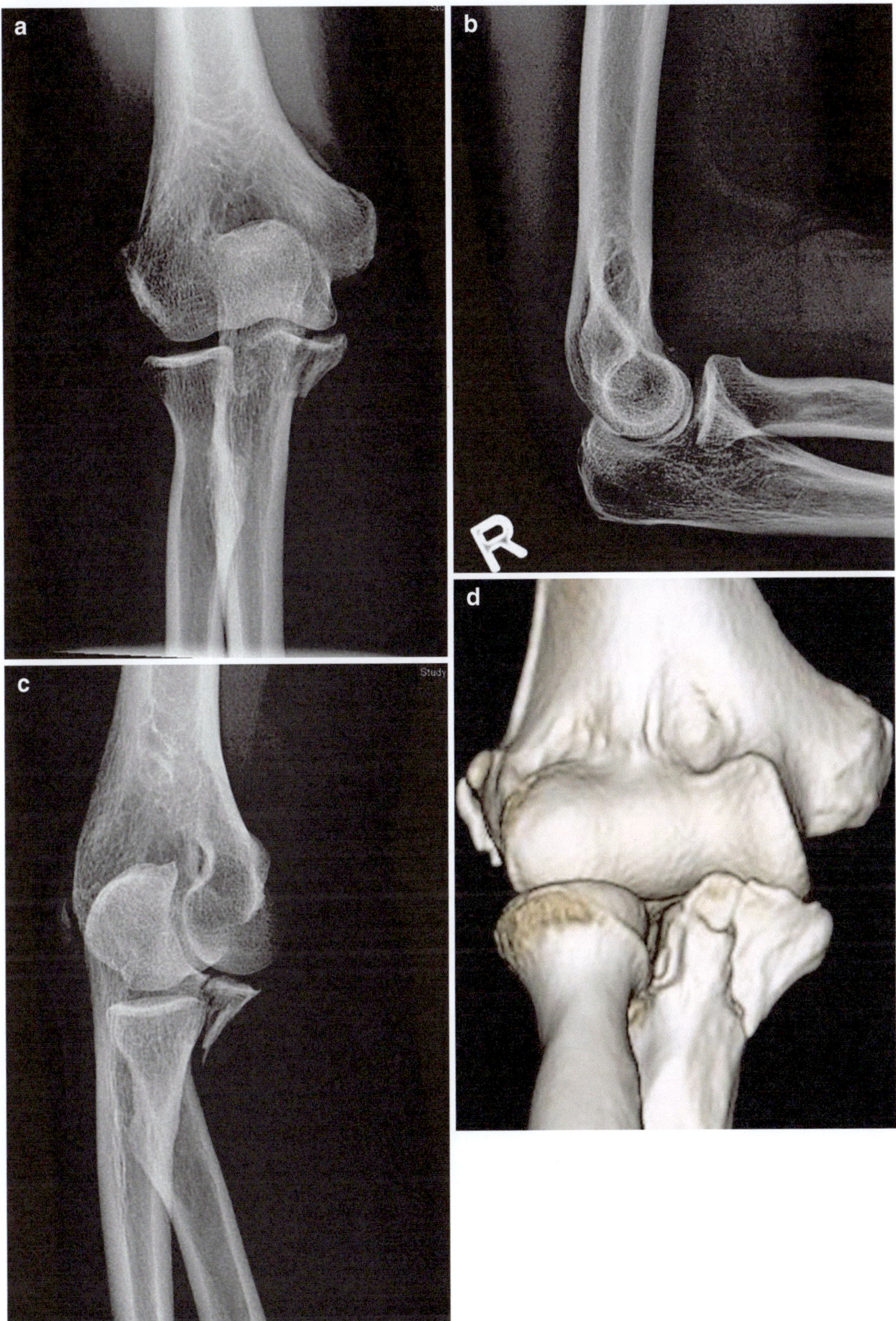

Fig. 5.11 Radiographs of a patient who sustained a right anteromedial coronoid facet fracture (**a–b**). Note the superimposed structures make the fracture difficult to diagnose on the lateral radiograph and the importance of oblique views and computed tomography (**c–f**). This patient was treated with a small profile plate to buttress the anteromedial coronoid fracture, and a K-wire was used to maintain the reduction of the coronoid tip fracture (**g–h**). The K-wire was placed retrograde through the fragment; the anterior tip was bent and the fragment pulled dorsally to reduce it, followed by bending the dorsal end of the K-wire to maintain the reduction. A suture anchor was used to repair the LCL

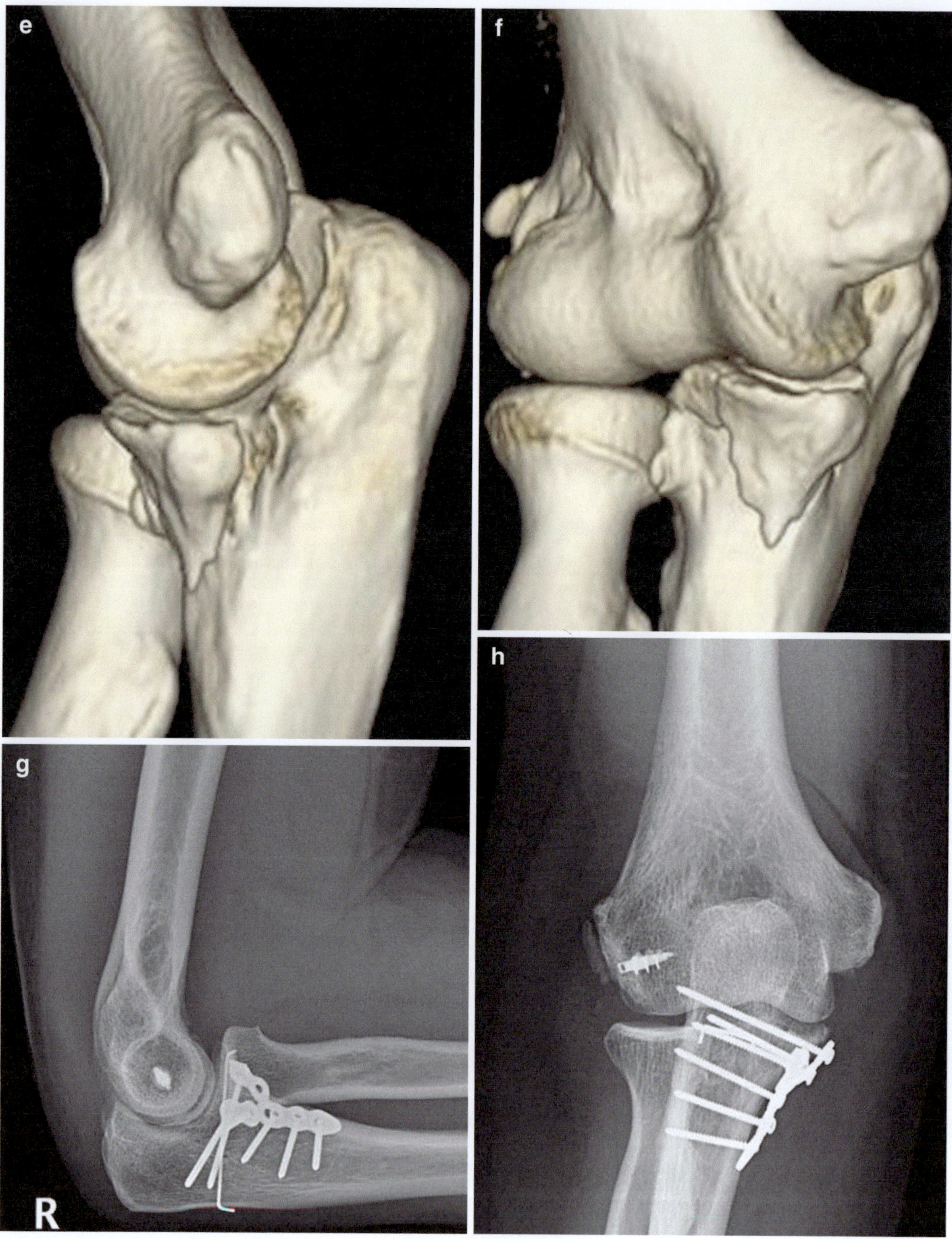

Fig. 5.11 (continued)

approached posteriorly along the subcutaneous border of the ulna. The fracture is identified and visualized with the least amount of bony stripping to maintain the blood supply to the fracture fragments. However, visualization is never sacrificed, as an anatomic reduction is critical for the management of this injury. With the elevation of the FCU off of the medial wall of the proximal ulna, coronoid fractures can be addressed if present.

Surgical Technique

We prefer to place the patient in a lateral decubitus position with the affected arm over an elbow positioner; however, supine positioning is also effective with the arm over the chest. If a radial head fracture is present, it can be dealt with through the olecranon or proximal ulna fracture and utilization of the Boyd approach by lifting the anconeus from the proximal ulna. Hence, the ulna should not be fixed before the radial head fracture is addressed. Once the ulnar fracture site is closed, this access to the radial head is limited. Fixation or replacement of the radial head will help stabilize the lateral side of the elbow, making it is easier to deal with the ulnar fracture. However, if the ulnar fracture involves the proximal radioulnar joint, or the length of the radial head cannot be accurately determined, it is best to fix the ulnar fracture first and then use a separate approach to address the radial head.

The coronoid fracture, if present, is generally approached next before fixing the ulna. The ulnar fracture may enhance visualization of the coronoid fragments. The fragments can be fixed with inter-fragmentary screw fixation or sub-articular threaded K-wire fixation for small articular fragments. Once the coronoid fracture is dealt with, the ulnar fracture is addressed. We prefer to use pre-contoured low-profile plates. One-third tubular and reconstruction plates are too weak and can jeopardize the fixation especially in the setting of early mobilization. The proximal aspect of the plate should be placed directly along the olecranon deep to the triceps tendon. Additional 1.5–2.0 mm plates can be used to secure smaller fracture fragments along the medial and lateral proximal ulna. It is important to anatomically reduce and stabilize fractures involving the sublime tubercle, supinator crest, and PRUJ, as they provide the attachments of the collateral ligaments (Fig. 5.12).

After the fracture fixation is complete, the elbow must be examined for ligamentous stability. Bado type II fractures often have associated LCL disruption. Although the ligaments are commonly intact after many Monteggia fractures, if there is residual instability, they must also be addressed.

Postoperatively, the patient's arm is placed in a volar long arm splint with the elbow in midflexion. This is done to allow the incision site to heal with the least amount of tension while avoiding wound pressure from a dorsally based splint. Once the wound has healed, the splint is discontinued and range of motion is commenced.

Results and Complications

In general the historical outcomes of Monteggia fractures have been unsatisfactory. However, with surgical treatment involving accurate reduction and stabilization of these fractures, the outcomes have improved. In a study by Bruce and colleagues in 1974, only five (24 %) of 21 adults treated for a Monteggia fracture had a good result. Sixteen (5 fair, 11 poor) or 76 % of 21 adults had fair or poor result [64]. In this study, four of the patients with fair or poor outcome had closed reduction, and four were treated with an intramedullary rod. None of the patients treated nonoperatively had good results.

In 1996, a multicenter study was carried out by Reynolds and colleagues assessing 67 patients with Monteggia fractures, all of whom were treated surgically [65]. They reported 54 % of patients with good to excellent results and 46 % had fair or poor results. Factors associated with poorer results were Bado types II and IV and olecranon fracture (i.e., Jupiter type IIA). Delayed healing was seen in ten patients and persistent dislocation of the radial head in seven.

In 2007, Konrad and colleagues presented their results on 47 patients with long-term follow-up. They demonstrated 34 patients (73 %) with good or excellent results and only 4 patients with poor results. Poor outcomes were associated with Bado type II fracture, Jupiter type IIA fracture, radial head fracture, coronoid fracture, and revision surgery [66].

These studies suggest that the results of operative treatment are improving as our understanding of Monteggia injuries advances. They also reveal the complexity and high rate of complications associated with these injuries. Posterior

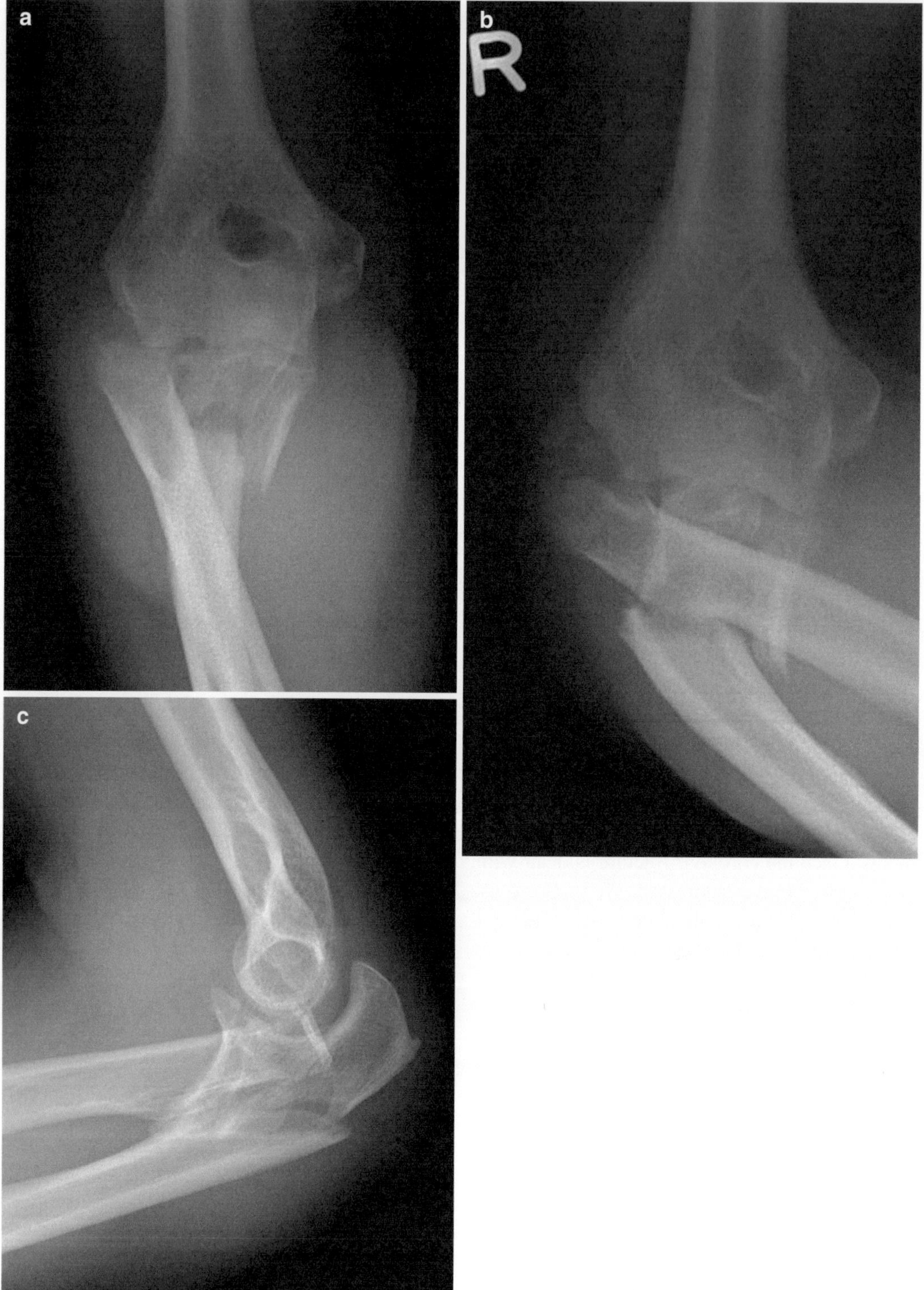

Fig. 5.12 Posterior Monteggia fracture-dislocation involving the proximal ulna and olecranon (**a–c**). Radiographs and 3-dimensional CT demonstrate the nature of the injury (**d–e**). This case was treated with triple plating of the proximal ulna and olecranon fracture as well as a radial head arthroplasty (**f–g**)

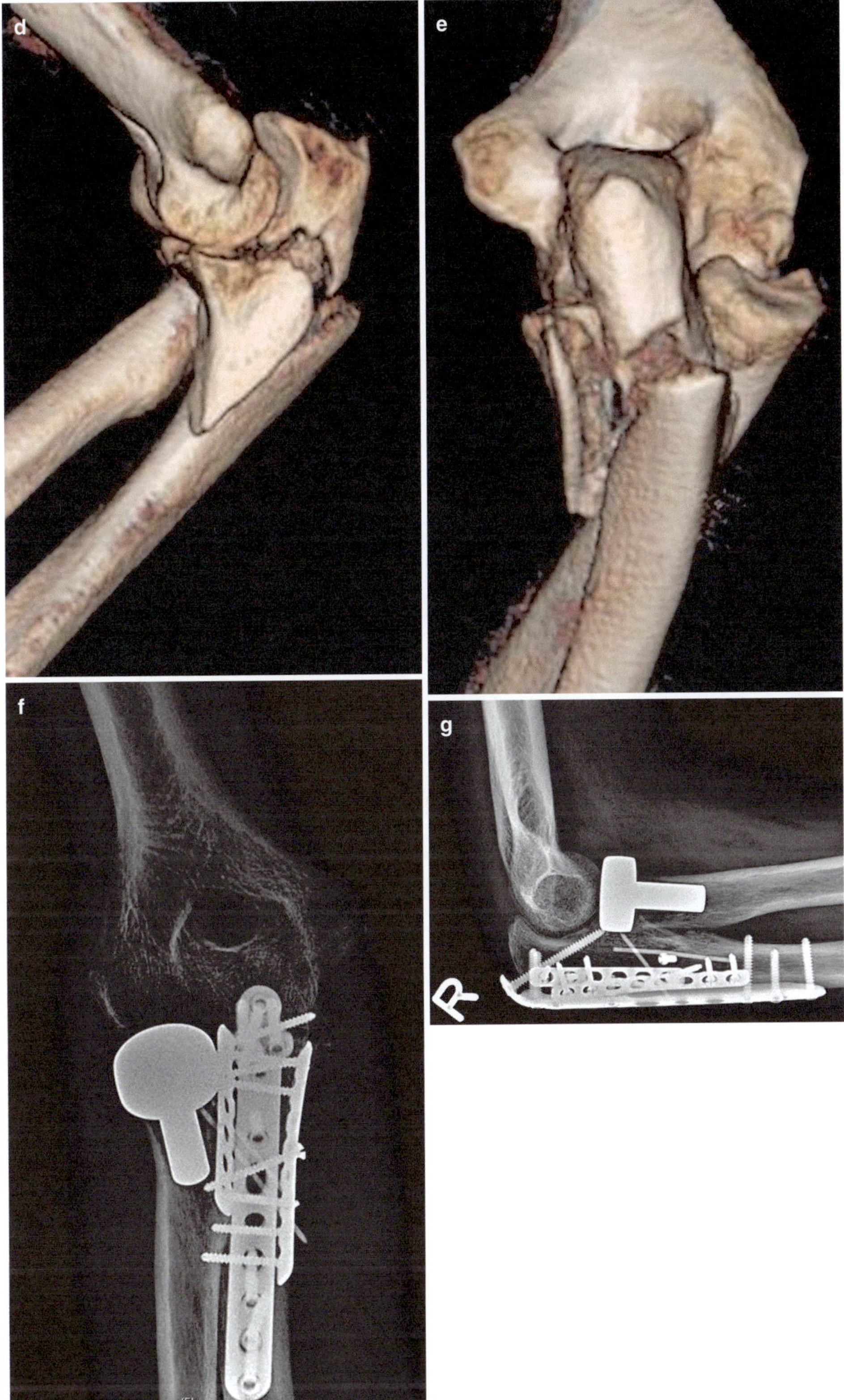

Fig. 5.12 (continued)

interosseous nerve injury is the most common neurologic injury seen with Monteggia fractures, although median and ulnar nerve injuries are also reported. Heterotopic ossification is a risk with surgical management of these fractures and can compromise motion in the elbow and forearm. Malunion is most commonly associated with Bado type II fractures and anterior comminution, which was not appreciated at the time of surgery. Ulnar malunion must be considered with any residual radial head subluxation or dislocation.

Trans-olecranon Fracture-Dislocation

Indications for Treatment

Trans-olecranon fracture-dislocation (TOFD) of the elbow involves fracture of the proximal ulna/olecranon, disruption of the ulnohumeral joint, along with dislocation of the radiocapitellar joint. In contrast to Monteggia injuries, with TOFD the proximal radioulnar joint (PRUJ) is intact but the ulnohumeral joint is disrupted. TOFD are divided into simple and complex based on the level of comminution in the greater sigmoid notch and proximal ulnar metaphysis [67]. They are also classified as being anterior or posterior [68]. The posterior TOFD has a similar injury pattern to posterior Monteggia. However, the mechanism of injury for anterior TOFD is most commonly a direct fall on the elbow, driving the distal humerus through the olecranon, and not an indirect force as is the case with most Monteggia fractures.

TOFD is often associated with larger coronoid fractures (Regan and Morrey Type III), radial head fractures, but typically intact collateral ligaments [67]. Many TFOD are open injuries and require early intervention for irrigation and debridement, followed by fixation if the wound is clean and soft tissues permitting. Such complex elbow injuries are usually treated operatively unless patient factors preclude this option.

All appropriate instrumentation along with an external fixator should be available prior to proceeding to the operating room. A CT scan of the elbow may be beneficial in fully characterizing the fracture and to help rule out other associated elbow fractures.

Preferred Surgical Approach

Similar to isolated olecranon fractures, a posterior approach is used to fix TOFD. As discussed earlier in this chapter, coronoid visualization can be carried out through the olecranon fracture or through a medial window by elevating the FCU from the medial proximal ulna. The latter approach requires release and protection of the ulnar nerve. The radial head injury can be dealt with through the fractured olecranon; otherwise, a separate lateral approach can be utilized as mentioned previously.

Surgical Technique

The coronoid fracture is visualized through the olecranon fracture or via a medial approach. Fixation of the coronoid can be obtained with antegrade or retrograde screws, plating, or trans-osseous sutures.

The radial head fracture can usually be addressed through the olecranon fracture. If radial head arthroplasty is required, reconstruction of the proximal radioulnar joint can assist in determining the correct implant size. Open reduction and internal fixation of a comminuted radial head fracture is usually difficult through the olecranon fracture; therefore, a separate lateral arthrotomy is necessary especially if a radial head/neck plate is required.

Finally the olecranon fracture is fixed with posterior plating using a contoured 3.5 mm low-profile plate. Prior to placement of the plate, any salvageable articular fragments are reduced and fixated via threaded K-wires or small intraosseous screws if possible (Fig. 5.13).

Fig. 5.13 Radiographs and CT of a 20-year-old male with a trans-olecranon fracture-dislocation of left elbow (**a–f**). Notice in this case the ulnohumeral joint is dislocated, and the proximal radioulnar joint is partially intact. His operation involved fixation of the radial head fracture, followed by fixation of the coronoid fractures with antegrade screws and medial plating, fixation of the olecranon fracture with 3.5 mm pre-contoured plate, and an LCL repair with a trans-osseous suture tied over a small plate (**g–h**)

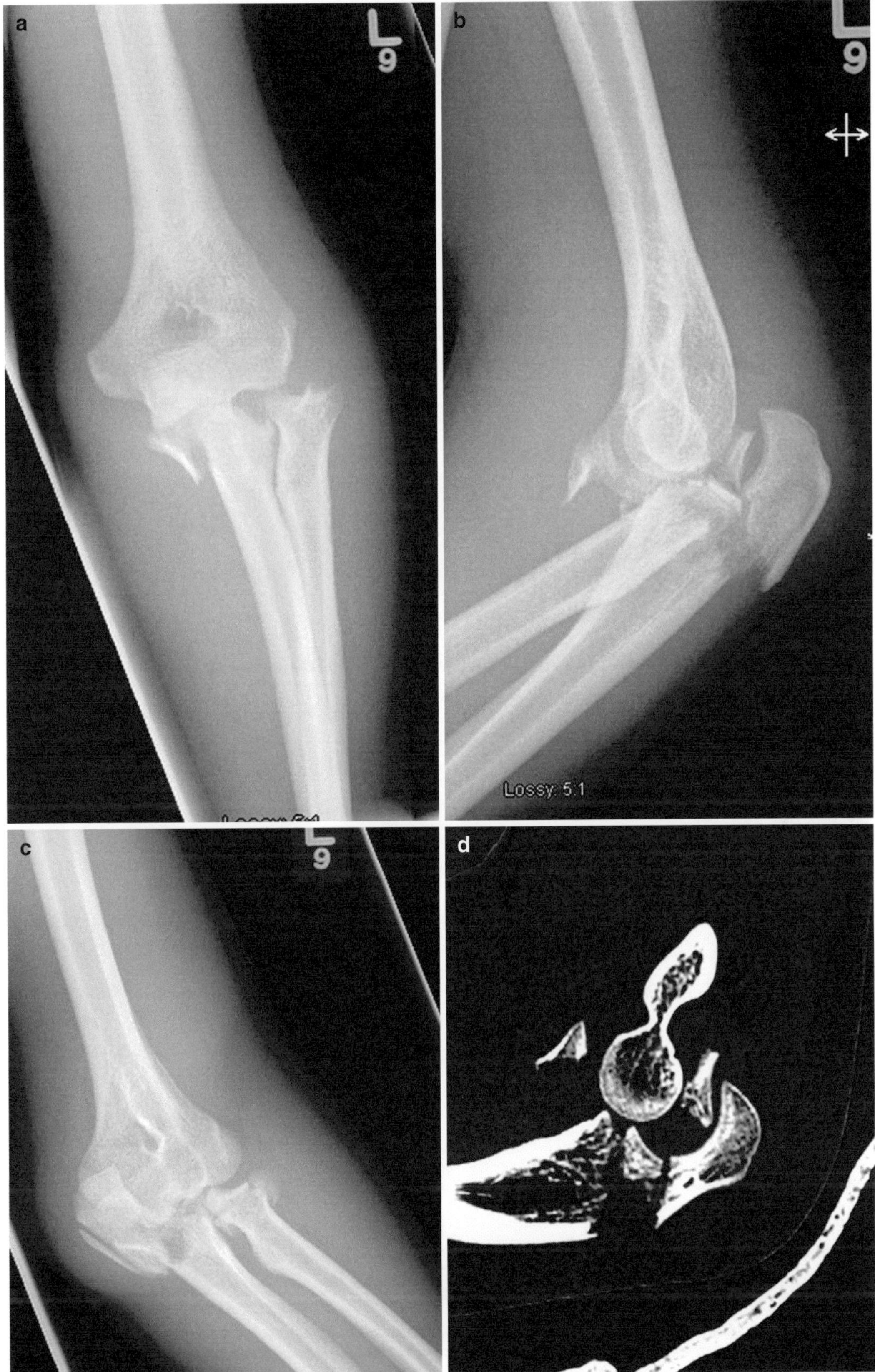
a
b
Lossy: 5:1
c
d

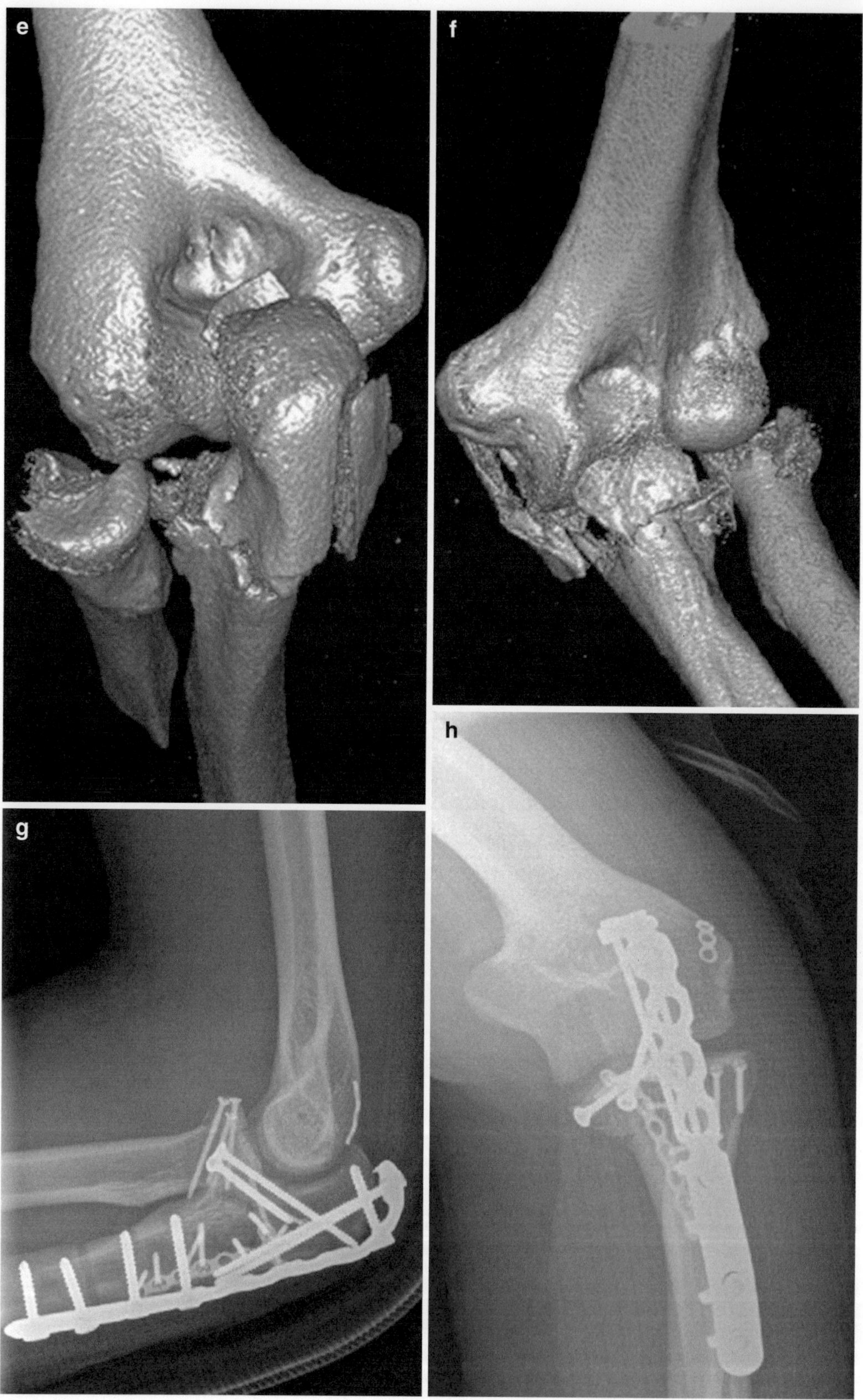

Fig. 5.13 (continued)

Ligamentous injuries can occur with TOFD; therefore, joint stability must always be assessed using fluoroscopy.

Results and Complications

There are very few studies reporting the outcomes of TOFDs. Although, this injury is not common, it has been confused with Monteggia fractures [67]. Ring et al. demonstrated good to excellent results in 15 of 17 (88 %) patients with an average of 25-month follow-up. Three patients had simple oblique fractures of the olecranon, and 14 had complex comminuted fractures. Patients with large coronoid fragments and extensive comminution of the trochlear notch had poorer outcomes unless adequate reduction and fixation was obtained. Elbow instability was not seen in any patient treated with surgical fixation. Two early hardware failures were secondary to the use of one-third tubular plate fixation, at which point they were changed to 3.5 mm dynamic compression plates.

Mouhsine and colleagues assessed 14 patients with TOFD including seven open fractures. Ten patients had complex comminuted olecranon fractures, five of whom had coronoid fractures. Elbow instability was not seen in any of the patients. At a mean follow-up of 3.6 years, they found ten patients (71 %) had good to excellent outcomes, and four patients (29 %) had fair to poor outcomes. Complications included early failure of fixation in three patients, delayed union in four patients, heterotopic ossification in one patient, and degenerative changes in four patients [69].

Although the literature is limited, patients with TOFD can do well when anatomic reduction and stable fixation of the trochlear notch and coronoid have been achieved.

Conclusion

Treatment of proximal ulna and radial head fracture-dislocations involves a clear understanding of the bony and soft tissue anatomy and pathoanatomy of the elbow. The history and physical exam are crucial in identifying the mechanism of injury and essential in recognition of injured structures. A critical appraisal of radiographs and advanced imaging when required will allow identification of fracture characteristics and injury patterns. The goals of treatment involve accurate reduction and fixation of the fractures, as well as ligament and soft tissue repairs as required, to allow stabilization of the elbow joint for early mobilization. Accurate diagnosis, prompt treatment, and rehabilitation of proximal ulna and radial head fracture-dislocations allow for the best outcomes.

References

1. Morrey BF. Current concepts in the treatment of fractures of the radial head, the olecranon, and the coronoid. Instr Course Lect. 1995;44:175–85.
2. van Riet RP, et al. Associated injuries complicating radial head fractures: a demographic study. Clin Orthop Relat Res. 2005;441:351–5.
3. Kaas L, et al. The incidence of associated fractures of the upper limb in fractures of the radial head. Strategies Trauma Limb Reconstr. 2008;3(2):71–4.
4. Regan W, Morrey B. Fractures of the coronoid process of the ulna. J Bone Joint Surg Am. 1989;71(9): 1348–54.
5. Veillette CJ, Steinmann SP. Olecranon fractures. Orthop Clin North Am. 2008;39(2):229–36, vii.
6. Amis AA, Miller JH. The mechanisms of elbow fractures: an investigation using impact tests in vitro. Injury. 1995;26(3):163–8.
7. Mason ML. Some observations on fractures of the head of the radius with a review of one hundred cases. Br J Surg. 1954;42(172):123–32.
8. Johnston GW. A follow-up of one hundred cases of fracture of the head of the radius with a review of the literature. Ulster Med J. 1962;31:51–6.
9. Broberg MA, Morrey BF. Results of treatment of fracture-dislocations of the elbow. Clin Orthop Relat Res. 1987;216:109–19.
10. Hotchkiss RN. Displaced fractures of the radial head: internal fixation or excision? J Am Acad Orthop Surg. 1997;5(1):1–10.
11. O'Driscoll SW, et al. Difficult elbow fractures: pearls and pitfalls. Instr Course Lect. 2003;52:113–34.
12. Essex-Lopresti P. Fractures of the radial head with distal radio-ulnar dislocation; report of two cases. J Bone Joint Surg Br. 1951;33B(2):244–7.
13. Forthman C, Henket M, Ring DC. Elbow dislocation with intra-articular fracture: the results of operative treatment without repair of the medial collateral ligament. J Hand Surg Am. 2007;32(8):1200–9.
14. Stoneback JW, et al. Incidence of elbow dislocations in the United States population. J Bone Joint Surg Am. 2012;94(3):240–5.
15. Mehlhoff TL, et al. Simple dislocation of the elbow in the adult. Results after closed treatment. J Bone Joint Surg Am. 1988;70(2):244–9.
16. Ring D, Quintero J, Jupiter JB. Open reduction and internal fixation of fractures of the radial head. J Bone Joint Surg Am. 2002;84-A(10):1811–5.

17. Boulas HJ, Morrey BF. Biomechanical evaluation of the elbow following radial head fracture. Comparison of open reduction and internal fixation vs. excision, silastic replacement, and non-operative management. Chir Main. 1998;17(4):314–20.

18. Goldberg I, Peylan J, Yosipovitch Z. Late results of excision of the radial head for an isolated closed fracture. J Bone Joint Surg Am. 1986;68(5):675–9.

19. Ikeda M, Oka Y. Function after early radial head resection for fracture: a retrospective evaluation of 15 patients followed for 3–18 years. Acta Orthop Scand. 2000;71(2):191–4.

20. Janssen RP, Vegter J. Resection of the radial head after Mason type-III fractures of the elbow: follow-up at 16 to 30 years. J Bone Joint Surg Br. 1998;80(2):231–3.

21. Dowdy PA, et al. The midline posterior elbow incision. An anatomical appraisal. J Bone Joint Surg Br. 1995;77(5):696–9.

22. Smith GR, Hotchkiss RN. Radial head and neck fractures: anatomic guidelines for proper placement of internal fixation. J Shoulder Elbow Surg. 1996; 5(2 Pt 1):113–7.

23. Smith AM, et al. Radius pull test: predictor of longitudinal forearm instability. J Bone Joint Surg Am. 2002;84-A(11):1970–6.

24. Athwal GS, et al. Determination of correct implant size in radial head arthroplasty to avoid overlengthening: surgical technique. J Bone Joint Surg Am. 2010;92(Suppl 1 Pt 2):250–7.

25. Van Glabbeek F, et al. Detrimental effects of overstuffing or understuffing with a radial head replacement in the medial collateral-ligament deficient elbow. J Bone Joint Surg Am. 2004;86-A(12):2629–35.

26. van Riet RP, et al. Validation of the lesser sigmoid notch of the ulna as a reference point for accurate placement of a prosthesis for the head of the radius: a cadaver study. J Bone Joint Surg Br. 2007;89(3):413–6.

27. Doornberg JN, et al. Reference points for radial head prosthesis size. J Hand Surg Am. 2006;31(1):53–7.

28. Frank SG, et al. Determination of correct implant size in radial head arthroplasty to avoid overlengthening. J Bone Joint Surg Am. 2009;91(7):1738–46.

29. Rowland AS, et al. Lateral ulnohumeral joint space widening is not diagnostic of radial head arthroplasty overstuffing. J Hand Surg Am. 2007;32(5):637–41.

30. Beingessner DM, et al. The effect of radial head excision and arthroplasty on elbow kinematics and stability. J Bone Joint Surg Am. 2004;86-A(8):1730–9.

31. Antuna SA, Sanchez-Marquez JM, Barco R. Long-term results of radial head resection following isolated radial head fractures in patients younger than forty years old. J Bone Joint Surg Am. 2010;92(3):558–66.

32. Zarattini G, et al. The surgical treatment of isolated mason type 2 fractures of the radial head in adults: comparison between radial head resection and open reduction and internal fixation. J Orthop Trauma. 2012;26(4):229–35.

33. Hume MC, Wiss DA. Olecranon fractures. A clinical and radiographic comparison of tension band wiring and plate fixation. Clin Orthop Relat Res. 1992;285:229–35.

34. Rouleau DM, Faber KJ, Athwal GS. The proximal ulna dorsal angulation: a radiographic study. J Shoulder Elbow Surg. 2010;19(1):26–30.

35. Izzi J, Athwal GS. An off-loading triceps suture for augmentation of plate fixation in comminuted osteoporotic fractures of the olecranon. J Orthop Trauma. 2012;26(1):59–61.

36. Hak DJ, Golladay GJ. Olecranon fractures: treatment options. J Am Acad Orthop Surg. 2000;8(4):266–75.

37. Gartsman GM, Sculco TP, Otis JC. Operative treatment of olecranon fractures. Excision or open reduction with internal fixation. J Bone Joint Surg Am. 1981;63(5):718–21.

38. Inhofe PD, Howard TC. The treatment of olecranon fractures by excision or fragments and repair of the extensor mechanism: historical review and report of 12 fractures. Orthopedics. 1993;16(12):1313–7.

39. Bell TH, et al. Contribution of the olecranon to elbow stability: an in vitro biomechanical study. J Bone Joint Surg Am. 2010;92(4):949–57.

40. Karlsson MK, et al. Comparison of tension-band and figure-of-eight wiring techniques for treatment of olecranon fractures. J Shoulder Elbow Surg. 2002;11(4):377–82.

41. Bailey CS, et al. Outcome of plate fixation of olecranon fractures. J Orthop Trauma. 2001;15(8):542–8.

42. Rommens PM, et al. Olecranon fractures in adults: factors influencing outcome. Injury. 2004;35(11): 1149–57.

43. Macko D, Szabo RM. Complications of tension-band wiring of olecranon fractures. J Bone Joint Surg Am. 1985;67(9):1396–401.

44. Parker JR, Conroy J, Campbell DA. Anterior interosseous nerve injury following tension band wiring of the olecranon. Injury. 2005;36(10):1252–3.

45. Morrey BF. The elbow and its disorders. Philadelphia: WB Saunders; 2000. p. 341–63.

46. Papagelopoulos PJ, Morrey BF. Treatment of nonunion of olecranon fractures. J Bone Joint Surg Br. 1994;76(4):627–35.

47. Doornberg JN, Ring D. Coronoid fracture patterns. J Hand Surg Am. 2006;31(1):45–52.

48. Steinmann SP. Coronoid process fracture. J Am Acad Orthop Surg. 2008;16(9):519–29.

49. McKee MD, et al. The pathoanatomy of lateral ligamentous disruption in complex elbow instability. J Shoulder Elbow Surg. 2003;12(4):391–6.

50. Pollock JW, et al. The influence of type II coronoid fractures, collateral ligament injuries, and surgical repair on the kinematics and stability of the elbow: an in vitro biomechanical study. J Shoulder Elbow Surg. 2009;18(3):408–17.

51. McKee MD, et al. Standard surgical protocol to treat elbow dislocations with radial head and coronoid fractures. Surgical technique. J Bone Joint Surg Am. 2005;87(Suppl 1(Pt 1)):22–32.

52. Pugh DM, McKee MD. The "terrible triad" of the elbow. Tech Hand Up Extrem Surg. 2002;6(1):21–9.
53. Pugh DM, et al. Standard surgical protocol to treat elbow dislocations with radial head and coronoid fractures. J Bone Joint Surg Am. 2004;86-A(6):1122–30.
54. O'Driscoll SW, et al. Elbow subluxation and dislocation. A spectrum of instability. Clin Orthop Relat Res. 1992;280:186–97.
55. Pollock JW, et al. The effect of anteromedial facet fractures of the coronoid and lateral collateral ligament injury on elbow stability and kinematics. J Bone Joint Surg Am. 2009;91(6):1448–58.
56. Doornberg JN, et al. The anteromedial facet of the coronoid process of the ulna. J Shoulder Elbow Surg. 2007;16(5):667–70.
57. Sanchez-Sotelo J, O'Driscoll SW, Morrey BF. Anteromedial fracture of the coronoid process of the ulna. J Shoulder Elbow Surg. 2006;15(5):e5–8.
58. Sanchez-Sotelo J, O'Driscoll SW, Morrey BF. Medial oblique compression fracture of the coronoid process of the ulna. J Shoulder Elbow Surg. 2005;14(1):60–4.
59. Doornberg JN, Ring DC. Fracture of the anteromedial facet of the coronoid process. J Bone Joint Surg Am. 2006;88(10):2216–24.
60. Ring D, Doornberg JN. Fracture of the anteromedial facet of the coronoid process. Surgical technique. J Bone Joint Surg Am. 2007;89(Suppl 2 Pt.2):267–83.
61. Adams JE, et al. Management and outcome of 103 acute fractures of the coronoid process of the ulna. J Bone Joint Surg Br. 2009;91(5):632–5.
62. Bado JL. The Monteggia lesion. Clin Orthop Relat Res. 1967;50:71–86.
63. Jupiter JB, et al. The posterior Monteggia lesion. J Orthop Trauma. 1991;5(4):395–402.
64. Bruce HE, Harvey JP, Wilson Jr JC. Monteggia fractures. J Bone Joint Surg Am. 1974;56(8):1563–76.
65. Reynders P, et al. Monteggia lesions in adults. A multicenter Bota study. Acta Orthop Belg. 1996;62 Suppl 1:78–83.
66. Konrad GG, et al. Monteggia fractures in adults: long-term results and prognostic factors. J Bone Joint Surg Br. 2007;89(3):354–60.
67. Ring D, et al. Transolecranon fracture-dislocation of the elbow. J Orthop Trauma. 1997;11(8):545–50.
68. Manidakis N, et al. Fractures of the ulnar coronoid process. Injury. 2012;43(7):989–98.
69. Mouhsine E, et al. Transolecranon anterior fracture dislocation. J Shoulder Elbow Surg. 2007;16(3):352–7.

Elbow Stiffness

Pierre Mansat and Nicolas Bonnevialle

Abstract

Elbow stiffness can be a very limiting condition. Interpretation of the etiology is crucial to decide the ideal indication of each patient. The status of the joint dictates the preferred treatment. Indications for operative and nonoperative treatment are reviewed. Detailed surgical technique for open and arthroscopic elbow capsulectomies is presented. The influence of the ulnar nerve on the outcome is discussed along with the complications and expected results of simple elbow stiffness. Complex cases requiring interposition or total joint arthroplasty are analyzed, and a preferred treatment algorithm is provided. Indications, techniques, and outcomes of each procedure are reviewed.

Keywords

Stiffness • Capsulectomy • Arthroplasty

Introduction

Of the numerous potential causes for elbow stiffness, the causes and pathophysiologic mechanisms dictate treatment and affect prognosis. Posttraumatic stiffness is one of the most frequent causes of this kind of contracture [1]; however, it can also occur in association with other causes, such as prolonged immobilization, congenital or developmental disease, osteoarthritis or inflammatory arthritis, burns, and head injury.

Several treatment options have been proposed for treatment of elbow contracture. Conservative treatment sometimes gives good results if the contracture is of short duration [2–12]; however, its efficacy is unpredictable. With failure of nonoperative treatment, surgical release may be indicated. Many surgical treatments can be proposed to treat stiff elbows. Surgical techniques will be chosen according to the type [13] and the severity of the stiffness [14–16]. Chronic extrinsic stiffness is usually managed by arthroscopic [17–30] or surgical release [31–50] with good results. When less than 50 % of the joint surface is involved in an intrinsic stiffness, the

P. Mansat, MD, PhD (✉) • N. Bonnevialle, MD, PhD
Orthopaedic and Traumatology Department,
University Hospital Toulouse,
Place du Dr BAYLAC, Toulouse 31059, France
e-mail: mansat.p@chu-toulouse.fr;
bonnevialle.n@chu-toulouse.fr

S. Antuña, R. Barco (eds.), *Essentials in Elbow Surgery*,
DOI 10.1007/978-1-4471-4625-4_6, © Springer-Verlag London 2014

same treatment can be proposed with less reliable results. However, when more than 50 % of the articular surface is involved, an interposition arthroplasty may be the treatment of choice in young patients [13, 51–56], whereas in older patients a total elbow arthroplasty has been considered the desirable option [57–61].

The Problem

The elbow is particularly prone to develop stiffness as a result of the high degree of congruency of the joint, the close continuity of the muscle to the capsule, the propensity for comminuted fractures, and the somewhat unique response of the joint capsule to trauma. Classifying the type and the severity of the stiffness is very important for preoperative planning and for estimation of prognosis.

Morrey described two types of contractures: extra-articular or extrinsic contractures and intra-articular or intrinsic [1] (Table 6.1).

Extrinsic contractures typically involve the periarticular soft tissue, without involvement of the articulating surface. Contracture may involve the capsulo-ligamentous structures or the muscular tissue. Ectopic ossifications following trauma, burn, or head injury are also considered extrinsic conditions. Bone may bridge across the joint or form in the capsule or muscle crossing the joint. Trauma is the major cause of soft tissue extrinsic stiffness, especially elbow dislocation with or without fracture. The brachialis muscle, that crosses the anterior capsule, tears with dislocation developing scar tissue or ectopic bone when healing, often associated with contracture of the capsule. Contracture of collateral ligament also contributes to elbow stiffness, and prolonged immobilization has been recognized also as a major contributor to postinjury contracture. In osteoarthritis, a mild inflammatory synovitis occurs with periarticular fibrosis and osteophytic new bone formation. The articular surface of the joint is intact, but osteophytes are present at the tip of the olecranon and at the tip of the coronoid process. Congenital stiffness is rare and is often associated with bony malformation, as well as soft tissue dysplasia.

Intrinsic or intra-articular contractures involve the intra-articular joint with a lesion of the cartilage surface or with intra-articular adhesions from a remodeling joint. Gross distorsion of the joint resulting from inadequate or failed reduction of an intra-articular fracture is another cause of intrinsic contracture. Finally, intra-articular fracture typically is associated with some degree of scarring around the joint. When both of these features contribute to the motion loss, it is considered a mixed process and portends a poorer prognosis.

The functional impact of the lost of motion depends on the extent and the specific position of the arc of motion that is affected. It is helpful to further grade the stiffness as very severe, severe, moderate, and minimal according to the arc of flexion. The stiffness is considered very severe when the total arc is less or equal to 30°, severe when the total arc is between 31° and 61°, moderate when the total arc is between 61° and 90°, and minimal when the total arc is greater than 90° [62]. Based on the functional arc of motion described by Morrey referable to the 30–130 functional arc [63], the distribution of the contracture has been classified by Allieu in four groups: within the functional arc of motion, in flexion, in extension, or in combined stiffness [15].

Finally, Jupiter et al. [16] distinguished the "simple stiff elbow" as characterized by mild to moderate contracture (<80° arc of motion) with no or minimal prior surgery, no prior nerve transposition, no internal fixation, minimal heterotopic ossification, and well-preserved bony

Table 6.1 Etiology of elbow stiffness

Extrinsic
Cutaneous or subcutaneous adhesion, capsular and collateral ligaments retraction
Muscular retraction (anterior/posterior)
Heterotopic ossification
Osteophytes at olecranon and/or coronoid
Intrinsic
Articular distorsion, joint malunion
Intra-articular adhesions
Cartilage involvement
Fibrosis at the coronoid and olecranon fossa obliteration
Loose bodies
Mixed

anatomy, from the "complex stiff elbow" that requires more expertise and has a higher surgical complication rate.

Patient Workup

Clinical Exam

The diagnosis of the contracture is not difficult and is usually made by a characteristic history and physical examination. Posttraumatic contracture of the elbow may occur at any age but frequently concerns young active patients around 40 years of age, with functional need and use of their elbow joint. Osteoarthritis on the other hand involves patients in the mid-50s and occurs predominantly in males. With extrinsic contracture, the patient's initial awareness is generally that of loss of full extension, with no limitation of their activity. The first complaint is pain in terminal extension; the mid-arc of motion is typically not painful, confirming the extrinsic nature of the stiffness. Occasionally, full flexion will also result in pain, and flexion contracture may develop progressively.

Intrinsic contracture on the other hand is often related to intra-articular fractures. The patient presents typically pain throughout the arc of motion with limitation of elbow motion. Clinical evaluation must analyze the local skin quality, the existence of previous incisions, or adhesions of the skin to bone. Passive and active range of motion must be measured in flexion-extension but also in pronation-supination. The sensory and motor function of the ulnar nerve should be assessed. Biologic evaluation of the inflammatory status may rule out an inflammatory process as well as an infection [64].

Imaging

Joint involvement is confirmed on plain radiographs. The anteroposterior view gives a good visualization of the joint line, but the lateral radiograph demonstrates osteophytes on the coronoid and at the tip of the olecranon even when the joint space is preserved. The details of the extent of the involvement are best observed with an arthro-CT [65] (Fig. 6.1). Sometimes, a 3D reconstruction precisely locates heterotopic bone formations and gives accurate information about the status of the articular surfaces. In our experience, MRI scanning adds no further

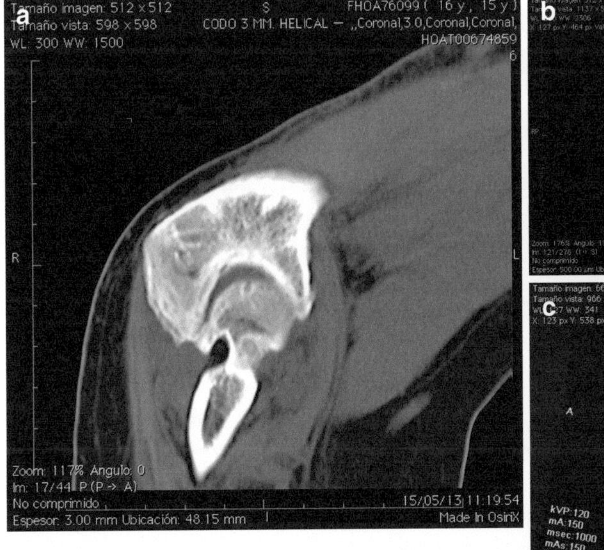
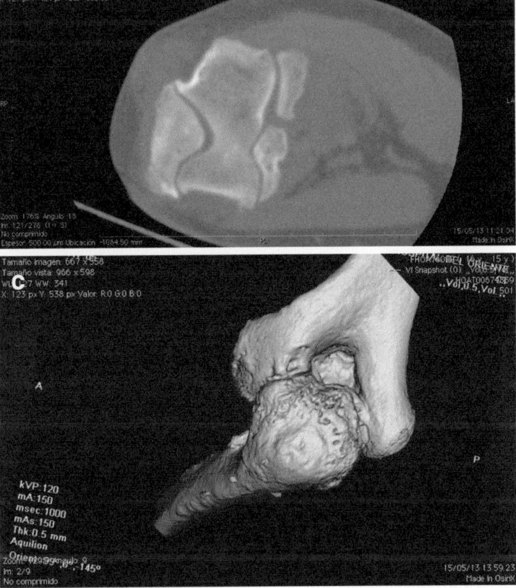

Fig. 6.1 (**a**) Lateral, (**b**) transverse, and (**c**) 3D CT scan images of an arthritic elbow

information for the diagnosis or preoperative planning.

The Simple Stiff Elbow

Conservative Treatment

The aim of treating the stiff elbow is to give the patient a pain-free, functional, and stable elbow. Several authors have reported good results after close treatment of the stiff elbow [2–12]. This nonoperative treatment includes physiotherapy, manipulation, and static and dynamic splinting. After elbow trauma or fracture, it is particularly important to recognize when the patient is not gaining motion on schedule. If the patient is progressing slowly, we strongly recommend the use of adjustable splints to restore flexion, extension, or both (Fig. 6.2). Several types of splints are available: the static splint, the hinged splint, the dynamic splint, and the adjustable static splint (turnbuckle device). We use usually the adjustable static splint because we believe inflammation occurs less with this device than with the dynamic brace [12]. The patient wears the device at all times, and the force of the splint is adjusted to the point of discomfort but no pain. As motion increases, two splints are often needed – one for flexion and the other for extension. The more severe contracture is corrected at night, and the opposite splint is worn during the day. Several reports have studied the result of this device [3–5, 8, 10, 11] (Table 6.2). Better results were obtained for moderate extrinsic stiffness of short duration.

Surgical Indications

The process is considered chronic or nonresponsive to nonoperative management at 6–12 months after injury. Indication for capsular release is very individual depending on the needs or occupation of the patient, in general, flexion contracture greater than 30° and flexion less than 110°. Surgical intervention follows only after a very careful discussion of the risks and benefits of surgery. An estimate of the likelihood that the procedure will satisfy specific patient needs is carefully addressed. The potential for improving motion at the expense of stability, strength, and pain is also specifically discussed.

Surgical Technique

Open Capsular Release: Column Procedure

Extrinsic contractures almost always involve the anterior capsule and less commonly the posterior capsule and extensor mechanism. Before surgery, a decision to approach the capsule from the lateral or medial aspect is made. If the ulnar nerve is to be addressed or there is extensive medial or coronoid arthrosis, the medial approach is of value. If the radiohumeral joint is involved or if a simple release is all that is required, which is the most common situation, the lateral "column procedure" is carried out.

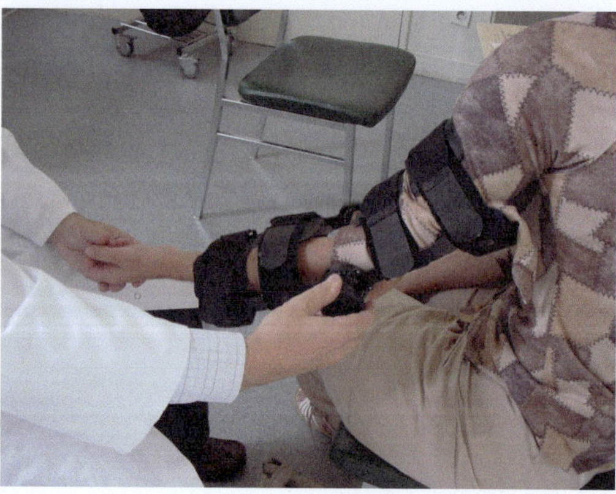

Fig. 6.2 Adjustable elbow splint

Table 6.2 Results of conservative treatment with splints

Authors	N	Arc of flex-ext		
		Preop	Postop	Gain
Static splints				
Bonutti [3]	20	79°	112°	33°
Doornberg [5]	29	71°	110°	39°
Green et McCoy [8]	15	62°	107°	45°
Ulrich [10]	37	81°	107°	26°
Dynamic splints				
Gallucci [11]	17	66°	107°	41°
Dickson [4]	1	10°	110°	100°

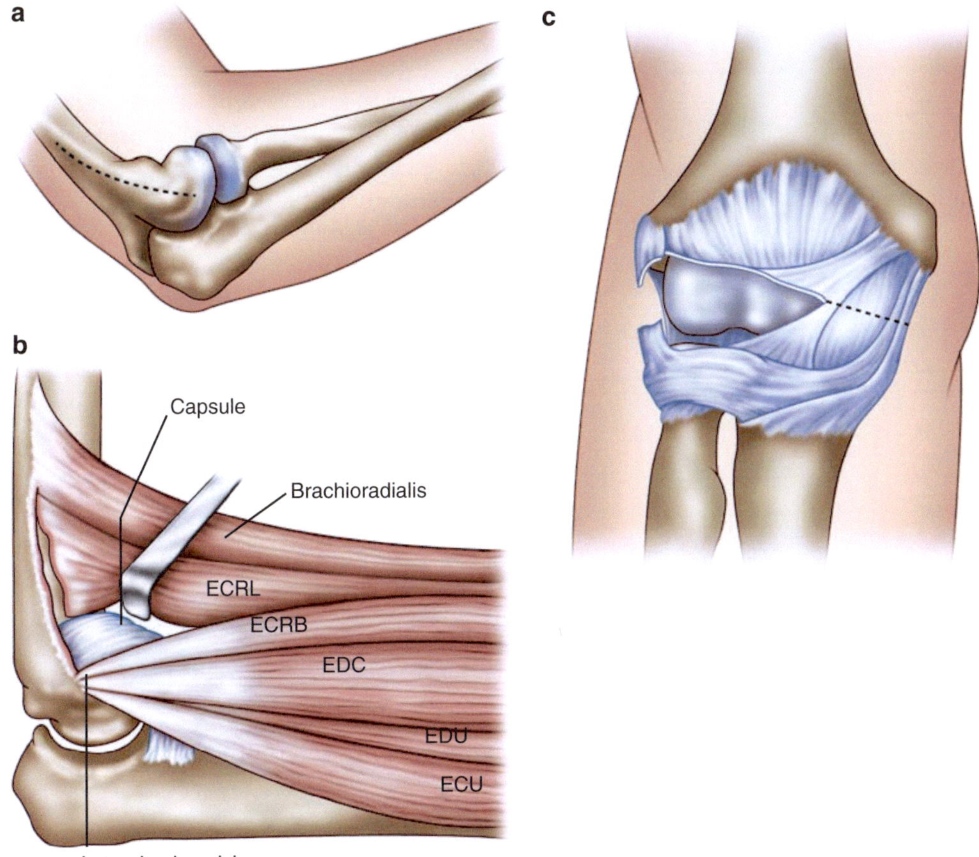

Fig. 6.3 The lateral column procedure: (**a**) incision on the proximal one-half of the Kocher incision; (**b**) the brachioradialis and ECRL are elevated from the humerus exposing the anterior capsule; (**c**) the capsulectomy is performed. *ECRL* extensor carpi radialis longus, *ECRB* extensor carpi radialis brevis, *EDC* extensor digitorum communis, *EDU* extensor digiti quintus proprius, *ECU* extensor carpi ulnaris

The column procedure consists of an open arthrolysis of the elbow through a limited lateral approach in order to release the anterior capsule safely, but also in order to release the triceps attachment and posterior capsule if needed. The exposure is also sufficient to remove coronoid or olecranon osteophytes if necessary. The proximal one-half of the Kocher incision is performed if no previous incision was present and if there are no ulnar nerve symptoms (Fig. 6.3a). The fleshy origin of the extensor carpi radialis longus and distal fibers of the brachioradialis are released from the humerus. The capsule is then entered anteriorly (Fig. 6.3b). The brachialis muscle is swept from the anterior capsule with a periosteal elevator. The anterior capsule is grasped and excised at least to the level of the coronoid (Fig. 6.3c). The medial-most aspect of the capsule often is difficult to visualize clearly but can be palpated. It is incised to complete the release. At this juncture, if extension is full or within 5° of normal and the radiographs reveal no olecranon spur, no additional release is needed. If extensive scarring has occurred and adhesions involve the posterior capsule, the triceps is elevated from the posterior aspect of the humerus. The posterior capsule is released, and the olecranon fossa is cleaned of soft tissue. Excision of the tip of the olecranon is done if osteophytes are present.

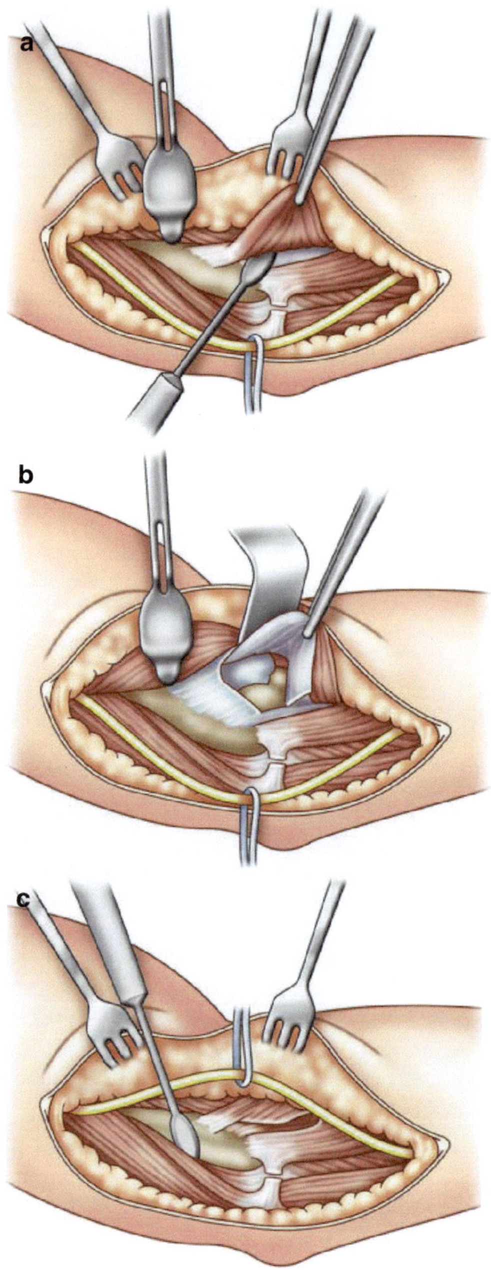

Fig. 6.4 The medial column approach: (**a**) after isolation of the ulnar nerve, the capsule is approached using the interval between the FCR and PT; (**b**) the anterior capsulectomy is performed; (**c**) the posterior aspect of the elbow is visualized by elevation of the triceps from the humerus

A medial approach may be preferred in the treatment of patients with posttraumatic elbow contractures [66, 67]. After isolation of the ulnar nerve, excellent exposure of the anterior aspect of the elbow can be achieved using the interval between flexor carpi radialis and the pronator teres (Fig. 6.4a, b). The posterior aspect of the elbow can be visualized by elevation of the triceps, and the posterior capsular tissues can be removed under vision (Fig. 6.4c). This approach is particularly useful in cases requiring excision of medial heterotopic bone, if there is an ulnar nerve neuropathy or if there is ossification of the medial collateral ligament.

Postoperatively, a brachial plexus block is done and maintained with a continuous pump through a percutaneous inserted catheter. Continuous passive motion (CPM) is begun the day of surgery and adjusted to provide as much motion as pain or the machine itself allows. At day 2, the plexus block is discontinued, and at day 3, the CPM machine is stopped. Adjustable splints are then prescribed for approximately 3 months. After 4 weeks, an arc of at least 80–100° is expected, and the amount of time that each splint is worn is decreased gradually.

Arthroscopic Debridement and Capsulectomy

With failure of nonoperative treatment a surgical release may be indicated. Some reports of this procedure being done through an arthroscopic approach have been published [17–30]. Arthroscopic capsular release of flexion contractures of the elbow is a procedure that in properly selected patients allows the surgeon to deal with extrinsic capsular and collateral ligament contracture as well as the intrinsic joint pathology. However, it is a technically demanding procedure requiring meticulous attention to detail and extensive experience in elbow arthroscopy to avoid complications [65]. The decreased capsular volume with elbow contractures reduces the ability of capsular distention to displace the neurovascular structures away from the portal sites, increasing the risk of nerve injury [68].

Eight portals are usually needed in order to position the scope and the shaver but also the retractors. Retractors are essential to move away tissue, muscles, and neurovascular structures in order for the shaver to get a great working space while decreasing the risk of neurovascular injury

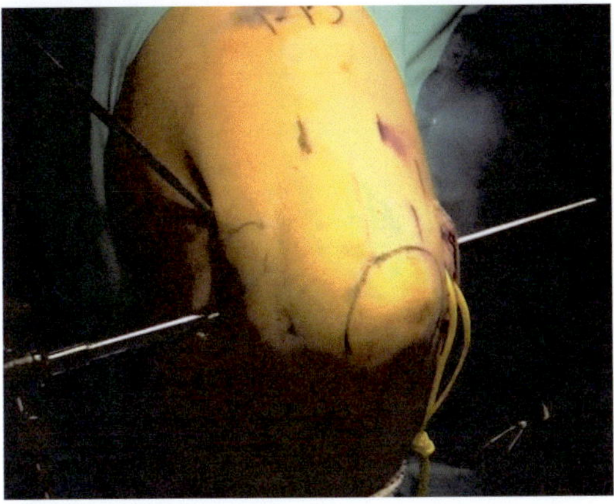

Fig. 6.5 Retractors help in improving the visualization and can be used from both sides of the joint

Table 6.3 Sequences of arthroscopic release of the elbow

1. Penetrate into the joint and establish the view
2. Create a space to work
3. Bone excision
4. Capsulectomy

(Fig. 6.5). The surgery must be systematized with different steps well described by O'Driscoll [69] (Table 6.3). After your portals have been performed, the anatomy must be recognized, a second portal is created, and the shaver is visualized. An inside-outside technique is usually recommended for the second portal placement. Then a working space is created with the retractors and the shaver. Usually, we start posteriorly for the debridement of the olecranon fossa and the excision of olecranon osteophytes (Fig. 6.6a). Then lateral gutter and medial gutter must be debrided. The ulnar nerve has a close relationship to the medial olecranon; while working medially, the surgeon should minimize the use of suction, use a hooded burr, and always keep the hooded portion oriented toward the ulnar nerve; as advocated by O'Driscoll [69], it is preferable to expose the nerve before performing the arthroscopic release to protect it while performing arthroscopic releases in this area (Table 6.4).

After entering the anterior compartment, retractors are used to strip tissue of the humerus and release scar tissue. Then the shaver is used to remove synovium and debris with the blade always away from the capsule and turned toward the joint (Fig. 6.6b); retractors retract the tissue anteriorly to leave more space for the shaver to work. Then the next step is bone removal with a 4.0 mm burr essentially at the tip of the coronoid and on the trochlea and coronoid fossa (Fig. 6.6c). The capsule is then stripped from the supracondylar ridge. Two retractors can be used, one lateral and one medial to open the space.

Then anterior capsulectomy is performed by first releasing the capsule along the supracondylar ridges, and then the capsule is cut from medial to lateral with wide duckbill basket punch where the interval between the capsule and the brachialis is well defined. A retractor is used to position and tension the capsule. The action of "bite and peel" is used which involves biting the capsule and then peeling it off the brachialis proximally (Fig. 6.6d). When the lateral edge of the brachialis is reached at the midpoint of the radial head, a strip of fat that encloses the radial nerve will be seen. This is a consistent anatomic landmark and the point at which the capsulotomy is stopped until the instruments are switched around. Then the capsulotomy is performed using a shaver facing into the joint and working from distal to proximal. With the scope in the anteromedial portal, all that is left to see of the capsule is a small triangle of tissue in front of the radial head and capitellum. This can either be left in place to protect the radial nerve or it can be dissected away from the overlying tissues. A knife-blade is used to release the capsule all way down the ECRB tendon preserving the collateral lateral ligament, as this is difficult to perform with a shaver.

Results and Complications

Open Release

The Mayo's experience has been reported in 1998 [31]. The total gain in flexion-extension was 43°. Greater improvement was obtained with severe or very severe stiffness and with combined flexion-extension type of contracture. The typical complication was loss of motion after surgery. Subsequent loss of the flexion arc after a period of improvement was seen in ten patients (26 %).

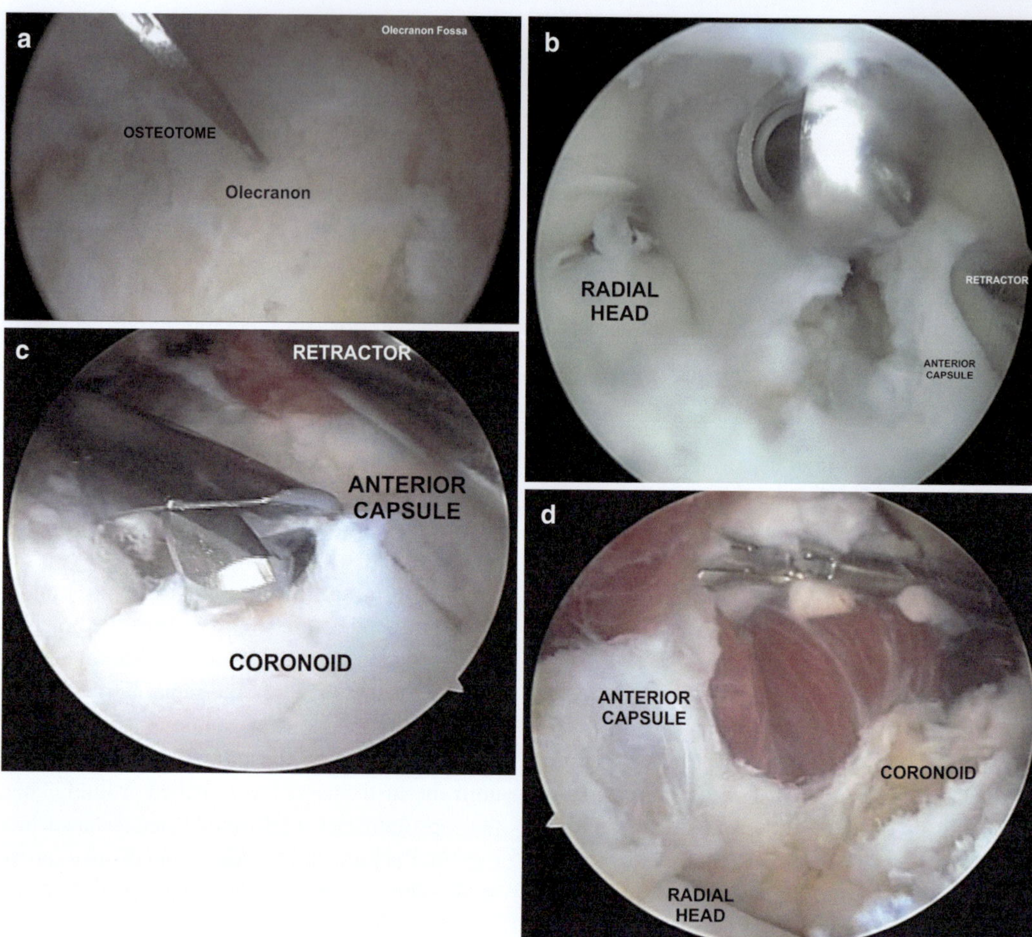

Fig. 6.6 Different steps of the arthroscopic release: (**a**) resection of the olecranon spur; (**b**) removal of the tissue and capsule from the coronoid and radial fossae; (**c**) resection of the osteophyte on the tip of the coronoid process; (**d**) anterior capsulectomy

Table 6.4 Indication of ulnar nerve release

1. Preoperative symptoms
2. Posteromedial osteophytes
3. Previous ulnar nerve surgery
4. Preoperative ROM $\leq 30°$ or flexion $\leq 90°$

Four ultimately lost the benefits from the procedure and averaged 25° less motion than before surgery. Postoperative management seemed to be very important with a splint program to preserve the motion gained at surgery.

Several reports [31–50] regarding the outcome of surgical arthrolysis reveal an absolute gain in flexion-extension arc between 30° and 60°. A functional arc of motion between 30° and 130° is obtained in more than 50 % of cases, and some improvement in motion has been reported in more than 90 % of the cases. Patient's satisfaction is often high (Table 6.5).

A most important emerging consideration of the proper treatment of the elbow stiffness is the vulnerability of the ulnar nerve. The most common cause of failure of treatment has been those patients in whom the preoperative ulnar nerve symptoms were not appreciated or addressed or those patients in whom ulnar nerve symptoms developed postoperatively without adequate treatment. This is attributed to traction neuritis caused by the abrupt increase in elbow flexion during the operation. Even in the absence of preoperative neurological symptoms, the nerve

Table 6.5 Results of open release

Authors	Year	N	Approach	Arc of flex-ext		
				Preop	Postop	Gain
Mansat [31]	1998	65	Lateral	49°	92°	43°
Cohen [32]	1998	22	Lateral	74°	129°	55°
Chantelot [33]	1999	23	Lateral ± posterior	52°	90°	38°
Wada [34]	2000	14	Medial	46°	110°	64°
Marti [35]	2002	47	Lateral ± medial	45°	99°	54°
Stans [36]	2002	37	Lateral	66°	94°	28°
Antuna [37]	2002	46	Posterior	79°	101°	22°
Heirweg [38]	2003	16	Lateral ± medial	47°	87°	40°
Aldridge [39]	2004	77	Anterior	59°	97°	38°
Cikes [40]	2006	18	Lateral ± medial	82°	122°	40°
Ring [41]	2006	46	Lateral ± medial	45°	103°	58°
Tan [42]	2006	52	Lateral ± medial	57°	116°	59°
Sharma [43]	2007	25	Lateral ± medial	55°	110°	55°
Tosun [44]	2007	30	Lateral and medial	35°	86°	51°
Gundlach [45]	2008	21	Lateral	69°	113°	44°
Ruch [46]	2008	14	Medial	53°	108°	55°
Lindenhovius [47]	2010	23	Lateral ± medial	51°	106°	55°
Park [48]	2010	42	Medial	55°	115°	60°
Kulkarni [49]	2010	26	Lateral ± medial	16°	102°	86°
Higgs [50]	2012	81	Lateral ± medial	69°	109°	40°

may be compromised subclinically and becomes symptomatic as elbow flexion increases after surgery. Therefore, all patients who have stiff elbows must be evaluated for the presence or absence of ulnar nerve symptoms. Antuna et al. [37] recommended that elbows with preoperative flexion limited to 90–100° in which we expect to improve the motion by 30° or 40° must be treated with inspection and often prophylactic decompression or translocation of the nerve depending on the appearance of the nerve once the surgical procedure is finished. Furthermore, all patients with preoperative ulnar nerve symptoms, even if they are mild, are treated with mobilization of the nerve. For Antuna et al. [37], manipulation of the elbow in the early postoperative period must be avoided if the nerve has not been decompressed or translocated. In our series, we found that about 10 % of patients have dysfunction of the nerve after release. Most of these problems resolve over a period of days or weeks. The radial nerve is also vulnerable, especially if excessive retraction is applied through the lateral approach. The other point of vulnerability is distal at the level of the posterior interosseous nerve [31].

Arthroscopic Release

In most of the studies reported in literature, a gain in motion was observed [17–30] (Table 6.6). The importance of the gain was dependent of the severity of the stiffness preoperatively and the integrity of the joint surfaces. If complications are uncommon, neurological injuries are reported [70, 71]. Most of nerve injuries are transitory, but definitive lesions have been described for all nerves around the elbow [72–76]. Three factors seem to limit the risk of neurological complications: the use of retractors to retract and protect the neurovascular structures during arthroscopic release, knowledge of the 3D anatomy of the elbow especially the localization of the nerves, and surgeon's recognition of own limits [77]. It was concluded that arthroscopic arthrolysis was not recommended in cases of severe fibrosis or bony ankylosis. This procedure is of limited value in patients with radiographic

Table 6.6 Results of arthroscopic release

Authors	Year	N	F/u (month)	Gain F/E (°)	Compl
Jones [17]	1993	12	25	67	1 PION
Redden [18]	1993	12	16		1 infection
Timmerman [19]	1994	19	2 m	29	0
Byrd [20]	1994	5	44	24	
Phillips [21]	1998	25	41	18	0
Savoie [22]	1999	24	32	81	
Kim [23]	2000	63	42	43	
Ball [24]	2002	14	12-29	42	1 infection
Nguyen [25]	2006	22	25	38	2 stiffness 1 superficial nerve
Kelly [26]	2007	24	67	32	0
Somanchi [27]	2008	22	25	19	1 stiffness
Adams [28]	2008	42	44	27	1 ulnar nerve 1 heterotopic ossif
Blonna [29]	2010	26		32	
Cefo [30]	2011	27	24	29	

evidence of severe posttraumatic arthritis and must be reserved for patients with extrinsic capsular retraction as well as limited osteophytes changes into the joint. However, arthroscopy of the arthritic elbow can be a valuable option, by removal of intra-articular debris, thickened synovial fluid, and inflamed synovium. Removal of bone spurs and loose bodies may relieve pain and restore motion and function, allowing more rapid rehabilitation.

The Complex Stiff Elbow

Indications

In some cases of severe extrinsic contracture involving the lateral and medial aspect of the elbow, a combined approach is preferred [78]. In intrinsic contracture with articular involvement, a distraction device may be needed. If more than 50 % of the articular surface has been violated and is not covered with hyaline cartilage, if significant adhesions cause avulsion of 50 % of the articular surface at surgical release, or if a malunion causes a refashioning of the articular surface, then interposition arthroplasty is indicated in the young patient, whereas a total elbow arthroplasty may be an option for the older patient.

Surgical Technique

Combined Lateral and Medial Approaches

The patient is usually positioned supine, supported by a hand table. The posterior joint must be accessible, and internal rotation or external rotation of the shoulder allows the surgeon to access to the lateral or medial compartment of the elbow. A posterior skin incision is used lateral to the tip of the olecranon. Two flaps are then elevated, one lateral up to the lateral column in order to have access to the lateral compartment and one medial to have access to the ulnar nerve and the medial column. The procedure is then performed as previously described [31, 66, 67, 78]. Fenestration of the olecranon fossa has been advocated by some authors to resect all the posterior osteophytes removing the posterior impingement with the tip of the olecranon [37] (Fig. 6.7).

Distraction Arthroplasty

If lateral collateral ligament has been released in cases with lateral ligament scarring or severe articular involvement, it is reattached through bone holes placed through the anatomic axis of rotation. However, this reconstruction is protected with a distraction device [48, 50]. Two to 3 mm of distraction is usually performed. The

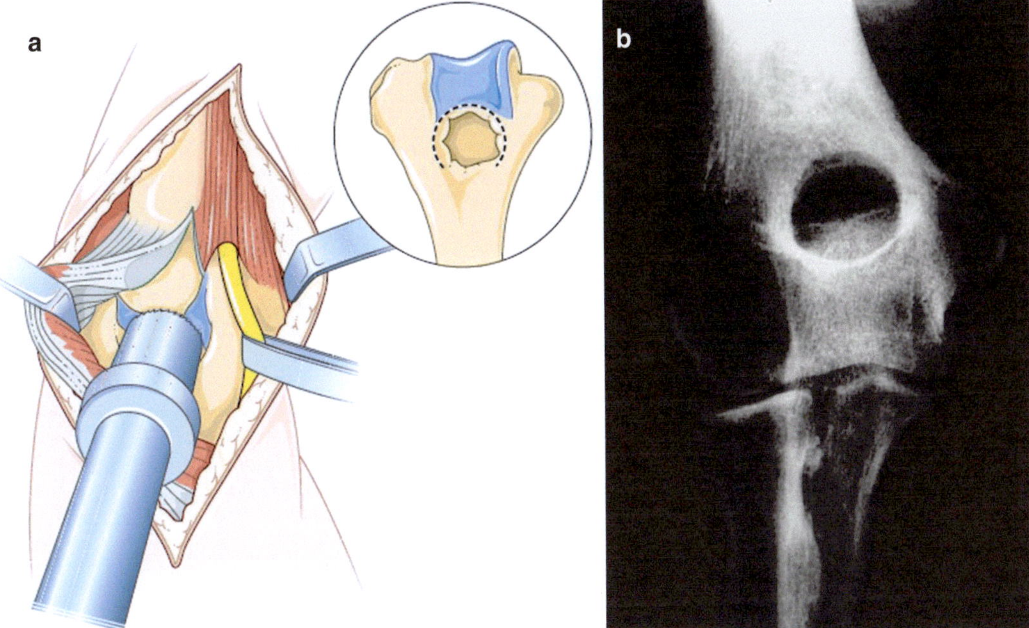

Fig. 6.7 Ulnohumeral arthroplasty with a trephine

elbow is moved to assure smooth motion with no impingement of the articular surfaces. At surgery, depending on the problem being treated, motion of at least 50–110° is possible with the distraction device. After 4 weeks, the patient is placed under anesthesia, and the device is removed. The elbow is then carefully examined to assess the firmness of the end points in flexion and in extension. Stability is also evaluated. Adjustable splints are then prescribed for a minimum of 6 weeks and often up to 3 months. The time in the splint is progressively decreased during the day, but the application of the splint continues at night for at least 3 months [13, 49, 51, 52].

Interpositional Arthroplasty

If more than 50 % of the articular surface has been violated and is not covered with hyaline cartilage, if significant adhesions cause avulsion of 50 % of the articular surface at surgical release, or if a malunion causes a refashioning of the articular surface, then interposition arthroplasty is indicated in the young patient, whereas a total elbow arthroplasty may be an option for older patient. Interposition arthroplasty at the elbow has been initially described for rheumatoid arthritis or for ankylosis [51, 54]. The results were often unpre-

dictable because of persistent pain and instability. Recently, the use of a distraction fixator allowed better healing of the collateral ligaments as well as a distraction of the joint surface to protect the interposition graft and to allow immediate passive motion.

Cutis, fascia lata, and Achilles tendon allografts are commonly used as interposition materials to resurface damaged joints. The joint is exposed through a Mayo modified Kocher approach with a midline posterior skin incision. The lateral collateral ligament is detached from its humeral origin, which allows for exposure of the joint. The radial head is preserved if the proximal radioulnar joint is intact. Minimal bone resection is performed with the goal of contouring the distal humerus to accept the graft. The graft is secured to the bone with trans-osseous nonabsorbable number 5 sutures. Part of the graft can be used to reconstruct the collateral ligaments. A distraction fixator is then applied, and the lateral ligament is repaired through drill holes in the lateral epicondyle (Fig. 6.8). A continuous axillary catheter is used to give good postoperative analgesia, and a continuous passive motion machine is used for 4 days. The external fixator is usually removed between 4 and 6 weeks

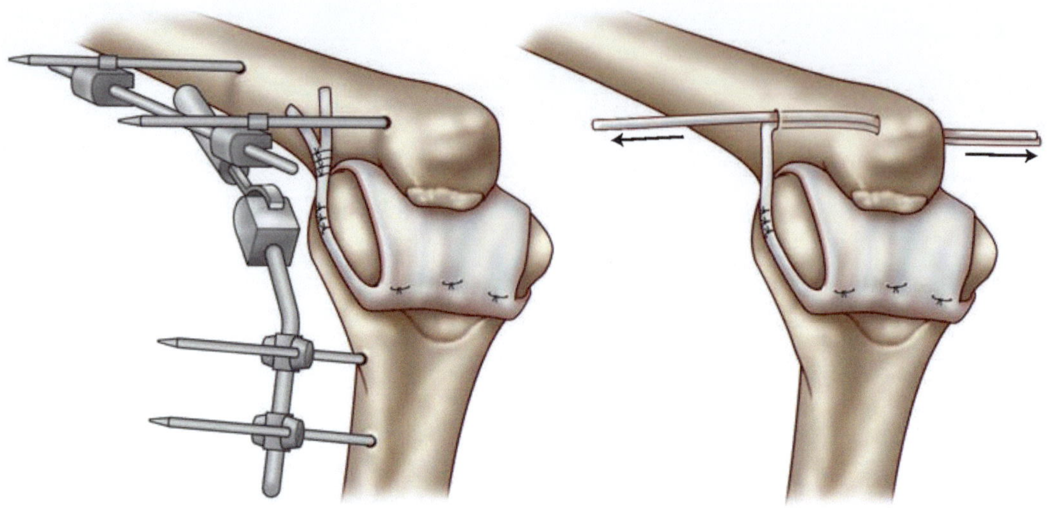

Fig. 6.8 Interpositional arthroplasty protected with an articulated external fixator

postoperatively. An articulated splint is maintained during 3 months.

Results published in literature have shown significant gain in motion with satisfactory results between 30 and 60 % of the cases [13, 53–56]. However, in some cases, because of persistence of pain, a total elbow can be indicated without alteration of the final results [57]. The main prognosis factor reported is the level of instability preoperatively. A satisfactory result was obtained in 80 % of the stable elbows versus 60 % if the elbow was unstable preoperatively. Distraction arthroplasty combined with interposition in patients who have extensive intra-articular changes appears to be effective in restoring a functional arc of motion of the elbow. The rate of complication after this procedure is high as would be anticipated from the extent of the lesions. The procedures are technically difficult, and experience is a prerequisite to success.

Elbow Arthroplasty

Patients older than 50 years with a painful reduction of elbow movement due to intra-articular deterioration interfering with activities of daily living can be treated with a total elbow arthroplasty [58–61].

The technique of total elbow arthroplasty for posttraumatic arthritis has been well described [59, 60]. Careful preoperative planning is necessary to avoid potential complications. The anatomical changes have to be addressed, as well as the bone morphology and the intramedullary canal size. Sometimes, a small-stemmed implant is needed. Careful exposure, prevention of vessel injury, and estimated options for skin closure need to be assessed preoperatively.

The patient is supine with a sandbag under the scapula. The Mayo (Bryan-Morrey) approach is used [60], and a posterior incision is performed. The ulnar nerve is carefully isolated and translocated using ocular magnification and a bipolar cautery. The triceps is then released from the olecranon and reflected laterally in continuity with the anconeus. Circumferential capsular and collateral ligaments are released to expose the distal humerus and to maximize postoperative motion and function. The anterior aspect of the capsule is completely excised and further reflected from the distal aspect of the humerus with a blunt periosteal elevator. The attachments of the flexors and extensors are released if contracted. In case of osseous ankylosis, a circular microsagittal saw or a small osteotome is used to reestablish the joint line. Care is taken to create the osteotomy as close as possible to the center of rotation of the ulnohumeral joint to maximize the biomechanical function of the

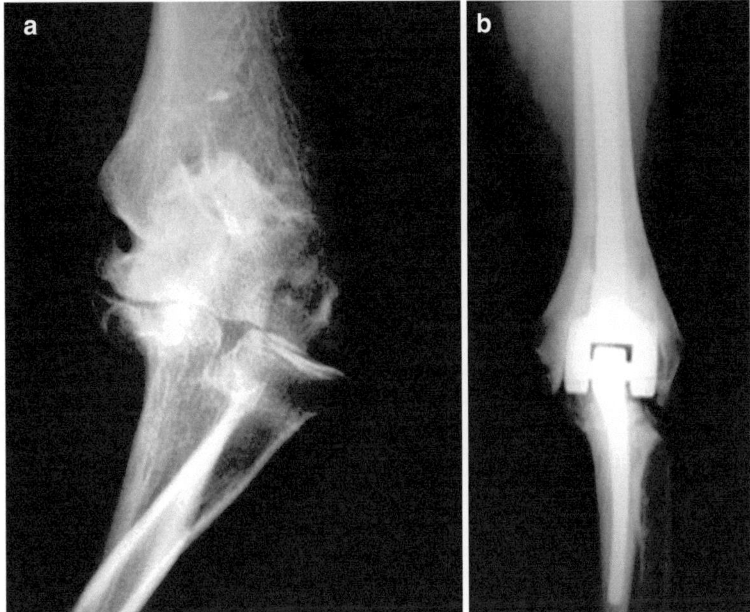

Fig. 6.9 Posttraumatic arthritis of the elbow (**a**) treated with a total elbow arthroplasty (**b**)

prosthetic elbow and to preserve a site for triceps attachment.

Care must be taken in grossly deformed elbows during preparation of the intramedullary canals. If the canal has been narrowed or obliterated by bone formation or because of malunion, it is necessary to recreate a new canal by using a small burr or cannulated flexible reamers. The surgeon must always stay centered on the humerus and on the ulna during the procedure. After the medullary canals have been prepared, a trial reduction allows resection of soft tissue contracture, which may include the flexor and extensor muscle origins. Antibiotic-impregnated cement is inserted with an intramedullary injection system. A bone graft is placed behind the anterior flange on the distal humerus, and the components are articulated. After careful hemostasis, the triceps is secured usually at 90° of flexion with number five non-absorbable sutures placed through drill holes in the proximal ulna.

The elbow is then placed in full extension with cold compressive dressing (CRYO CUFF AIRCAST®) and an extension splint, and then it is elevated in a vertical position for 24 h. Then the dressing is changed at 2–3 days, and the patient is allowed to move his elbow as tolerated.

No formal physical therapy is required. Strength exercises are avoided. A system of flexion and extension braces is used if motion remains limited or was difficult to obtain at surgery. The patient is advised not to lift more than 0.5–1 kg over the next 3 months and no more than 1 kg on a repetitive basis or 5 kg as a single event (Fig. 6.9a, b).

Results and Complications

Replacement for the stiff elbow is the least predictable and has the lowest overall rate of success and highest complication rate, compared to other diagnosis. Nonetheless, this experience must be placed in the context of alternative intervention options. The non-custom semiconstrained total elbow arthroplasty seems to be a useful option for patients older than 60 years with intrinsic stiffness involving more than 50 % of the articular surface with ankylosed or very stiff elbow with considerable improvement of motion. However, limitation of the flexion arc of less than 60° remains a problem for some (40 %). Due to the nature of the underlying pathology, complications, including reoperation, are frequent but can be lessened by careful preoperative planning and surgical technique.

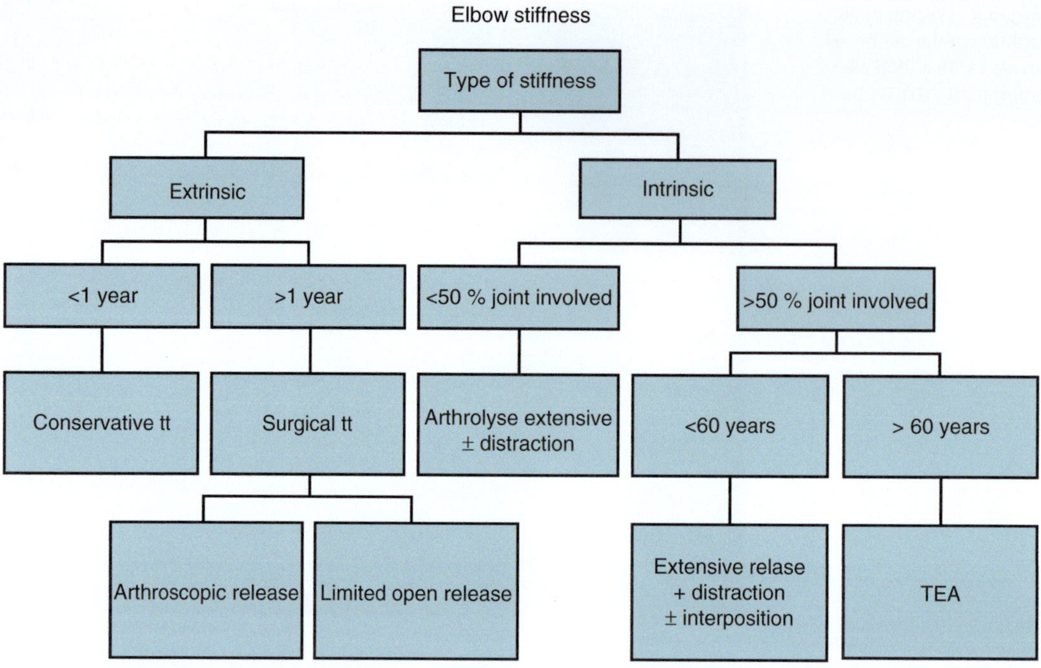

Fig. 6.10 Decision algorithm for a stiff elbow

Conclusion

Elbow contractures are a common complication of trauma and a significant cause of disability because of the inability to position the hand in space. An adequate classification and a careful patient selection are necessary for choosing optimal treatment. Several treatment options have been proposed for treatment of elbow contracture. Initial treatment should be nonoperative consisting of splinting and physical therapy. Turnbuckle splinting may be useful in patients who have failed a conventional therapy program. Conservative treatment sometimes gives good results if the contracture is of short duration; however, its efficacy is unpredictable.

Established elbow contractures that interfere with a patient's activities can be treated operatively by an open or arthroscopic release. The choice of surgical approach depends on the localization of the pathology and the surgeon's preference. Chronic extrinsic stiffness is usually managed by arthroscopic or surgical release with good results. When less than 50 % of the joint surface is involved in an intrinsic stiffness, the same treatment can be proposed with less reliable results.

Distraction arthroplasty is useful in the severe intrinsic contractures, especially in the perioperative unstable elbow. Extensive release through a posterior approach to the joint may reestablish a functional range of motion in the pain-free contracted elbow. Finally, a total elbow replacement yields good results in older patients with a low functional demand on the elbow, suffering an intrinsic painful contracture of the elbow joint (Fig. 6.10).

References

1. Morrey BF. The posttraumatic stiff elbow. Clin Orthop. 2005;431:26–35.
2. Balay B, Setiey L, Vidalain JP. Les raideurs du coude. Traitement orthopédique et chirurgical. Acta Orthop Belg. 1975;41:414–25.
3. Bonutti PM, Windau JE, Ables BA, Miller BG. Static progressive, stretch to reestablish elbow range of motion. Clin Orthop. 1994;303:128–34.
4. Dickson RA. Reversed dynamic slings. A new concept in the treatment of posttraumatic elbow flexion contractures. Injury. 1976;8:35–8.
5. Doornberg JN, Ring D, Jupiter JB. Static progressive splinting for posttraumatic elbow stiffness. J Orthop Trauma. 2006;20:400–4.

6. Duke JB, Tessler RH, Dell PC. Manipulation of the stiff elbow with patient under anesthesia. J Hand Surg Am. 1991;16:19–24.

7. Gelinas JJ, Faber KJ, Patterson SD, King GJW. The effectiveness of turnbuckle splinting for elbow contractures. J Bone Joint Surg Br. 2000;82:74–8.

8. Green DP, McCoy H. Turnbuckle orthotic correction of elbow-flexion contractures after acute injuries. J Bone Joint Surg Am. 1979;61:1092–5.

9. Mac Kay-Lyons M. Low-load, prolonged stretch in treatment of elbow flexion contractures secondary to head trauma: a case report. Phys Ther. 1989;69:292–6.

10. Ulrich SD, Bonutti PM, Seyler TM, Marker DR, Morrey BF, Mont MA. Restoring range of motion via stress relaxation and static progressive stretch in post-traumatic elbow contractures. J Shoulder Elbow Surg. 2010;19:196–201.

11. Gallucci GL, Boretto JG, D´Avalos MA, Donndorff A, Alfie VA, De Carli P. Dynamic splint for the treatment of stiff elbow. J Shoulder Elbow. 2011;3:52–5.

12. Morrey BF. Splints and bracing at the elbow. In: Morrey BF, editor. The elbow and its disorders. 3rd ed. Philadelphia: W. B. Saunders; 2000. p. 150–4.

13. Morrey BF. Post-traumatic contracture of the elbow. Operative treatment, including distraction arthroplasty. J Bone Joint Surg Am. 1990;72:601–18.

14. Estève P, Valentin P, Deburge A, Kerboull M. Raideurs et ankyloses post-traumatiques du Coude. Rev Chir Orthop. 1971;57(Suppl I):25–86.

15. Allieu Y. Raideurs et Arthrolyses du Coude. Rev Chir Orthop. 1989;75(Suppl I):156–66.

16. Jupiter JB, O'Driscoll SW, Cohen MS. The assessment and management of the stiff elbow. Instr Course Lect. 2003;52:93–111.

17. Jones GS, Savoie III FH. Arthroscopic capsular release of flexion contractures (arthrofibrosis) of the elbow. Arthroscopy. 1993;9:277–83.

18. Redden JF, Stanley D. Arthroscopic fenestration of the olecranon fossa in the treatment of osteoarthritis of the elbow. Arthroscopy. 1993;9:14–6.

19. Timmerman LA, Andrews JR. Arthroscopic treatment of posttraumatic elbow pain and stiffness. Am J Sport Med. 1994;22:230–5.

20. Byrd JWT. Elbow arthroscopy for arthrofibrosis after type I radial head fractures. Arthroscopy. 1994;10:162–5.

21. Phillips BB, Strasburger S. Arthroscopic treatment of arthrofibrosis of the elbow joint. Arthroscopy. 1998;14:38–44.

22. Savoie FH, Nunley PD, Field LD. Arthroscopic management of the arthritic elbow: indications, technique, and results. J Shoulder Elbow Surg. 1999;8:214–9.

23. Kim SJ, Shin SJ. Arthroscopic treatment for limitation of motion of the elbow. Clin Orthop. 2000;375:140–8.

24. Ball CM, Meunier M, Galatz LM, Calfee R, Yamaguchi K. Arthroscopic treatment of post-traumatic elbow contracture. J Shoulder Elbow Surg. 2002;11:624–9.

25. Nguyen D, Proper SI, MacDermid JC, King GJ, Faber KJ. Functional outcomes of arthroscopic capsular release of the elbow. Arthroscopy. 2006;22:842–9.

26. Kelly EW, Bryce R, Coghlan J, Bell S. Arthroscopic débridement without radial head excision of the osteoarthritic elbow. Arthroscopy. 2007;23:151–6.

27. Somanchi BV, Funk L. Evaluation of functional outcome and patient satisfaction after arthroscopic elbow arthrolysis. Acta Orthop Belg. 2008;74:17–23.

28. Adams JE, Wolff III LH, Merten SM, Steinmann SP. Osteoarthritis of the elbow: results of arthroscopic osteophyte resection and capsulectomy. J Shoulder Elbow Surg. 2008;17:126–31.

29. Blonna D, Lee GC, O'Driscoll SW. Arthroscopic restoration of terminal elbow extension in high-level athletes. Am J Sports Med. 2010;38:2509–15.

30. Cefo I, Eygendaal D. Arthroscopic arthrolysis for posttraumatic elbow stiffness. J Shoulder Elbow Surg. 2011;20:434–9.

31. Mansat P, Morrey BF. The column procedure: a limited lateral approach for extrinsic contracture of the elbow. J Bone Joint Surg Am. 1998;80:1603–15.

32. Cohen MS, Hastings H. II Post-traumatic contracture of the elbow: operative release using a lateral collateral ligament sparing approach. J Bone Joint Surg Br. 1998;80:805–12.

33. Chantelot C, Fontaine C, Migaud H, Remy F, Chapnikoff D, Duquennoy A. Etude rétrospective de 23 arthrolyses du coude pour raideur post-traumatique: facteurs prédictifs du résultat. Rev Chir Orthop. 1999;85:823–7.

34. Wada T, Ishii S, Usui M, Miyano S. The medial approach for operative release of posttraumatic contracture of the elbow. J Bone Joint Surg Br. 2000;82:68–73.

35. Marti RK, Kerkhoffs GM, Maas M, Blankevoort L. Progressive surgical release of a posttraumatic stiff elbow. Technique and outcome after 2–18 years in 46 patients. Acta Orthop Scand. 2002;73:144–50.

36. Stans AA, Maritz NG, O'Driscoll SW, Morrey BF. Operative treatment of elbow contracture in patients twenty-one years of age or younger. J Bone Joint Surg Am. 2002;84:382–7.

37. Antuna SA, Morrey BF, Adams RA, O'Driscoll SW. Ulnohumeral arthroplasty for primary degenerative arthritis of the elbow: long-term outcome and complications. J Bone Joint Surg Am. 2002;84:2168–73.

38. Heirweg S, De Smet L. Operative treatment of elbow stiffness: evaluation and outcome. Acta Orthop Belg. 2003;69:18–22.

39. Aldridge 3rd JM, Atkins TA, Gunneson EE, Urbaniak JR. Anterior release of the elbow for extension loss. J Bone Joint Surg Am. 2004;86:1955–60.

40. Cikes A, Jolles BM, Farron A. Open elbow arthrolysis for posttraumatic elbow stiffness. J Orthop Trauma. 2006;20:405–9.

41. Ring D, Adey L, Zurakowski D, Jupiter JB. Elbow capsulectomy for posttraumatic elbow stiffness. J Hand Surg Am. 2006;31:1264–71.

42. Tan V, Daluiski A, Simic P, Hotchkiss RN. Outcome of open release for posttraumatic elbow stiffness. J Trauma. 2006;61:673–8.

43. Sharma S, Rymaszewski LA. Open arthrolysis for post-traumatic stiffness of the elbow: results are durable over the medium term. J Bone Joint Surg Br. 2007;89:778–81.

44. Tosun B, Gundes H, Buluc L, Sarlak AY. The use of combined lateral and medial releases in the treatment

of post-traumatic contracture of the elbow. Int Orthop. 2007;31:635–8.

45. Gundlach U, Eygendaal D. Surgical treatment of post-traumatic stiffness of the elbow: 2-year outcome in 21 patients after a column procedure. Acta Orthop. 2008;79:74–7.

46. Ruch DS, Shen J, Chloros GD, Krings E, Papadonikolakis A. Release of the medial collateral ligament to improve flexion in post-traumatic elbow stiffness. J Bone Joint Surg Br. 2008;90:614–8.

47. Lindenhovius AL, Doornberg JN, Ring D, Jupiter JB. Health status after open elbow contracture release. J Bone Joint Surg Am. 2010;92:2187–95.

48. Park MJ, Chang MJ, Lee YB, Kang HJ. Surgical release for posttraumatic loss of elbow flexion. J Bone Joint Surg Am. 2010;92:2692–9.

49. Kulkarni GS, Kulkarni VS, Shyam AK, Kulkarni RM, Kulkarni MG, Nayak P. Management of severe extra-articular contracture of the elbow by open arthrolysis and a monolateral hinged external fixator. J Bone Joint Surg Br. 2010;92:92–7.

50. Higgs ZC, Danks BA, Sibinski M, Rymaszewski LA. Outcomes of open arthrolysis of the elbow without post-operative passive stretching. J Bone Joint Surg Br. 2012;94:348–52.

51. Judet R, Judet T. The Use of a hinge distraction apparatus after arthrolysis and arthroplasty. Rev Chir Orthop. 1978;64:353–65.

52. Gausepohl T, Mader K, Pennig D. Mechanical distraction for the treatment of posttraumatic stiffness of the elbow in children and adolescents. J Bone Joint Surg Am. 2006;88:1011–21.

53. Froimson AI, Silva JE, Richey D. Cutis arthroplasty of the elbow joint. J Bone Joint Surg Am. 1976;58:863–5.

54. Ljung P, Jonsson K, Larsson K, Rydholm U. Interposition arthroplasty of the elbow with rheumatoid arthritis. J Shoulder Elbow Surg. 1996;5:81–5.

55. Cheng SL, Morrey BF. Treatment of the mobile, painful arthritic elbow by distraction interposition arthroplasty. J Bone Joint Surg Br. 2000;82:233–8.

56. Larson AN, Morrey BF. Interposition arthroplasty with an Achilles tendon allograft as a salvage procedure for the elbow. J Bone Joint Surg Am. 2008;90:2714–23.

57. Blaine TA, Adams R, Morrey BF. Total elbow arthroplasty after interposition arthroplasty for elbow arthritis. J Bone Joint Surg Am. 2005;87:286–92.

58. Figgie MP, Inglis AE, Mow CS, Figgie 3rd HE. Total elbow arthroplasty for complete ankylosis of the elbow. J Bone Joint Surg Am. 1989;71:513–20.

59. Schneeberger AG, Adams RA, Morrey BF. Semi-constrained total elbow replacement for the treatment of post-traumatic osteoarthrosis. J Bone Joint Surg Am. 1997;79:1211–22.

60. Mansat P, Morrey BF. Semiconstrained total elbow arthroplasty for stiff or ankylosed elbow. J Bone Joint Surg Am. 2000;82:1260–8.

61. Peden JP, Morrey BF. Total elbow replacement for the management of the ankylosed or fused elbow. J Bone Joint Surg Br. 2008;90:1198–204.

62. Morrey BF, Askew LJ, Chao EY. A biomechanical study of normal functional elbow motion. J Bone Joint Surg Am. 1981;63:872–7.

63. Charalambous CP, Morrey BF. Current concepts review: posttraumatic elbow stiffness. J Bone Joint Surg Am. 2012;94:1428–37.

64. Zubler V, Saupe N, Jost B, Pfirrmann CW, Hodler J, Zanetti M. Elbow stiffness: effectiveness of conventional radiography and CT to explain osseous causes. Am J Roentgenol. 2010;194:W515–20.

65. Morrey BF. Complications of elbow arthroscopy. AAOS Instr Course Lect. 2000;49:255–8.

66. Mansat P, Morrey BF. Extrinsic contracture: lateral and medial column procedures. In: Morrey BF, editor. The elbow and its disorders. 4th ed. Philadelphia, Saunders/Elsevier; 2009. p. 487–98.

67. Mansat P, André A, Bonnevialle N. Extrinsic contracture release: medial "over the top" approach. In: Wiesel S, editor. Operative techniques in orthopaedic surgery, vol. 3, chapter 44. Wolters Kluwer, Philadelphia, Lippincott Williams & Wilkins; 2010. p. 3413–9.

68. Gallay SH, Richards RR, O'Driscoll SW. Intraarticular capacity and compliance of stiff and normal elbows. Arthroscopy. 1993;9:9–13.

69. O'Driscoll SW. Arthroscopic osteocapsular arthroplasty. In: Yamagushi K, King GJW, McKee MD, O'Driscoll SWM, editors. Advanced reconstruction – elbow. The American Academy of Orthopaedic Surgeons; Rosemont, Illinois. 2007. p. 59–68.

70. Kelly EW, Morrey BF, O'Driscoll SW. Complications of elbow arthroscopy. J Bone Joint Surg Am. 2001; 83:25–34.

71. Savoie III FH, Field LD. Arthrofibrosis and complications in arthroscopy of the elbow. Clin Sports Med. 2001;20:123–9.

72. Haapaniemi T, Berggren M, Adolfsson L. Complete transection of the median and radial nerves during arthroscopic release of post-traumatic elbow contracture. Arthroscopy. 1999;15:784–7.

73. Hahn M, Grossman JA. Ulnar nerve laceration as a result of elbow arthroscopy. J Hand Surg Br. 1998;23:109.

74. Dumonski ML, Arciero RA, Mazzocca AD. Ulnar nerve palsy after elbow arthroscopy. Arthroscopy. 2006;22:577.e1–3.

75. Gay DM, Raphael BS, Weiland AJ. Revision arthroscopic contracture release in the elbow resulting in an ulnar nerve transection: a case report. J Bone Joint Surg Am. 2010;92:1246–9.

76. Park JY, Cho CH, Choi JH, Lee ST, Kang CH. Radial nerve palsy after arthroscopic anterior capsular release for degenerative elbow contracture. Arthroscopy. 2007;23:1360.e1–3.

77. Marshall PD, Fairclough JA, Johnson SR, Evans EJ. Avoiding nerve damage during elbow arthroscopy. J Bone Joint Surg Br. 1993;75:129–31.

78. Mansat P, Bonnevialle N, Werner B. Indikationen und operationstechniken für kombinierte mediale und laterale eingriffe bei schwerer extrinsischer ellenbogensteife [Indications and technique of combined medial and lateral column procedures in severe extrinsic elbow contractures.] Orthopäde. 2011;40:307–15.

Chronic Elbow and Forearm Instability

Matthias Vanhees, Frederik Verstreken, and Roger P. van Riet

Abstract

Elbow instability may be medial or lateral and presents as an acute or chronic problem. Traumatic or iatrogenic insufficiency of the lateral collateral ligament is reviewed, with emphasis on the clinical presentation, diagnostic exam, and appropriate imaging tests. Current trends on lateral elbow instability treatment are reviewed including both open and arthroscopic techniques. Medial instability is more prevalent among throwing athletes and may be associated with a valgus overload syndrome. Key aspects of the pathoanatomy, diagnosis, and treatment of this entity are reviewed.

Keywords

Lateral elbow instability • Medial elbow instability • Posterolateral rotatory instability

All figures are the property of MoRe Foundation. Permission has been granted to use these figures.

M. Vanhees, MD
Orthopedic and Traumatology, AZ Monica/MoRe Foundation, Stevenslei 20, Antwerp 2100, Belgium

F. Verstreken, MD
Orthopedic and Traumatology, AZ Monica/MoRe Foundation, Stevenslei 20, Antwerp 2100, Belgium

Orthopedic and Traumatology, University Hospital Antwerp, Wilrijkstraat 10, Antwerp 2650, Belgium

R.P. van Riet, MD, PhD (✉)
Orthopedic and Traumatology, AZ Monica/MoRe Foundation, Stevenslei 20, Antwerp 2100, Belgium

Orthopedic and Traumatology, Erasme University Hospital Brussels, Route De Lennik 808, Brussels 1070, Belgium
e-mail: drrogervanriet@azmonica.be

Epidemiology

Elbow dislocations are common with a rate of 6–13 injuries per 100,000 people [18]. They are more frequent in males [7], and 60 % occurs in the non-dominant extremity [19]. Simple elbow dislocation treated by closed reduction may develop into chronic instability in 35–45 % of cases [10, 28]. Sports-related elbow dislocations occur in 10–50 % of the total number of elbow dislocations [22]. Fractures about the elbow can also lead to chronic instability: even treated terrible triad injuries will remain unstable in 5 % of patients [12, 35].

A special type of instability is the valgus overload syndrome in which the medial collateral ligament (MCL) is stretched to the point that it

S. Antuña, R. Barco (eds.), *Essentials in Elbow Surgery*,
DOI 10.1007/978-1-4471-4625-4_7, © Springer-Verlag London 2014

becomes dysfunctional or tears. It is a common injury in throwing athletes.

The Problem

Chronic elbow instability can be divided into three types: medial, lateral, and longitudinal instability. Medial instability most commonly affects the throwing athlete as a result of repetitive microtrauma to the MCL (valgus overload syndrome). Chronic medial instability can also occur after simple dislocations, as was stated earlier [10].

Posterolateral rotatory instability (PLRI) is the most frequent pattern of chronic lateral instability caused by laxity or avulsion of the lateral ulnar collateral ligament (LUCL) [31]. Longitudinal radioulnar instability (LRUD), also known as the Essex-Lopresti lesion, is caused by an axial load that leads to a radial head fracture, a rupture of the interosseous membrane (IM), and a lesion of the distal radioulnar joint (DRUJ) [9].

Patient Workup

Clinical Exam

The patient should be asked about the origin of the injury. Was there an acute traumatic event or provoking activity? The patient remembers feeling or hearing a "pop" in case of an MCL avulsion. Pain and functional impairment will often be mentioned spontaneously, but it should always be included in the history taking. Patients will frequently not present with instability as their primary complaint, but a thorough questioning should be performed about complaints of instability while loading the elbow. The history will not only guide to the origin of the complaint but also to the direction and type of instability.

Inspection of the elbow may reveal a medial or lateral hematoma. Obvious deformity may be present in the case of a fracture or persistent dislocation. The position of any previous surgical scars should be noted as well as possible muscle atrophy. Range of motion (ROM) and strength of biceps and triceps should be tested as well as resisted wrist extension and flexion.

A thorough neurovascular exam is done to rule out median nerve (anterior interosseous nerve) or radial nerve (posterior interosseous nerve) pathology. The ulnar nerve should be located (inside or outside the cubital tunnel) by palpating the nerve in flexion and extension, and its motor function is tested and noted. This is not only important to rule out nerve damage from the trauma but is also important should nerve symptoms occur following a surgical intervention.

First, static valgus and valgus stress should be applied in different degrees of flexion and extension while holding the forearm in pronation or supination to relax and tighten the dynamic structures [34]. The anterior bundle of the MCL is the primary constraint to valgus stress with the elbow flexed between 30° and 90°, whereas the posterior and anterior bundle of the MCL share the load in 120° of flexion [5]. The anterior capsule becomes more important with the elbow extended. The same is true for the resistance to varus stress, but the articulation is more important to resist varus than it is to resist valgus. Approximately 75 % of resistance to varus stress comes from the articulation when the elbow is flexed 90° [29].

Specific clinical tests are very useful to determine medial compartment instability. The milking test is used for dynamic assessment of the ligament. The ulnohumeral joint space is palpated, and the examiner grasps the ipsilateral thumb, while the elbow is flexed fully. The test is positive if pain occurs around the medial ligament and the joint space opens [48]. Finally, the moving stress test is the most precise test in predicting injury to the MCL, with a sensitivity of 100 % and a specificity of 75 %. Valgus stress is applied to the fully flexed elbow while the elbow is moved to extension by the examiner constantly maintaining valgus stress (Fig. 7.1). For a positive test, pain should be felt at the MUCL and it should be most intense at 120° and 70° of flexion (painful arc) [33].

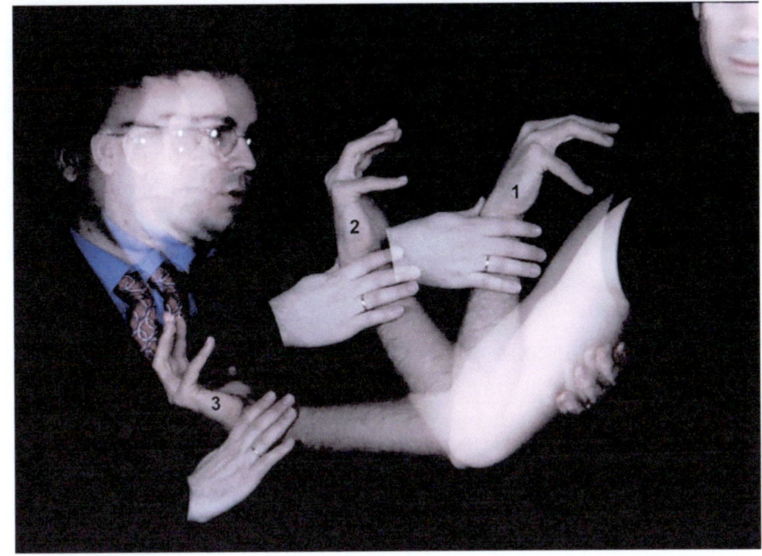

Fig. 7.1 Moving valgus stress test: to perform this test, the examiner applies and maintains a constant moderate valgus torque to the fully flexed elbow and then extends the elbow. The test is positive if the medial elbow pain is reproduced at the medial collateral ligament and is at maximum between 120° and 70° (Used with permission of Samuel Antuna)

Several tests have also been described to evaluate the lateral compartment of the elbow. The pivot shift test is performed by supinating the forearm. A valgus force is applied to the elbow, while the elbow is flexed from full extension. For this test to be positive, the elbow should subluxate as it is flexed and subsequently reduce at about 40° of flexion. Because of laxity of the LUCL, subluxation of the ulnohumeral joint and secondary dislocation of the radiohumeral joint will occur [31]. The pivot shift test is sometimes hard to perform in an awake patient and apprehension may prevent the elbow to subluxate; apprehension can therefore be a sign of posterolateral rotatory instability (Fig. 7.2). Other tests have been developed. The push-up sign, chair test, and tabletop tests are variations to the more or less the same tests. The push-up sign is performed by having the patient performing active push-ups with the arms abducted to more than shoulder width. The test is positive as apprehension or subluxation occurs at near full extension [36]. The chair sign is more sensitive and is performed by a seated patient with the elbows flexed in 90° with the forearms supinated. Using the armrests of the chair, push-up is again performed by the patient. The sensitivity of the two tests

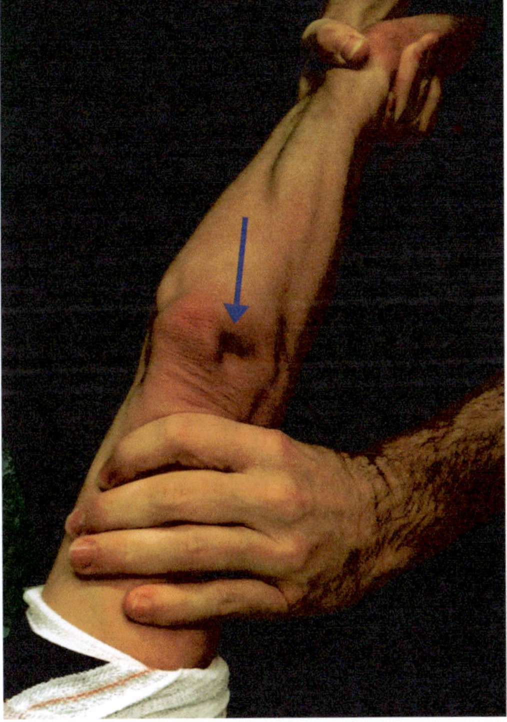

Fig. 7.2 The pivot shift test is performed by supinating the forearm while applying an axial compression and a valgus load. The radial head will subluxate posteriorly in a positive test and a dimple (*blue arrow*) will appear. The forearm will reduce with further extension and flexion (Used with permission of the MoRe Foundation)

individually is 87,5 % and increases to 100 % when combined [36]. Finally, the tabletop test relocation is performed by pushing up of a table, but this test consists of two parts. If apprehension or subluxation occurs, the test is repeated while the examiner stabilizes the radiohumeral joint by pushing the radial head anteriorly. This test is positive if this relocation alleviates the symptoms [3].

One of the most useful tests for the detection of subtle PLRI is the posterior drawer test. The examiner palpates the lateral joint space while rotating the forearm relative to the humerus. The radial head will rotate posteriorly in a positive test. It is important not to pronate or supinate during this test as the palpating finger will be pushed posteriorly due to the noncircular shape of the radial head instead of detecting a true posterior subluxation [32].

None of these tests is 100 % accurate. It is therefore important to use more than one single test. We have found the posterior drawer test to be the most sensitive. In a small patient group that was treated arthroscopically for subtle PLRI, patients were examined in clinic, using the posterior drawer, tabletop, and pivot shift tests. Two out of three tests were positive in all patients, with the posterior drawer being the most sensitive.

Examination under anesthesia to determine the indication for surgery is not current in our practice but could be used in cases of suspected instability symptoms that are difficult to reproduce during clinical examination in the outpatient service. Examination under anesthesia is however always performed preoperatively but this has so far not changed our indication.

Imaging

Plain radiographs should always be done both in the acute setting, in the emergency room, if a fracture or a dislocation is suspected but also following a closed reduction, as fractures may only become apparent once the elbow has been reduced. Standard radiographs (anteroposterior and lateral) are also a necessary adjunct in the workup of chronic instability to look for bony anomaly and malunion or nonunion of fractures or dysplasia. Stress views and continuous fluoroscopy during physical examination are a possibility, but we do not use it in our current practice.

Magnetic resonance imaging (MRI) is useful to detect soft tissue injuries. MCL or LUCL injuries will often be visible in acute ruptures, but are sometimes hard to detect in chronic instability, where scar tissue may have formed [13]. Bony lesions of the humerus, radial head, or coronoid process can also be diagnosed on MRI, but in cases where bony abnormalities are predominant, computed tomography (CT) scans will be more appropriate.

CT is especially helpful in acute cases in order to evaluate displacement and number of fragments. Anteromedial facet fractures of the coronoid process, for example, are almost impossible to detect on plain radiographs and can easily be diagnosed on CT images. CT is also useful in chronic cases where bony insufficiency is suspected (Fig. 7.3), as well as in the evaluation of osteophyte formation or calcification of the ligaments, as this will guide the treatment but also determine the prognosis.

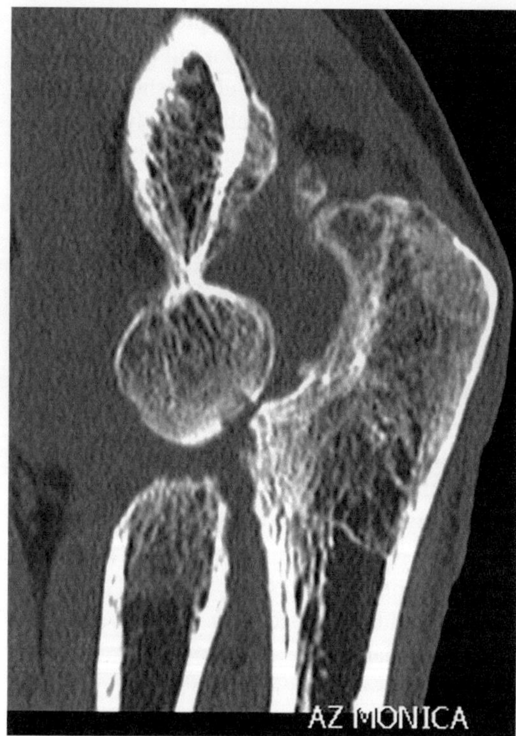

Fig. 7.3 CT scan showing gross chronic instability following a radial head resection. Progressive instability is caused due to a bony deficiency of the coronoid process (Used with permission of the MoRe Foundation)

Lateral Instability

The Origin

Traumatic elbow injuries with osseous (radial head or coronoid) and/or soft tissue (primarily LUCL) involvement are mostly responsible for chronic lateral instability in our patient population. Secondary referrals to our practice often involve failed open reduction of internal fixation of fractures or failed conservative treatment of instability. Instability following previous release of the common extensor tendon [27] is also relatively common as a cause for lateral instability and subsequent referral.

Indications

LCL injuries after simple dislocation generally do not require surgery and can be treated with a short period of, or preferably, no immobilization followed by a hinged brace for 6 weeks. Traumatic lateral elbow instability with displaced fractures of radial head and/or coronoid is an indication for surgery. The indication is usually made depending on the fracture instead of the ligamentous injury [20].

Acute surgery of simple dislocations is also indicated when closed reduction is not possible or if the elbow remains grossly unstable following reduction. A relative indication for surgery is professional or sports activities of the patient. A high level athlete will often require surgery, even after a simple dislocation.

Most patients will have a good result following a simple dislocation, but a small number of patients will have symptomatic laxity or even instability following conservative treatment. When conservative treatment fails, and recurrent lateral instability develops with functional impairment in activities of daily living, delayed surgical reconstruction is justified. Gross instability is treated with a ligament reconstruction using a tendon graft. This is done using an open technique. More subtle instability with functional impairment and pain can be treated with an arthroscopic plication of the LCL complex.

Surgical Approach

Both the arthroscopic and open surgical options are done under tourniquet control. The patient is placed in lateral decubitus for the arthroscopic technique, and supine position with the arm on a side table for the open technique. The arthroscopic approach to plicate the LCL complex is essentially identical to the standard arthroscopic technique, which is outside the scope of this chapter.

The modified Kocher approach is used for LUCL reconstruction. The interval between the anconeus and the extensor carpi ulnaris (ECU) is found by identifying the fatty streak between the two muscle bellies and is used to expose the entire LCL complex. The ECU is reflected anteriorly, and the anconeus posteriorly. Proximally, the common extensor tendon is released from the lateral epicondyle. If there is still a remainder of LCL attached to the epicondyle, care is taken not to damage this remnant, and the capsule is opened anterior to the remnant. Usually, the entire LCL complex has been avulsed of the bone, and the lateral epicondyle is stripped of soft tissue (Fig. 7.4). The radiocapitellar joint is inspected for degenerative changes. An excellent view of the lateral side of the capitellum is necessary later in the procedure. A more extensive anterior release can be performed in patients with a fixed flexion deformity. Distally, the interval is followed all the way to the ulna. Blood vessels are invariably found at the distal end of the dissection and should be coagulated in order to prevent a

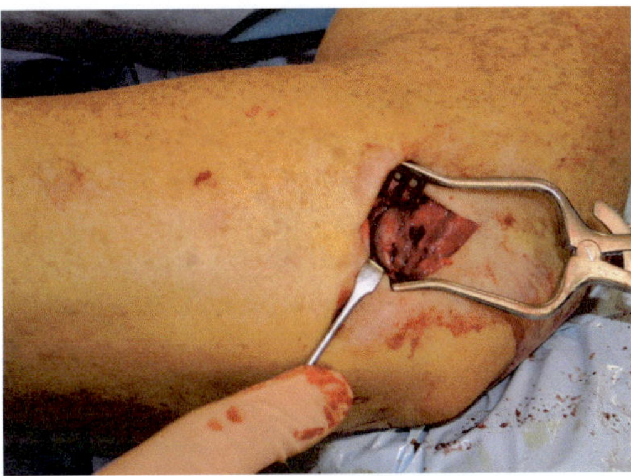

Fig. 7.4 The capitellum is in clear view as the lateral structures were stripped from the lateral epicondyle in this patient (Used with permission of the MoRe Foundation)

large hematoma postoperatively. The lateral side of the ulna is exposed. The LUCL inserts on a small tubercle on the proximal border of the supinator crest. The supinator crest is palpated, and the tubercle is exposed on the ulna at the base of the radial head.

Surgical Technique

Open Technique

Once the tubercles on the supinator crest and the lateral epicondyle have been exposed, the ligament reconstruction is done. A variety of grafts and fixation methods can be used. Grafts that are commonly used include the palmaris longus, hamstrings or triceps autograft, or an extensor hallucis longus or hamstring allograft. All of these grafts have been shown to be strong enough to be used, and the choice therefore depends on the preference of the surgeon [4]. The most common technique to fix the graft is the docking technique, where the graft is fixed through bone tunnels. Other fixation methods include bone anchors, interference screws, endobutton or transosseous sutures, or any combination.

We preferably use an extensor hallucis allograft. There is no donor site morbidity, and the extensor hallucis tendon graft is relatively constant in width and length, which is not always the case with palmaris longus autograft or allograft. A guide pin is drilled through supinator tubercle on the lateral cortex of the ulna. Care is taken not to drill through the second, medial cortex in order to avoid iatrogenic ulnar nerve damage. The guide pin is then overdrilled with a cannulated 4.5 mm endobutton drill, again taking care not to drill through the medial cortex (Fig. 7.5). The humeral insertion of the LCL complex is then determined. The capitellum is a sphere and the insertion of the LCL is situated at the center of this sphere. The guide pin is drilled from this center to the posterior cortex of the humerus. The guide pin should not exit in the olecranon fossa, as this will impair extension once the second implant is placed. The guide pin should also not be directed too far medially as this again may pierce the ulnar nerve. The sur-

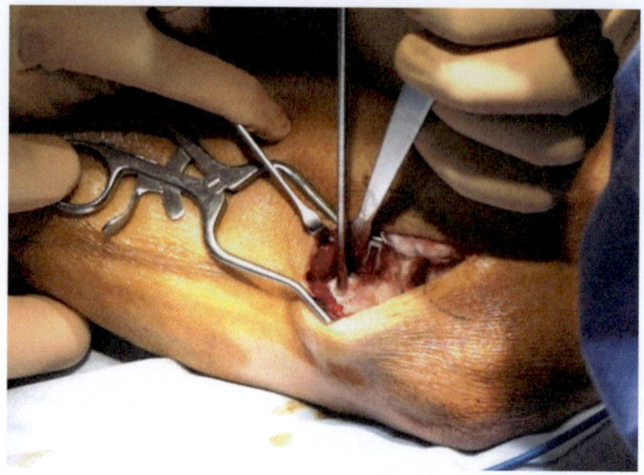

Fig. 7.5 The first cortex is over a guidewire, drilled with a 4.5 mm drill to create a bone tunnel in the ulna at the insertion of the LUCL (Used with permission of the MoRe Foundation)

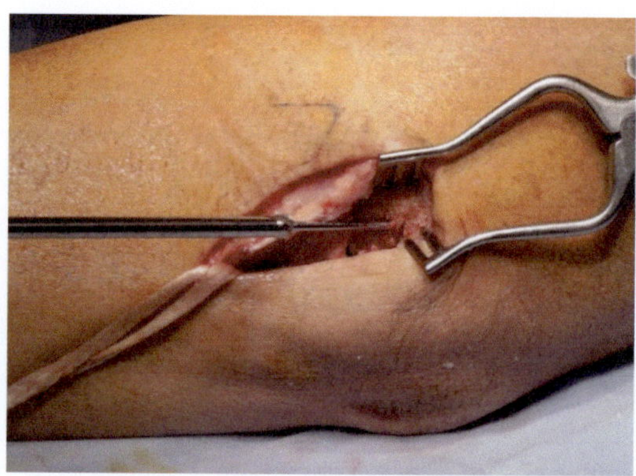

Fig. 7.6 The first cortex of the lateral epicondyle is over-drilled with a 6 mm drill, thus creating a tunnel for the graft. The far humeral cortex is only drilled with a 4.5 mm drill bit, so the button can advance through both cortices and the graft can be tensioned and fixed securely (Used with permission of the MoRe Foundation)

geon can decide to release the lateral part of the triceps and intermuscular septum to get a good visualization of the posterior humeral cortex and drill the guide pin under direct view. The first cortex at the lateral epicondyle is overdrilled with a 6 mm cannulated drill (Fig. 7.6). The second cortex is drilled with the 4.5 mm endobutton drill. A ZipLoop implant (Biomet, Warsaw, IN, USA) is then inserted into the ulna. As the second cortex is intact, this can be somewhat difficult as the implant cannot be pulled through but has to be pushed in. The tendon allograft is then pulled through the loop until one third of the graft is in the loop. The loop is then tightened. A second

ZipLoop is then inserted into the humerus. This is done in the standard fashion with the use of the guide pin and shuttle suture of the implant. Once the implant is brought through the second cortex, the implant is flipped and secured on the posterior cortex of the humerus. If needed, this position can be confirmed visually or with the use of fluoroscopy. The longer limb of the graft is then brought through the loop and tightened as much as possible when the loop is closed. The closing of the loop pulls the graft into the humeral tunnel, while the graft is tightened even further (Fig. 7.7). Although the graft is then already securely fixed between both loops, we prefer to double the ulnar and humeral limbs of the graft and suture all limbs together with a non-resorbable suture, together with the lateral capsule and overlying extensor tendons. The fascia and skin are closed in layers (Fig. 7.8).

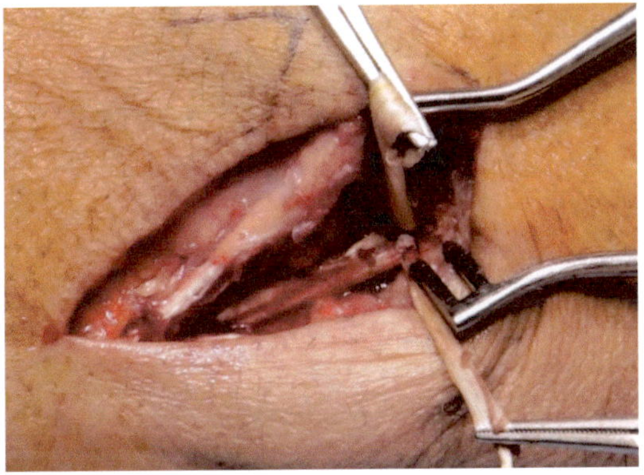

Fig. 7.7 The graft is pulled into the lateral epicondyle (Used with permission of the MoRe Foundation)

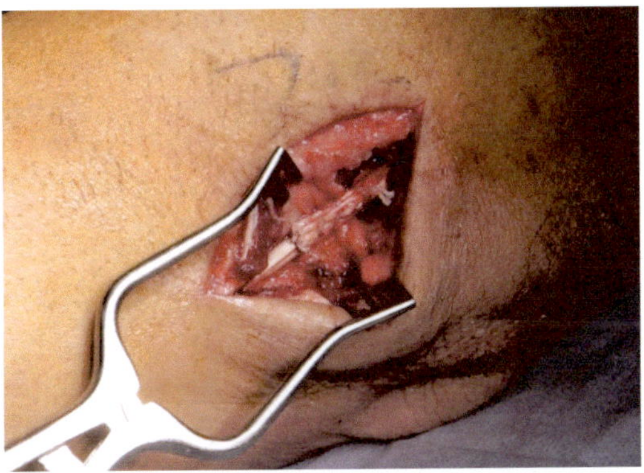

Fig. 7.8 All limbs of the graft are sutured together for additional fixation (Used with permission of the MoRe Foundation)

Arthroscopic Technique

A standard arthroscopic technique is used to inspect the joint. Concomitant lesions can be treated accordingly. After a thorough inspection of all compartments, the scope is brought into the posterior radial gutter. A soft spot portal is made, and a synovectomy is performed to increase the view. The lateral epicondyle is palpated, and a spinal needle is inserted from the insertion of the LCL complex on the lateral epicondyle into the posterior radial gutter. The tip is brought into view, and a number 2 PDS suture is shuttled trough the needle (Fig. 7.9). A grasper pulls the PDS out of the soft spot portal and the needle is removed. The subcutaneous border of the ulna and the radial head are then palpated. The origin of the LUCL is located approximately at the base on the radial head. The spinal needle is then inserted from the subcutaneous border of the ulna into the radial gutter, and a PDS is shuttled into the joint (Fig. 7.10). This limb is then again pulled out from the soft spot portal and both limbs are tied. A loop is then made in ulnar free end of the suture, and a second PDS is pulled up to its midportion through the loop. The humeral free end of the suture is then pulled out until the double PDS appears. The initial shuttle suture is then removed,

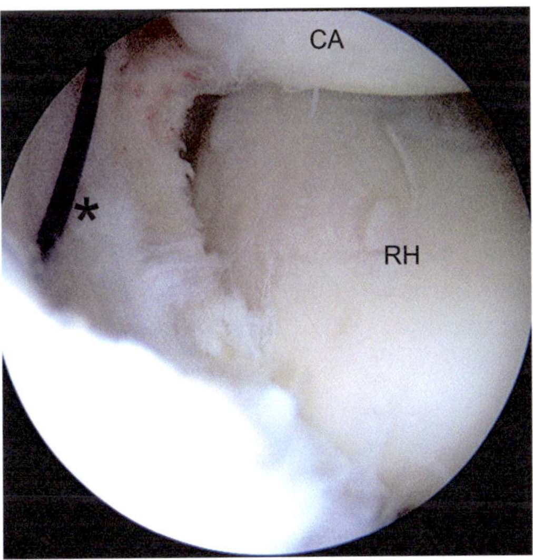

Fig. 7.9 Arthroscopic view from the posterolateral portal. Radial head (*RH*) and capitellum (*CA*) can be seen, as well as the PDS suture (*) on the lateral side. This suture is used to plicate the lateral collateral ligament complex (Used with permission of the MoRe Foundation)

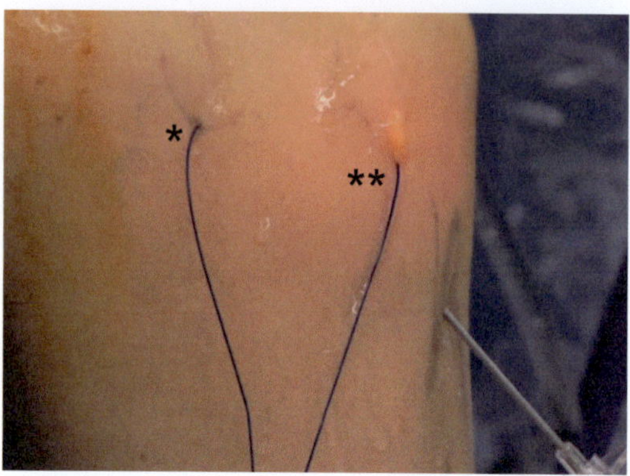

Fig. 7.10 Lateral view of the elbow. The first limb of the suture has been inserted into the joint from the origin of the LCL complex at the lateral epicondyle (*). It was pulled out through the soft spot portal (**). The second limb is inserted with a spinal needle at the insertion of the LUCL. Care is taken to stick to the bone in order to avoid neurovascular complications. This limb will also be pulled out of the soft spot portal so both limbs can be joined to imbricate the LCL complex (Used with permission of the MoRe Foundation)

and all four ends of the double suture are subcutaneously brought out of the soft spot portal. Both sutures are then tightened and tied individually.

Postoperatively, a removable splint is applied for 24 h to reduce the risk of any unforeseen movements when the patient wakes up from the anesthesia or during the time the peripheral nerve block is still active. A dynamic elbow brace is applied on the first postoperative day. Flexion is allowed immediately, and at the first 2 weeks, extension is blocked at 60°. From 2 to 4 weeks, extension is allowed to 30°, and the following 2 weeks full extension is allowed in the brace. Physiotherapy is usually delayed as most patients regain their motion in the brace. A physiotherapist will however supervise the return to sport specific activities. A full return to sports is usually allowed around 3–6 months postoperatively.

Results and Complications

Recently, two studies have been published looking at the outcome of reconstruction of the LUCL after posterolateral elbow instability. Lin et al. found that 13 of 14 patients (93 %) had a good to excellent result at a mean follow-up time of 49 months after surgery, based on the Mayo Elbow Performance Score (MEPS) [25]. Jones et al. reported an average follow-up of 7 years after reconstruction in 8 patients. They found that all included patients had a good to excellent result, with a mean MEPS score of 87.5 [17].

The most common complication after reconstruction of the LUCL is occasional or persistent instability. This is most common in preoperative severe elbow instability [17, 25]. Early results of the arthroscopic technique are equally positive. We have now used this technique for a little over 2 years and nearly 20 patients. Overall results are good to excellent in our ongoing study with significant improvement in stability, Mayo Elbow Performance Score, and Dash scores. There have been no complications in our patient cohort.

Medial Instability

The Origin

Chronic medial instability can be caused by trauma or overuse. Medial collateral ligament ruptures are usually treated conservatively with good results but a group of patients may develop medial instability. Valgus instability in overhead or throwing athletes is a different entity and is caused by chronic overuse of the MCL. The MCL stretches and becomes insufficient to withstand the extreme forces placed on the medial side of the elbow with a tennis serve, for example. The medial tip of the olecranon may touch the side of the olecranon fossa and reactive osteophytes may form. In a subsequent stage, degenerative changes of the radiohumeral joint will occur as well.

Indications

Low-demand patients will most often recover with conservative treatment, because most daily activities will not load the elbow in valgus. Even throwing athletes have a 42 % chance to return to the same level of sports after conservative treatment [37]. Surgery may be indicated in high-demand athletes and manual laborers with persistent symptoms of instability and pain, despite at least 6 months of adequate conservative treatment including strengthening of the flexor-pronator group.

Surgical Approach

Reconstruction of the MCL can be performed with several techniques using different approaches and graft materials.

The MCL can be approached through several planes. Jobe was the first to describe a figure-of-eight reconstruction with bony tunnels in the medial epicondyle and the ulna. This technique also included a takedown of the common flexor origin and an ulnar nerve transposition [16]. Unfortunately, postoperative ulnar nerve symptoms are common with this technique.

The Hotchkiss "over the top" technique [15] and the flexor carpi ulnaris split [38] have decreased the incidence of this complication. Patients often have ulnar nerve symptoms preoperatively [6] but these resolve in the majority of cases, even without an anterior transposition of the nerve. Our preferred operative technique is the FCU split approach, with the ulnar nerve left in situ and usually not released.

Surgical Technique

Choice of graft and fixation is similar to the lateral side and depend on the preference of the surgeon [4]. Again, we prefer to use an extensor hallucis longus allograft to avoid donor site morbidity and anatomical variations that sometimes results in a disappointing autograft.

Jobe described a figure-of-eight reconstruction with bony tunnels in the medial epicondyle and the ulna [16].

As on the lateral side, we prefer an endobutton (Smith & Nephew, Warsaw, IN, USA) or ZipLoop technique (Biomet). Details of this technique are similar to the technique described earlier on the lateral side. The ulnar nerve needs to be located and protected at all times for both the ulnar and humeral tunnels. The ulnar tunnel is made on the sublime tubercle of the ulna. This can easily be palpated and visualized. The button is advanced through the first cortex of the ulna and the graft is fixed to the button. A second button is advanced from the isometric point on the humerus, just anterior and distal to the base of the medial epicondyle. The button is advanced from medial, through the second cortex of the humerus on the posterolateral side, avoiding the olecranon fossa. One or both strands of the graft are then passed through the loop of the button and tensioned, and when the loop is tightened, the graft is fixed and tensioned even more. The limbs can then be sutured onto themselves so that a double or four-strand reconstruction is achieved.

Combined Medial and Lateral Instability

The Origin

In rare cases it may be necessary to reconstruct both the lateral and medial collateral ligaments with a graft. These patients will have severe varus and valgus instability, leading to recurrent dislocations.

Indications

If gross instability of the elbow exists, a circumferential graft [44] may be necessary.

Surgical Approach

A posterior incision is made, and thick skin and subcutaneous flaps are developed medially and laterally. The medial and lateral approaches are identical to the individual approaches described earlier.

Surgical Technique

A guidewire is drilled through the humeral axis of rotation from medial to lateral. Once the position of the pin is confirmed and satisfactory, the pin is overdrilled using a 4.5 mm cannulated drill. A suture is passed through the tunnel, using a suture retriever. The ulnar insertions of the anterior band MCL and LUCL are determined as described earlier. The guidewire is then drilled from medial

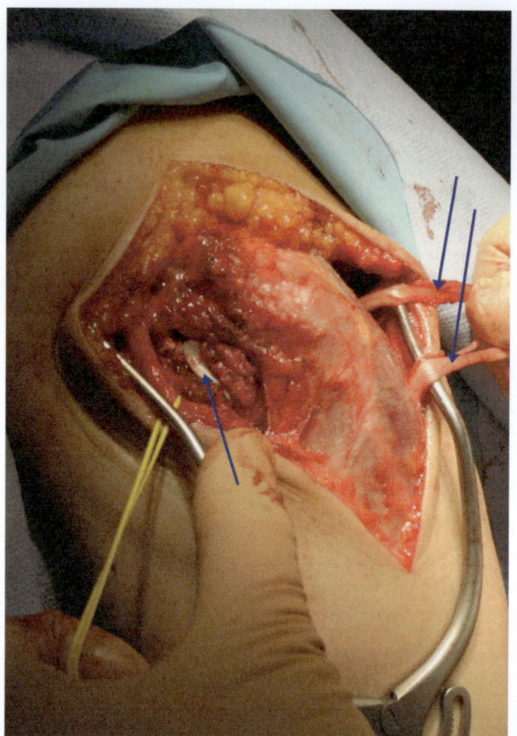

Fig. 7.11 Posterior view of the elbow. The ulnar nerve is marked with a vessel loop. The *blue arrows* indicate the graft. The limbs are pulled through the ulnar and humeral tunnels from medial to lateral (Used with permission of the MoRe Foundation)

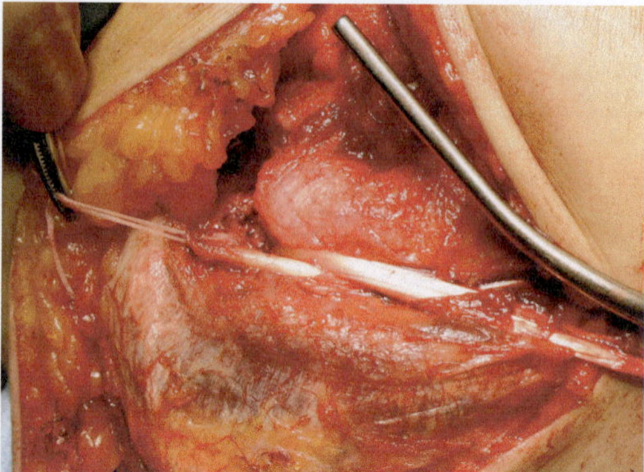

Fig. 7.12 Lateral view of the elbow. Both graft limbs are tensioned and sutured onto themselves on the lateral side in order to avoid ulnar nerve symptoms from the bulk of the graft (Used with permission of the MoRe Foundation)

to lateral again, connecting both insertions. This is again overdrilled and the suture is passed through the tunnel. The tendon graft is stitched with a non-resorbable suture, and this trailing suture is pulled through the tunnels, followed by the graft (Fig. 7.11). The graft is tensioned laterally (Fig. 7.12) and the limbs are sutured. Interference screws can be used to avoid rotation of the graft in the tunnels (Fig. 7.13). A second loop can be made if it is deemed necessary to also reconstruct the posterior band of the MCL.

Postoperative Protocol

The postoperative protocol is similar for all reconstructions described. A removable splint is applied for the first 24 h to reduce the risk of any unforeseen movements when the patient wakes up from the anesthesia or during the time the peripheral nerve block is still active. A dynamic elbow brace

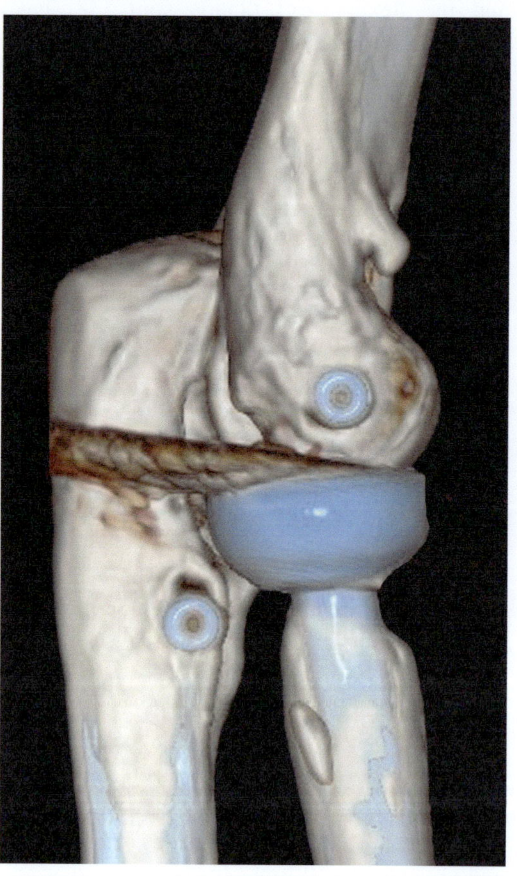

Fig. 7.13 Interference screws can be used to further secure the graft and to avoid rotation of the graft in the tunnels. Note the presence of radial head prosthesis in this postoperative CT scan (Used with permission of the MoRe Foundation)

is applied on the first postoperative day. Flexion is allowed immediately, and at the first 2 weeks, extension is blocked at 60°. From 2 to 4 weeks, extension is allowed to 30°, and the following 2 weeks full extension is allowed in the brace. Physiotherapy is usually delayed as most patients regain their motion in the brace. A physiotherapist will however supervise the return to sport specific activities. A full return to sports is usually allowed around 3–6 months postoperatively.

Results and Complications

Several clinical studies have been executed to evaluate patients after MCL reconstruction. The patient population mostly consists of baseball players, as they are prone to this type of injury. The MCL reconstruction techniques had excellent results in 83–95 % with a mean return to play of 13 months [8, 23, 24, 42]. Ulnar nerve symptoms remain the major complication of this reconstruction, although this complication has decreased from 20 % with detachment of the flexors to 6 % with the muscle-splitting approach. The incidence of ulnar nerve symptoms decreases even further if the ulnar nerve is left in situ, instead of performing the classic transposition [49].

Preexisting arthritic changes will of course dictate the outcome of the treatment even in cases where a strong reconstruction was obtained. This is obviously also the case for isolated medial or lateral instability.

Longitudinal Forearm Instability

The Origin

Peter Essex-Lopresti was the first to describe longitudinal radioulnar dissociation (LRUD). LRUD consists of the combination of a radial head fracture, injury to the interosseous membrane (IOM), and a lesion of the distal radioulnar joint (DRUJ) [9]. It is an important but uncommon pathology following axial compression injuries of the forearm, occurring in only 3 % of all radial head fractures [45]. Diagnosis is difficult, as only 25 % of patients with this lesion will be correctly diagnosed

initially [43]. If longitudinal stability is not restored, proximal migration of the radius may occur, causing secondary wrist and elbow problems [43].

Indications

Patients with a history of a fall on the outstretched hand, which were diagnosed with a radial head fracture, are the population at risk for a LRUD. Pain and swelling along the forearm, pain at the wrist with pronation and supination, and tenderness and instability at the DRUJ are all possible clinical signs of LRUD that warrant further investigation (radiographs, ultrasound, or MRI). Radiographs of the wrist may show proximal migration of the radius. MRI and ultrasound have both been shown to be of use to diagnose an acute rupture of the IOM [11, 26].

When these investigations confirm an Essex-Lopresti lesion and the radial head fracture is displaced or comminuted, then a surgical intervention will be unavoidable (Fig. 7.14). Primary reconstruction of the radial head is preferred, but if this is not possible, a radial head replacement should be used in cases of an acute LRUD injury.

Chronic cases of LRUD are difficult to treat and become symptomatic if the radial head was excised as part of the initial treatment. Studies have shown that following radial head excision, up to 2 mm of radial migration is physiologic and mostly asymptomatic [30]. In patients with LRUD however, proximal migration may progress further and lead to ulnar abutment syndrome or abutment of the radial stump on the capitellum (Fig. 7.15). Several surgical options exist for these patients depending on the severity of the symptoms, chronicity, and the extent of proximal migration. Often, a combination of surgical techniques may be required. A radial head prosthesis is the first choice. Capitellar osteopenia may predispose to capitellar resorption or wear, and in these cases it may be better to also replace the capitellum. Reconstruction of the IOM and DRUJ may be combined in cases of severe LRUD. In chronic cases, the interosseous membrane (IOM), and more specifically the central band of the IOM, can be reconstructed with a bone-patellar tendon-bone auto- or allograft. Several techniques have been described to stabi-

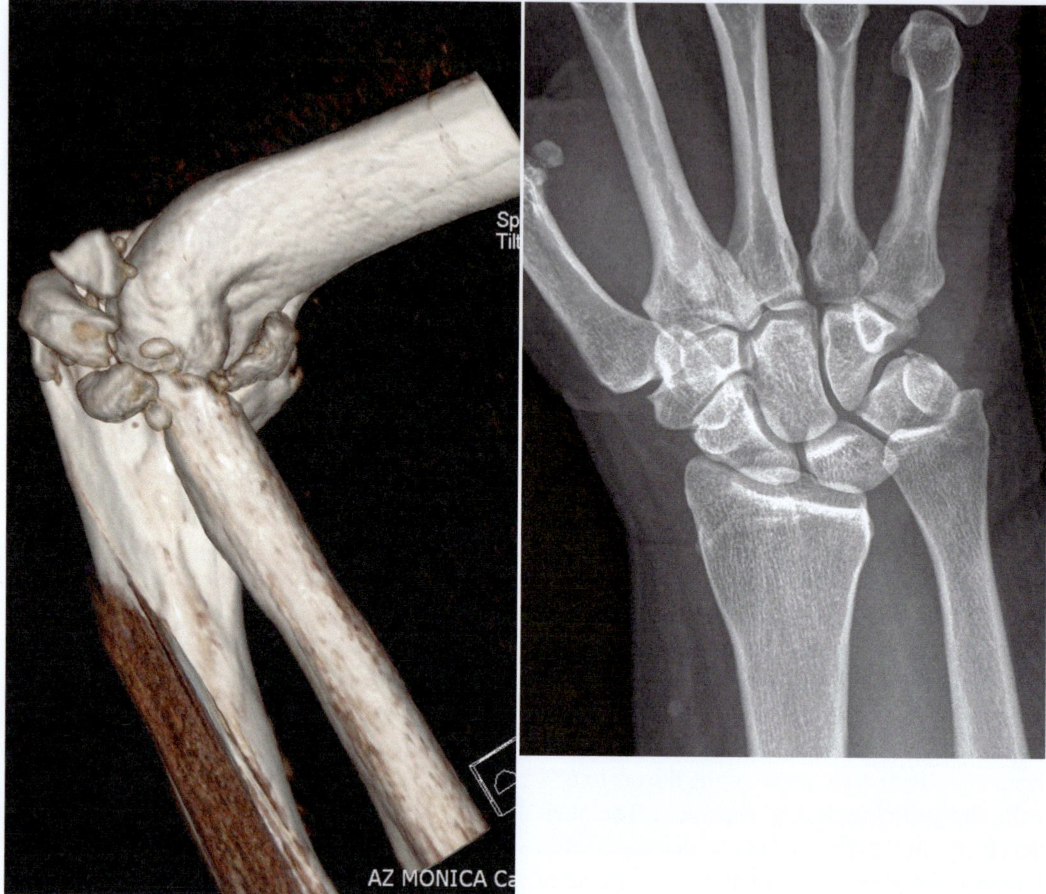

Fig. 7.14 Acute trauma to the forearm and elbow with fracture of the radial head, rupture of the interosseous membrane, and disruption of the distal radioulnar joint ligaments. A classic presentation for an acute Essex-Lopresti injury (Used with permission of the MoRe Foundation)

lize the DRUJ [21], but the one described by Adams and Berger is probably the most commonly used technique [1]. This technique is basically an anatomic reconstruction of the dorsal and palmar radioulnar ligaments with a tendon graft. Finally, an ulnar shortening osteotomy may have to be added, as restoration of normal ulnar variance may not be possible in these chronic cases.

Surgical Approach: Radial Head

A 3 cm lateral incision is made, starting from the lateral epicondyle, extending distally. The lateral collateral ligament is palpated but is often torn as part of the injury [45]. An extensor split is made sharply, anterior to the LCL. The annular liga-

ment is incised longitudinally and the radial head is brought into view. The view is even greater if the LCL was torn at the time of injury. The LCL can be released sharply from the lateral epicondyle if additional exposure is needed, e.g., if a radiocapitellar replacement is implanted.

Surgical Technique: Radial Head

In acute cases, an open reduction and internal fixation can be performed using two headless cannulated screws. Care is taken so that the screws do not penetrate the far cortex as this will limit pronation and supination and cause proximal radioulnar arthritis. If it is not possible to reconstruct the radial head, all fragments are excised and any

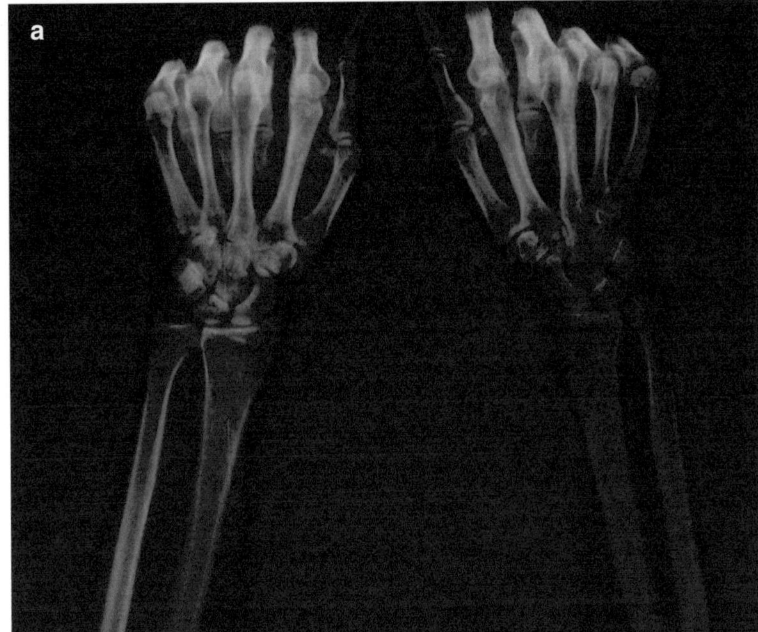

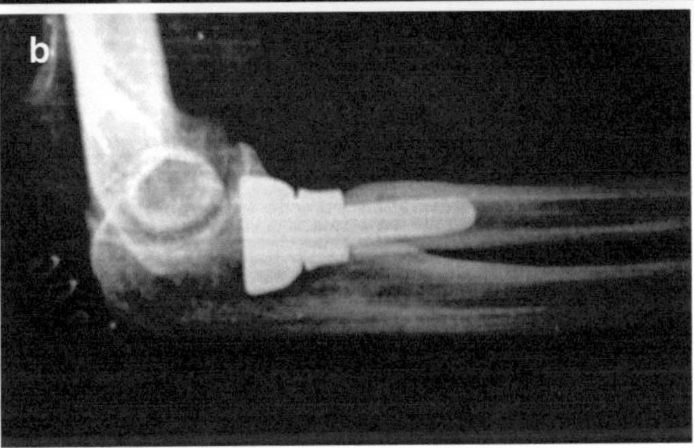

Fig. 7.15 (**a**) AP radiographs of the wrist in a patient with a chronic injury to the interosseous membrane that became clinically apparent a few months after a radial head resection. Note subtle proximal migration of the right radius. Patient had wrist pain and mild discomfort along the dorsal aspect of the forearm. (**b**) Patient was treated with implantation of a radial head replacement and her symptoms improved (Used with permission of Samuel Antuna)

remaining radial head is removed with an oscillating saw. Longitudinal stability is examined using the radius pull test [41]. A positive test, more than 2 mm proximal motion of the radius relative to the ulna, is indicative of LRUD, and the radial head should be replaced by a metal prosthesis in these cases. Another option is to repair or reconstruct the IOM, but this is not indicated in acute cases in our opinion. The specific technique to replace the radial head depends on the type of prosthesis used but the basic technique remains the same. The radial canal is prepared using rasps and this determines the size of the stem component. The size of the head component is determined by the size of the native radial head. A trial component is inserted and the height of the prosthesis is determined, using the lesser sigmoid notch as a landmark. The radial head should be flush with the proximal edge of the lesser sigmoid notch [47]. Further bone can be removed from the neck if necessary. If the capitellum is osteopenic or severe posttraumatic arthritis of the capitellum is apparent, the capitellum can be replaced as well. Instruments and technique depend on the manufacturer. The capitellar component is cemented into place. The definitive radial head is then placed and all lateral structures are sutured. We prefer to use a bone anchor if the LCL was torn as part of the fracture or if it was released. Both the LCL and common extensors are sutured tightly.

Surgical Approach: IOM

Two incisions are required for the reconstruction of the IOM. First, one small longitudinal incision is made at the distal 2/3 of the ulna, and another small longitudinal incision is made at the proximal 1/3 of the radius. At this point only the skin is incised. Further dissection towards the radial and ulnar bone is continued, making sure to stay volar to the extensor tendons.

Surgical Technique: IOM

A hemostat is passed from ulna to radius. It is important to stay under the extensor tendons and to protect both anterior and posterior interosseous nerves. The hemostat should exit radially between the brachioradialis and the extensor carpi radialis. The radial dorsal sensory nerve is identified and protected before passing the hemostat at the radial side.

The bony ends of the bone-patellar-bone auto- or allograft need to be adjusted to the size of radius and ulna. The angle between the tendon graft and the longitudinal axis of the ulna should be about 21° [2, 39].

The graft is inserted, using the hemostat, and it is fixed at the ulna first. The forearm is then place into slight supination before the graft is fixed to the radius. Before closure, pronation and supination are tested.

Surgical Approach: DRUJ

A 4 cm incision is made between the fifth and sixth extensor compartments, starting at the level of the ulnar styloid. The fifth extensor compartment is opened leaving the distal portion intact. The extensor digiti minimi is retracted ulnarly, and the capsule of the DRUJ is incised. The articular surface of the DRUJ becomes clearly visible. Care is taken not to open the extensor carpi ulnaris sheath, as this is important for the stability of the ulnocarpal joint [1].

Surgical Technique: DRUJ

The tunnel in the distal radius is drilled first. A guidewire is placed proximal to the lunate fossa and radial to the sigmoid notch and advanced parallel to these articular surfaces. Fluoroscopy is used to confirm that the guidewire does not run through subchondral bone. A 4 mm cannulated drill is used to create the tunnel in the distal radius. The palmaris longus autograft is already advanced through this tunnel.

Next, the ulnar tunnel is created by placing the guidewire between the fovea and the ulnar neck and advancing obliquely in the proximal direction. The aimed exit point is palmar to the extensor carpi ulnaris. Again a cannulated drill is used to create the tunnel. The free limbs of the graft are advanced through the ulnar tunnel. At the ulnar neck, a hemostat is passed from dorsal to volar, staying close to the ulna. One graft limb is grasped and pulled dorsally. Care is taken not to entrap any nerves or vessels. The 2 graft limbs are tensioned and sutured against the ulnar neck [1]. Alternatively, a suture anchor can be used.

Surgical Approach: Ulnar Shortening Osteotomy

A longitudinal incision is made at the subcutaneous border of the ulna. The incision is started 3–4 cm from the tip of the ulnar styloid and extends approximately 8 cm proximally. The subcutaneous border and flexor carpi ulnaris muscle are exposed by blunt dissection in order to protect the sensory branches of the ulnar nerve.

Surgical Technique: Ulnar Shortening Osteotomy

The flexor carpi ulnaris (FCU) fascia is incised sharply close to its insertion on the ulna, but leaving a cuff for later repair. The volar surface of the ulna is exposed by blunt elevation of the FCU. Care is taken not to disturb the periosteum as this may cause unnecessary devascularization of the bone. The amount of shortening is determined preoperatively, based on imaging of the wrist. The goal is to obtain a congruent distal radioulnar joint with approximately minus 1 mm ulnar variance. Several commercially available systems are available, with drilling and cutting guides that allow a precise shortening osteotomy and stable plate fixation. Techniques using a transverse, oblique, or step-cut osteotomy have been reported, and neither of them has proven to be superior as far as healing time is concerned. We therefore prefer a transverse osteotomy, as it is technically easy, allows minimal devascularization of the bone, and can be made very precisely with the now commercially available double bladed saw blades. The use of a new saw blade and rinsing with cold saline when making the saw cuts will help to minimize heat generation and additional damage to the bone. When good bone apposition and stable fixation with a plate is obtained, postoperative immobilization is not necessary in our experience. A meta-analysis of papers published on ulnar shortening showed an average healing time of 10.3 weeks, but this is dependent on the criteria that are used. We allow return to full activities when bridging callus formation is observed on radiographs.

Results and Complications

In general, results of metal radial head prostheses are good in the majority of patients [40].

The most common complications after treatment with radial head prosthesis are stiffness, recurrent instability, aseptic loosening, and degenerative changes at the elbow, including capitellar wear [46].

Heijink et al. published a series of eight patients treated with a monobloc metallic radial head for an Essex-Lopresti injury. Five patients suffered from recurrent instability, and needed revision surgery, illustrating the difficulty in obtaining a satisfactory result in these chronic cases [14].

Adams et al. reported a series of 16 patients undergoing an ulnar shortening osteotomy and reconstruction of the central band using a bone patella bone graft. Ninety-four percent stated that wrist discomfort had improved. Grip strength had improved 31 % comparing to preoperative values. Ulnar variance was diminished by an average of 1.5 mm at final follow-up. The most common complaint was located at the donor site of the autograft tendon. Therefore, allograft can be a good alternative [2].

Adams et al. stated that the DRUJ reconstruction restored stability and relieved symptoms in 12 out of 14 patients at 1–4 years of follow-up, all achieving near full pronation and supination. Two patients developed recurrence of DRUJ instability. Also, two patients had transient paresthesias and reduced sensibility in the distribution of the dorsal cutaneous branch of the ulnar nerve, but these symptoms resolved within 4 months after surgery [1].

Conclusion

Elbow instability cannot be considered to be a single entity. Both bony and soft tissue considerations play a role. Different techniques to reconstruct lateral and medial structures have been described but in essence both sides are similar. An excellent knowledge of elbow's anatomy is necessary to avoid disastrous complications, such as nerve damage.

In chronic cases, direct ligament repair is difficult, and a reconstruction using a ligament graft is recommended in most cases. Both auto- and allografts may be used, depending on the surgeon's preference. Fixation of the graft can be achieved by different means as well. We prefer to use an extensor hallucis allograft and fix the graft through bone tunnels and a bone-button technique. Results of both medial and lateral reconstructions are usually satisfactory with an acceptable complication rate.

In rare cases of severe medial and lateral instability, both medial and lateral ligaments need to be reconstructed. When necessary, reconstruction of both the medial and lateral side is performed simultaneously, using a circular graft technique, where the graft is sutured on itself and one or two interference screws to obtain additional fixation. Although results are satisfactory in this difficult patient group, complication and reoperation rates are somewhat higher and this procedure should be considered to be a salvage procedure.

Longitudinal instability is complex, and results of surgical treatment are less predictable and can be disappointing. As in other cases of elbow instability, early detection is key to obtain the best results. Once the diagnosis is made, a decision can be made on the treatment plan, and if surgery is needed. Soft tissue injury resulting in LRUD often does not need surgery but when combined with bony instability, surgery is indicated. Acute radial head replacement is simple and will avoid severe complications in patients with LRUD. Once secondary changes occur at the elbow, forearm, or wrist, it is very difficult to restore function and stop the degenerative process.

References

1. Adams BD, Berger RA. An anatomic reconstruction of the distal radioulnar ligaments for posttraumatic distal radioulnar joint instability. J Hand Surg Am. 2002;27(2):243–51. S0363502302983917 [pii].
2. Adams JE, Culp RW, Osterman AL. Interosseous membrane reconstruction for the Essex-Lopresti injury. J Hand Surg. 2010;35(A):129–36.
3. Arvind CH, Hargreaves DG. Tabletop relocation test: a new clinical test for posterolateral rotatory instability of the elbow. J Shoulder Elbow Surg. 2006;15(6):707–8. doi:10.1016/j.jse.2006.01.005. S1058–2746(06)00075–9 [pii].
4. Baumfeld JA, van Riet RP, Zobitz ME, Eygendaal D, An KN, Steinmann SP. Triceps tendon properties and its potential as an autograft. J Shoulder Elbow Surg. 2010;19(5):697–9. doi:10.1016/j.jse.2009.12.001. S1058–2746(09)00555–2 [pii].
5. Callaway GH, Field LD, Deng XH, Torzilli PA, O'Brien SJ, Altchek DW, Warren RF. Biomechanical evaluation of the medial collateral ligament of the elbow. J Bone Joint Surg Am. 1997;79(8):1223–31.
6. Conway JE, Jobe FW, Glousman RE, Pink M. Medial instability of the elbow in throwing athletes. Treatment by repair or reconstruction of the ulnar collateral ligament. J Bone Joint Surg Am. 1992;74(1):67–83.
7. DeLee JC, Drez D, Miller MD. DeLee & Drez's orthopaedic sports medicine: principles and practice. 3rd ed. Philadelphia: Saunders (Elsevier); 2009. ISBN 978-1-4160-3143-7.
8. Dodson CC, Thomas A, Dines JS, Nho SJ, Williams 3rd RJ, Altchek DW. Medial ulnar collateral ligament reconstruction of the elbow in throwing athletes. Am J Sports Med. 2006;34(12):1926–32. doi:10.1177/0363546506290988.0363546506290988 [pii].
9. Essex-Lopresti P. Fractures of the radial head with distal radio-ulnar dislocation; report of two cases. J Bone Joint Surg Br. 1951;33B(2):244–7.
10. Eygendaal D, Verdegaal SH, Obermann WR, van Vugt AB, Poll RG, Rozing PM. Posterolateral dislocation of the elbow joint. Relationship to medial instability. J Bone Joint Surg Am. 2000;82(4):555–60.
11. Failla JM, Jacobson J, van Holsbeeck M. Ultrasound diagnosis and surgical pathology of the torn interosseous membrane in forearm fractures/dislocations. J Hand Surg Am. 1999;24(2):257–66. doi:10.1053/jhsu.1999.0257. S0363–5023(99)82539–8 [pii].
12. Forthman C, Henket M, Ring DC. Elbow dislocation with intra-articular fracture: the results of operative treatment without repair of the medial collateral ligament. J Hand Surg Am. 2007;32(8):1200–9. doi:10.1016/j.jhsa.2007.06.019. S0363–5023(07)00629–6 [pii].
13. Grafe MW, McAdams TR, Beaulieu CF, Ladd AL. Magnetic resonance imaging in diagnosis of chronic posterolateral rotatory instability of the elbow. Am J Orthop (Belle Mead NJ). 2003;32(10):501–3; discussion 4.
14. Heijink A, Morrey BF, van Riet RP, O'Driscoll SW, Cooney 3rd WP. Delayed treatment of elbow pain and dysfunction following Essex-Lopresti injury with metallic radial head replacement: a case series. J Shoulder Elbow Surg. 2010;19(6):929–36. doi:10.1016/j.jse.2010.03.007. S1058–2746(10)00119–9 [pii].
15. Hotchkiss RN, Kasparyan NG. The medial "Over the top" approach to the elbow. Tech Orthop. 2000;15(2):105–12.
16. Jobe FW, Stark H, Lombardo SJ. Reconstruction of the ulnar collateral ligament in athletes. J Bone Joint Surg Am. 1986;68(8):1158–63.
17. Jones KJ, Dodson CC, Osbahr DC, Parisien RL, Weiland AJ, Altchek DW, Allen AA. The docking technique for lateral ulnar collateral ligament reconstruction: surgical technique and clinical outcomes. J Shoulder Elbow Surg. 2012;21(3):389–95. doi:10.1016/j.jse.2011.04.033. S1058–2746(11)00202–3 [pii].
18. Josefsson PO, Johnell O, Wendeberg B. Ligamentous injuries in dislocations of the elbow joint. Clin Orthop Relat Res. 1987;221:221–5.
19. Josefsson PO, Nilsson BE. Incidence of elbow dislocation. Acta Orthop Scand. 1986;57(6):537–8.
20. Kaas L, van Riet RP, Turkenburg JL, Vroemen JP, van Dijk CN, Eygendaal D. Magnetic resonance imaging in radial head fractures: most associated injuries are not clinically relevant. J Shoulder Elbow Surg. 2011;20(8):1282–8. doi:10.1016/j.jse.2011.06.011. S1058–2746(11)00270–9 [pii].
21. Kakar S, Carlsen BT, Moran SL, Berger RA. The management of chronic distal radioulnar instability. Hand Clin. 2010;26(4):517–28. doi:10.1016/j.hcl.2010.05.010. S0749–0712(10)00044–2 [pii].
22. Kenter K, Behr CT, Warren RF, O'Brien SJ, Barnes R. Acute elbow injuries in the National Football League. J Shoulder Elbow Surg. 2000;9(1):1–5. S1058274600994795 [pii].
23. Kodde IF, Rahusen FT, Eygendaal D. Long-term results after ulnar collateral ligament reconstruction

of the elbow in European athletes with interference screw technique and triceps fascia autograft. J Shoulder Elbow Surg. 2012;21(12):1656–63. doi:10.1016/j.jse.2012.07.010.

24. Koh JL, Schafer MF, Keuter G, Hsu JE. Ulnar collateral ligament reconstruction in elite throwing athletes. Arthroscopy. 2006;22(11):1187–91. doi:10.1016/j.arthro.2006.07.024. S0749–8063(06)00902–9 [pii].

25. Lin KY, Shen PH, Lee CH, Pan RY, Lin LC, Shen HC. Functional outcomes of surgical reconstruction for posterolateral rotatory instability of the elbow. Injury. 2012;43(10):1657–61. doi:10.1016/j.injury.2012.04.023. S0020–1383(12)00168–4 [pii].

26. McGinley JC, Roach N, Hopgood BC, Limmer K, Kozin SH. Forearm interosseous membrane trauma: MRI diagnostic criteria and injury patterns. Skeletal Radiol. 2006;35(5):275–81. doi:10.1007/s00256–005–0069-x.

27. McKee MD, Schemitsch EH, Sala MJ, O'Driscoll SW. The pathoanatomy of lateral ligamentous disruption in complex elbow instability. J Shoulder Elbow Surg. 2003;12(4):391–6. doi:10.1016/mse.2003. S1058274603000272. S1058274603000272 [pii].

28. Mehlhoff TL, Noble PC, Bennet JB. Simple dislocations of the elbow in the adult: results after closed treatment. J Bone Joint Surg Am. 1988;70:244–9.

29. Morrey BF, An KN. Articular and ligamentous contributions to the stability of the elbow joint. Am J Sports Med. 1983;11(5):315–9.

30. Morrey BF, Chao EY, Hui FC. Biomechanical study of the elbow following excision of the radial head. J Bone Joint Surg Am. 1979;61(1):63–8.

31. O'Driscoll SW, Bell DF, Morrey BF. Posterolateral rotatory instability of the elbow. J Bone Joint Surg Am. 1991;73(3):440–6.

32. O'Driscoll SW, Jupiter JB, King GJW, Hotchkiss RN, Morrey BF. The unstable elbow. J Bone Joint Surg Am. 2000;82(A-5):724–38.

33. O'Driscoll SW, Lawton RL, Smith AM. The "moving valgus stress test" for medial collateral ligament tears of the elbow. Am J Sports Med. 2005;33(2):231–9.

34. Park MC, Ahmad CS. Dynamic contributions of the flexor-pronator mass to elbow valgus stability. J Bone Joint Surg Am. 2004;86-A(10):2268–74. 86/10/2268 [pii].

35. Pugh DM, Wild LM, Schemitsch EH, King GJ, McKee MD. Standard surgical protocol to treat elbow dislocations with radial head and coronoid fractures. J Bone Joint Surg Am. 2004;86-A(6):1122–30.

36. Regan W, Lapner PC. Prospective evaluation of two diagnostic apprehension signs for posterolateral instability of the elbow. J Shoulder Elbow Surg. 2006;15(3):344–6. doi:10.1016/j.jse.2005.03.009. S1058–2746(05)00111–4 [pii].

37. Rettig AC, Sherrill C, Snead DS, Mendler JC, Mieling P. Nonoperative treatment of ulnar collateral ligament injuries in throwing athletes. Am J Sports Med. 2001;29(1):15–7.

38. Ring D, Doornberg JN. Fracture of the anteromedial facet of the coronoid process. Surgical technique. J Bone Joint Surg Am. 2007;89(Suppl 2 Pt.2):267–83. doi:10.2106/JBJS.G.00059. 89/2_suppl_2/267 [pii].

39. Skahen JR, Palmer AK, Werner FW, Fortino MD. The interosseous membrane of the forearm: anatomy and function. J Hand Surg. 1997;22(A):981–5.

40. Smets S, Govaers K, Jansen N, van Riet RP, Schaap M, Van Glabbeek F. The floating radial head prosthesis for comminuted radial head fractures: a multicentric study. Acta Orthop Belg. 2000;66(4):353–8.

41. Smith AM, Urbanosky LR, Castle JA, Rushing JT, Ruch DS. Radius pull test: predictor of longitudinal forearm instability. J Bone Joint Surg Am. 2002; 84-A(11):1970–6.

42. Thompson WH, Jobe FW, Yocum LA, Pink MM. Ulnar collateral ligament reconstruction in athletes: muscle-splitting approach without transposition of the ulnar nerve. J Shoulder Elbow Surg. 2001;10(2):152–7. doi:10.1067/mse.2001.112881. S1058–2746(01)10913–4 [pii].

43. Trousdale RT, Amadio PC, Cooney WP, Morrey BF. Radio-ulnar dissociation. A review of twenty cases. J Bone Joint Surg Am. 1992;74(10):1486–97.

44. van Riet RP, Bain GI, Baird R, Lim YW. Simultaneous reconstruction of medial and lateral elbow ligaments for instability using a circumferential graft. Tech Hand Up Extrem Surg. 2006;10(4):239–44.

45. van Riet RP, Morrey BF, O'Driscoll SW, Van Glabbeek F. Associated injuries complicating radial head fractures: a demographic study. Clin Orthop Relat Res. 2005;441:351–5.

46. van Riet RP, Sanchez-Sotelo J, Morrey BF. Failure of metal radial head replacement. J Bone Joint Surg Br. 2010;92(5):661–7. doi:10.1302/0301–620X.92B5.23067.

47. van Riet RP, van Glabbeek F, de Weerdt W, Oemar J, Bortier H. Validation of the lesser sigmoid notch of the ulna as a reference point for accurate placement of a prosthesis for the head of the radius: a cadaver study. J Bone Joint Surg Br. 2007;89(3):413–6. doi:10.1302/0301–620X.89B3.18099. 89-B/3/413 [pii].

48. Veltri DM, O'Brien SJ, Field FP, editors. The milking maneuver: a new test to evaluate the MCL of the elbow in the throwing athlete. Presented at the 10th open meeting of the American Shoulder and Elbow Surgeons Specialty Day, New Orleans, 17 Feb 1994.

49. Vitale MA, Ahmad CS. The outcome of elbow ulnar collateral ligament reconstruction in overhead athletes: a systematic review. Am J Sports Med. 2008;36(6):1193–205. doi:10.1177/0363546508319053.

The Arthritic Elbow

8

Charlie Talbot and David Stanley

Abstract

Elbow arthritis may be the end stage of different aetiologies. Key clinical aspects and diagnostics strategies for primary osteoarthritis of the elbow, rheumatoid arthritis and posttraumatic conditions are reviewed. Arthroscopic and open procedures are discussed. Total elbow arthroplasty has proved to be an optimal solution for patients with severe joint damage. However, an adequate indication and a delicate surgical technique are essential to reduce the rate of complications. This chapter will provide the reader a simple but thoughtful approach to the arthritic elbow.

Keywords

Arthritis • Total elbow arthroplasty • Arthroscopy

Epidemiology

Elbow arthritis is relatively rare and often asymptomatic. It is characterised by loss of elbow motion and pain. It can be classified as predominantly posttraumatic, degenerative or inflammatory.

Posttraumatic arthritis results from articular fractures of the elbow that are either incompletely reconstructed or associated with a chondral injury. The incidence of posttraumatic arthritis is lower than that of degenerative or rheumatoid arthritis. Degenerative arthritis of the elbow commonly affects the dominant arm of men after the fourth decade of life, particularly in those who carry out manual labour. Symptomatic elbow osteoarthritis affects around 2 % of the population, although racial differences in prevalence have been reported [1]. Rheumatoid arthritis is an inflammatory immune-mediated arthropathy of unknown aetiology. It affects women more than men in a ratio of between 2 and 4:1 and is present in 0.5–2 % of the population [2]. The improved medical management of inflammatory arthropathy with disease-modifying medication has significantly reduced the number of rheumatoid

C. Talbot, MBChB, MSc(Eng), FRCS(Tr&Orth)
Department of Orthopaedic Surgery,
Harrogate & District NHS Foundation Trust,
Lancaster Park Road, Harrogate,
North Yorkshire HG2 7SX, UK
e-mail: charlie.talbot@hdft.nhs.uk

D. Stanley, MB BS, BSc (Hons), FRCS (✉)
Orthopaedic Department, Sheffield Teaching
Hospitals NHS Foundation Trust, Herries Road,
Sheffield, South Yorkshire S5 7AU, UK
e-mail: dave.stanley@sth.nhs.uk

S. Antuña, R. Barco (eds.), *Essentials in Elbow Surgery*,
DOI 10.1007/978-1-4471-4625-4_8, © Springer-Verlag London 2014

patients who require operative intervention. If however symptoms persist despite adequate medical therapy, surgical treatment is often of benefit.

The Problem

Elbow arthritis occurs most commonly either secondary to trauma, as a result of degenerative change, or due to progressive inflammatory disease (most commonly rheumatoid arthritis). Additional pathologies such as psoriasis, haemophilia, infection and neuropathic conditions can similarly lead to arthritic change in the joint.

The aetiology of osteoarthritis is not, as yet, fully understood. Primary osteoarthritis of the elbow is more common in manual workers [3]; and whilst repetitive trauma is undoubtedly an important factor, there are additional factors such as genetic make-up that influence the development of the disease.

Nonoperative management is appropriate for patients with early symptoms, whilst surgery is reserved for more advanced disease. Surgical options include joint-sparing procedures (arthroscopic or open debridement, including removal of osteophytes and capsular release), arthroplasty (interposition or replacement) and fusion. Treatment should be individualised but can broadly be divided into those suitable for degenerative and posttraumatic arthritis and those more suited to inflammatory disease.

Patient Workup

History

Posttraumatic and osteoarthritic patients usually have one of three types of presentation. Most commonly they complain of aching in the joint with loss of full elbow extension and at times loss of flexion. Forearm rotation and loading the joint whilst gripping (the grip and grind test) can exacerbate the symptoms due to degenerative changes in the radiocapitellar joint. A second frequent presentation is acute episodes of pain with associated mechanical symptoms of locking

or impingement. In extension the olecranon and its fossa abut (posterior impingement), whilst in flexion the coronoid and its fossa impact causing sharp anterior impingement pain. Loose bodies may be present and despite often being tethered to the capsule can cause elbow "locking" if they get trapped between the articular surfaces. A less common primary presentation is with ulnar nerve symptoms although these may occur as part of the patients' other symptoms in up to 50 % of those with elbow arthritis [4].

Patients with inflammatory arthropathy complain of swelling, loss of motion, pain and deformity if the disease is advanced. These patients are often on disease-modifying therapies, and it is important to specifically ask about the patients' drug history.

Clinical Examination

Adequate exposure is key to a good examination of the elbow. Inspection should assess the state of the soft tissues (particularly in the posttraumatic, previously operated elbow) as well as the carrying angle (though this may not be fully assessed in the presence of a flexion contracture). Range of motion (flexion/extension and forearm rotation) is assessed, and both full active and passive ranges are recorded. With passive end range movement impingement, discomfort may be elicited. Mid-arc pain is consistent with loss of cartilage. With the elbow extended, the medial and lateral epicondyles should line up with the tip of the olecranon, whilst in 90° of flexion, the three bony landmarks create an equilateral triangle. Loss of this configuration may indicate fracture, malunion, dislocation, congenital or structural abnormality. The grip and grind test will assess radiocapitellar disease. In rheumatoid elbows, swelling is often present, and in combination with pain and loss of movement, elbow stability should be evaluated.

In all patients a careful neurological examination is essential and the clinician should specifically record the sensory and motor function of the ulnar nerve as it is this nerve that is at particular risk in elbow arthritis.

Imaging

Plain anteroposterior and lateral radiographs will usually confirm the diagnosis. In osteoarthritis the characteristic changes of osteophytes at the olecranon and coronoid tips and the radial head can be seen, along with thickening of the olecranon fossa. The radiocapitellar joint narrows relatively late in idiopathic osteoarthritis and is more commonly seen in inflammatory arthropathies. Loose bodies may be noted but can be difficult to isolate, and therefore cross-sectional imaging with computerised tomography (CT) or magnetic resonance imaging (MRI) may be required to locate the loose fragments and also assess for sites of impinging osteophytes. Imaging inflammatory arthropathies will confirm the characteristic joint destruction and erosion, which can be marked. In cases of posttraumatic elbow arthritis, imaging may reveal arthrosis alone or deformity from joint incongruity or mal-united or mal-reduced fractures.

Posttraumatic Arthritis

Indications

Posttraumatic arthritis affects both men and women who have sustained elbow trauma, particularly comminuted intra-articular distal humerus fractures. The resultant degenerative changes are progressive although the speed at which symptoms occur is variable. In patients with unnoticed chondral damage at the time of injury or in those with poorly or nonanatomically reconstructed intra-articular fractures, symptoms are likely to develop rapidly and may require surgical intervention. In addition, patients who sustain an injury to their medial ulnar collateral ligament will, with time, experience a valgus overload of the elbow resulting in posteromedial impingement with osteophyte formation on the posteromedial olecranon and humerus. Following trauma elbow stiffness may also occur which remains unresponsive to nonoperative measures. Loss of motion following trauma can be due to either soft tissue or

osseous abnormalities within or around the joint. Intra-articular joint incongruity from mal-united fractures, articular adhesions and posttraumatic arthritis along with capsular thickening and extra-articular soft tissue contracture or heterotopic bone formation can all result in elbow stiffness following trauma.

Surgical options should be individualised to the patients needs and depend on the cause of the posttraumatic arthritic pain and its likely associated stiffness.

In general terms, if the elbow has a reasonably well-preserved joint space, but with osteophyte formation, either arthroscopic or open joint preservation surgery is offered. Arthroscopy is generally reserved for less severe cases, i.e. multiple intra-articular loose bodies, coronoid and olecranon osteophytes but no significant alteration to the bony anatomy and limited joint stiffness. The radial head is excised if there is established radiocapitellar degeneration combined with positive clinical signs. The ulnar nerve is transposed or decompressed if ulnar nerve symptoms are present. However, if there is significant joint destruction, then interposition or replacement arthroplasty is offered. Interposition is suitable for younger (<65-year-olds), higher-demand patients with a stable joint, and in the older, lower-demand patient total elbow arthroplasty can be considered.

In our practice arthroscopy is used for early disease with loose body formation and osteophytes at the tip of the olecranon and coronoid process. With more advanced disease with significant stiffness, an arthrolysis is undertaken with excision of the anterior or posterior capsule depending on which movement (flexion or extension) is limited.

Interposition arthroplasty is undertaken in young patients when the articular surfaces are damaged and deformed. This procedure however in our hands is unreliable, and we find it impossible to predict which patients will achieve a good outcome and which will continue to have symptoms of pain and discomfort.

Total elbow arthroplasty in posttraumatic arthritis is limited to elderly patients who agree to use their elbow with caution. Heavy activities will result in early failure of the arthroplasty and the need for revision surgery.

Surgical Techniques

Arthroscopic Debridement

Arthroscopic debridement has gained popularity, but it does require intimate anatomical knowledge of the elbow and its surrounding neurovascular structures, as well as the technical ability to perform the procedure. The benefits of arthroscopic treatment over the more established open techniques are reduced soft tissue trauma, smaller scars, faster rehabilitation and reduced length of hospital stay. Arthroscopy also allows the surgeon to address all underlying pathologies. Patient outcomes are similar, if not better, than open techniques.

Arthroscopy is contraindicated if there is severe degenerative change, extreme stiffness of the joint, several heterotopic ossifications, significant joint incongruity or surgeon inexperience. The best results are obtained in patients with either loose bodies or those with mild osteophytosis and mild stiffness. Good outcomes are reported for arthroscopic arthrolysis of the elbow [5, 6]. Whilst range of movement can be gained in the flexion-extension axis, forearm rotation is unlikely to be improved through arthroscopy alone.

We perform elbow arthroscopy in the lateral position with the patient under general anaesthesia and with a high arm tourniquet. The anterior compartment is generally examined first using the anteromedial viewing portal, and assessment of the articular surfaces is made. Loose bodies and osteophytes from the coronoid tip and the anterior humerus are removed using an arthroscopic burr, via a lateral portal. The posterior compartment is then entered, and osteophytes from the olecranon tip and the fossa are similarly excised (Fig. 8.1). If a capsular release is to be performed for loss of extension, we preferentially start in the posterior compartment to avoid significant swelling developing after the anterior capsule has been excised. If the patient has loss of flexion, the anterior compartment is debrided and loose bodies removed after which the posterior compartment of the

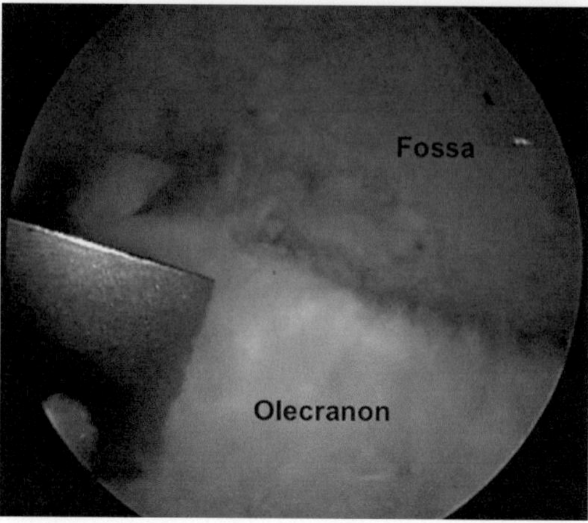

Fig. 8.1 Arthroscopic view of the posterior compartment of the elbow. Olecranon osteophytes can be removed with osteotomes

elbow is entered and the capsule excised from the posterior humerus. We use either an arthroscopic soft tissue shaver or an arthroscopic punch. Great care must be taken to avoid the radial nerve as it lies anterior to the radial head in a strip of fat. Assessment of range of motion can be repeatedly checked to gauge the amount of excision/release that is required, and a gentle manipulation may provide some extra range of movement at the end of the procedure.

The medial and lateral gutters are inspected, with particular care to avoid the ulnar nerve on the medial side, and again loose bodies are removed if present. If a significant increase in the range of elbow movement is anticipated, release or anterior transposition of the ulnar nerve is mandatory as without it ulnar nerve symptoms are likely to occur postoperatively.

Postoperative analgesia is achieved with a regional block. A bulky dressing is applied, and if there have been significant increases in range of motion achieved, continuous passive motion may be employed. The majority of patients however are allowed to freely mobilise the elbow. The bulky dressing is discarded at 5 days to facilitate range of motion exercises.

Interposition Arthroplasty

Interposition arthroplasty of the elbow was introduced in an attempt to address the resultant instability following an excisional arthroplasty for a painful elbow ankylosis. By removing less bone and maintaining a fulcrum between the distal humerus and the olecranon and keeping the collaterals, better stability was achieved. In Europe, interposition was used more extensively for patients with rheumatoid arthritis, though advances in total elbow arthroplasty have seen its decline. More recently it has also been advocated for posttraumatic arthritis in young patients. The procedure involves interposition of soft tissues between the articular surfaces of the elbow.

We infrequently perform an elbow interpositional arthroplasty. However, when we do, we position the patient in the lateral decubitus position, with a high arm tourniquet. We incorporate previous scars; otherwise, we perform a longitudinal posterior midline incision and utilise a Shahane-Stanley approach to the joint [7]. This enables the joint to be dislocated. A variety of grafts have been advocated for the interposition material. These include dermis, fascia and allograft Achilles tendon. Our personal choice at present is to use Graft Jacket although allograft Achilles tendon has the advantage that it can also be used to reconstruct deficient collateral ligaments if significant instability is present.

After exposure of the joint surfaces, bony spurs are removed from around the joint and the interposition material fixed to the distal humerus either using sutures through bony tunnels or with bone anchors. The joint is then reduced and soft tissue closure performed. We then apply an external fixator (DJD external fixator) across the joint and distract the joint surfaces by 2–3 mm. The fixator is locked for 1 week after which progressive active gentle flexion and extension of the joint is permitted. The fixator is removed after 6 weeks. Figure 8.1 shows radiographs of postoperative patient following a previous interposition arthroplasty.

Hemiarthroplasty

Lateral resurfacing of the elbow, or radiocapitellar replacement, was introduced to address isolated primary or secondary radio-humeral arthritis [8]. The lateral compartment of the elbow is commonly involved in elbow trauma. Radial head fracture, capitellum fracture, Monteggia-type injuries and the terrible triad can all result in chondral injury and posttraumatic lateral compartment arthritis. The perceived benefit of lateral resurfacing is not only to address the patient's current underlying pathology, and therefore pain, but also to preserve bone in younger patients should further surgery be required in the future. There are however concerns regarding overstuffing of the radiocapitellar joint and subsequent development of ulnohumeral degeneration.

Pooley [8] reported short-term results using this implant and had 6 excellent, 3 good and 1 fair result using the Mayo Elbow Performance Index (MEPI). One implant had to be removed as a result of a deep infection. More recently, a multicentre trial reviewed 20 patients at a mean of 22 months postoperatively, and MEPI scores were excellent in 12, good in 2 and fair and poor in 3 each. As such, there may be role for uni-compartmental replacement arthroplasty in patients with symptomatic isolated posttraumatic radiocapitellar arthritis.

Total Elbow Replacement

Total elbow replacement reliably treats pain from arthritic elbows but is really only suited to lower-demand patients, typically those with advanced rheumatoid arthritis. Figure 8.2 shows a typical posttraumatic arthritic elbow managed with a total elbow arthroplasty. In higher-demand patients with excessive use, early loosening and implant failure occur. Total elbow replacement is discussed in more detail in the section on inflammatory arthritis.

Elbow Fusion

This procedure is poorly tolerated by patients due to the functional restriction that occurs. It restricts the majority of necessary daily living activities, and shoulder wrist and hand motion cannot compensate for the loss of elbow movement.

If an elbow arthrodesis is the only option for limb salvage, then the procedure can be undertaken either with internal or external fixation. Internal fixation with plating is probably most commonly used, but if this is performed, it is essential to consider whether soft tissue closure

Fig. 8.2 (**a**) Posttraumatic arthritis with a mal-/non-united fracture of the distal humerus. (**b**) Reconstruction was not possible in this elderly patient and a total elbow arthroplasty was performed

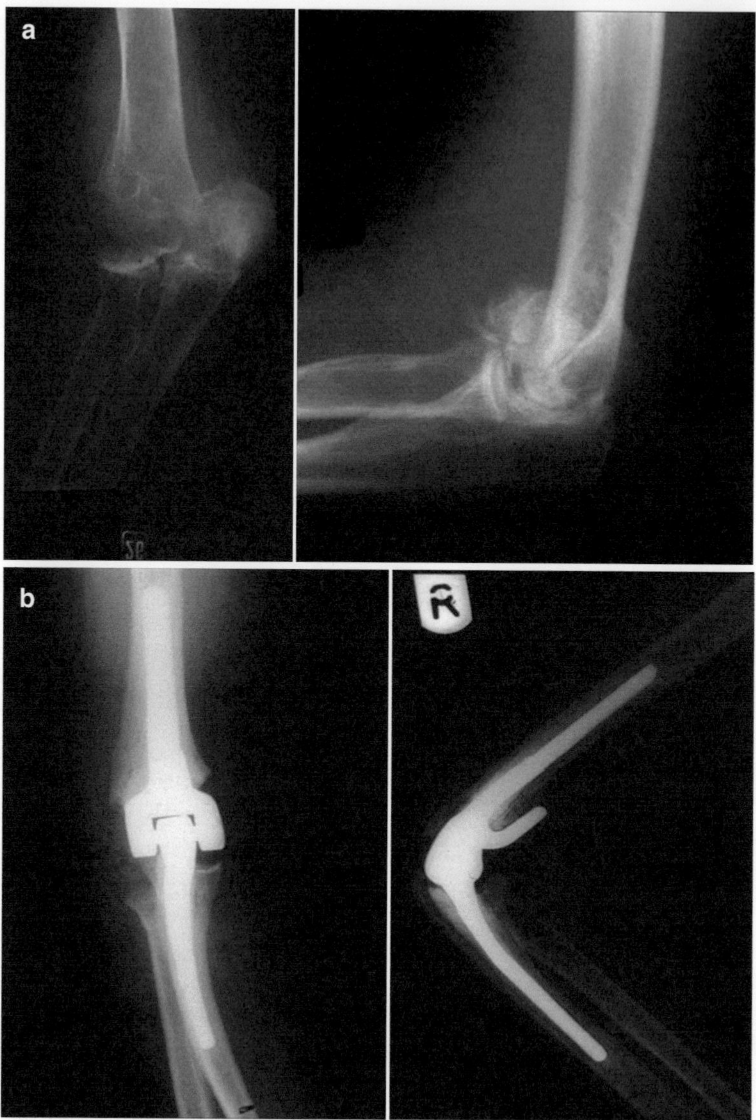

will be possible at the end of the procedure. If there is doubt, then an opinion from a plastic and reconstruction surgeon should be obtained.

Results and Complications

There are few reports on the outcome of interpositional arthroplasty of the elbow and the results are mixed, with instability being a troublesome complication. Nolla et al. [9] reported on a series of 13 patients, including 4 women (mean age 41 years) who underwent the procedure for posttraumatic arthritis: the results were 1 excellent, 4 good, 4 fair and 4 poor. Larson et al. [10] similarly reported mixed results in 34 patients: 13 patients had a good or excellent result, 14 had a fair result, 11 had a poor result and the remaining seven underwent revision. The group subsequently reported the outcomes of failed interposition arthroplasty [11]. Five of nine patients were subjectively satisfied and four had continued manual work. All series report an improvement in pain, but patients are not pain-free following interposition. Interposition is therefore a salvage procedure that should be reserved for a few patients in whom conservative treatment has failed and replacement arthroplasty is contraindicated, and even then patients need to be aware of the unpredictability of the results. Conversion to total elbow arthroplasty has been reported with encouraging results in a small series [12] and may be an option for the failing or failed interposition arthroplasty.

There are few reports of lateral resurfacing of the elbow. This technique has similar complications to other forms of arthroplasty. Specifically overstuffing of the joint is a risk and will increase contact pressures of the medial ulnohumeral articulation, with characteristic "opening" of the lateral ulnohumeral articulation seen on anteroposterior radiographs.

The complications of total elbow replacement are discussed in the section on inflammatory arthritis. When performed for posttraumatic arthritis, there is a risk that the potentially greater functional demands in this situation may result in an increased rate of aseptic loosening.

Elbow arthrodesis is not without complication and achieving union is a major concern. There are reports of between 56 and 100 % union rates in small series [13]. Internal fixation with or without external fixation achieves higher union rates than external fixation alone, with union occurring at an average of 6 months.

Primary Osteoarthritis of the Elbow

Indications

The mainstay of treatment in early disease is nonoperative with nonsteroidal anti-inflammatory medication (NSAIDs), activity modification, intra-articular injections and avoidance adaptation. Physiotherapy is rarely indicated and may actually exacerbate symptoms. If conservative treatment fails to resolve the patient's symptoms, surgical management should be considered. Patients with end range impingement signs will respond well to debridement in comparison to those with mid-range pain secondary to more extensive cartilage degeneration.

Surgical Techniques

Arthroscopic Debridement

Arthroscopic debridement of the elbow for primary osteoarthritis is similar to that for post-traumatic arthritis. Loose bodies and osteophytes can be removed in combination with a capsular release and if necessary excision of the radial head. Good results have been published with good overall patient satisfaction and improved pain scores [14, 15].

In addition to debridement and loose body removal, arthroscopic modifications of the ulno-humeral arthroplasty have also been described that include fenestration of the olecranon fossa membrane to negate the chance of impingement of the coronoid in flexion and olecranon in extension.

Ulnohumeral Arthroplasty

There are a number of reports that have advocated the use of the Outerbridge-Kashiwagi (OK) procedure, or ulnohumeral arthroplasty, with respect to improving pain and even range of movement of the elbow, in mild to moderate degenerative arthritis [16–19]. Kashiwagi [20] first reported the OK technique and attributed it to Outerbridge. Morrey [17] subsequently modified the procedure, which he termed the ulnohumeral arthroplasty. The procedure allows debridement of the elbow joint through a posterior incision and fenestration of the olecranon fossa membrane to gain access to the anterior compartment of the joint. Loose bodies, osteophytes and the thickened olecranon fossa membrane that cause impingement and pain can be excised.

We perform the procedure under tourniquet control with the patient supine and a sandbag under the ipsilateral shoulder. The arm is positioned across the chest, and an 8 cm posterior longitudinal incision is made from the tip of the olecranon proximally. The triceps is split in the line of its fibres and the posterior capsule opened. Loose bodies in the posterior compartment are removed along with any associated osteophytes on the tip of the olecranon or the fossa itself. A trephine of a similar size to the fossa is used to fenestrate the membrane, allowing access to the anterior of the elbow joint; the trephine must not compromise the medial or lateral column of the distal humerus for fear of fracture. Flexion and extension of the joint will reveal any loose bodies that require removal. Maximum flexion will bring osteophytes at the coronoid tip into view, which can be removed through the fenestration (Fig. 8.3). A thorough washout is performed to ensure all loose material is removed. The wound is closed over a small suction drain and a bulky dressing is applied. The drain and bulky bandage are removed within 24 h, and range of motion exercises are encouraged in the early postoperative period. Morrey [17] employs a postoperative regime of continuous passive motion under a continuous brachial plexus block for a period of 2–3 days and a flexion-extension orthosis to maintain the operative gain in elbow movement.

Tsuge and Mizuseki [21] described a more radical open debridement of the elbow joint for arthritis. This also utilised a posterior approach and required dissection of the ulnar nerve with release of the posterior portion of the ulnar collateral ligament as well as the radial collateral ligament to facilitate dislocation of the joint. Loose bodies and osteophytes were then removed, and the radial head reshaped to improve forearm prono-supination. Postoperatively continuous passive motion was continued for 7 days.

Results and Complications

There are numerous reports of the efficacy of arthroscopic debridement for primary elbow arthritis [14, 15, 22–24]. Ogilvie-Harris reported good outcomes following debridement and removal of loose bodies [23]. More recent studies have looked at the results of arthroscopic ulnohumeral arthroplasty. Kelly et al. [14] reported 24 "better" or "much better" outcomes in 25 patients who underwent arthroscopic modified ulnohumeral arthroplasty, with 14 excellent and seven good outcomes according to the elbow rating system of Andrews and Carson. The patients had an average 21° improvement in range of motion. Redden and Stanley [24] below showed improved

symptoms in 12 patients, though no significant improvements in range of motion. Adding anterior and posterior capsular releases has been advocated to improve range of motion [25].

Open debridement with ulnohumeral arthroplasty has similar good results [16–19]. Morrey [17] reported excellent results in 87 % of 15 patients followed for a mean of 33 months. Other studies have shown that improvement in symptoms appears to be maintained in the long term [26]. Cohen et al. [27] compared open and arthroscopic techniques, and whilst both were

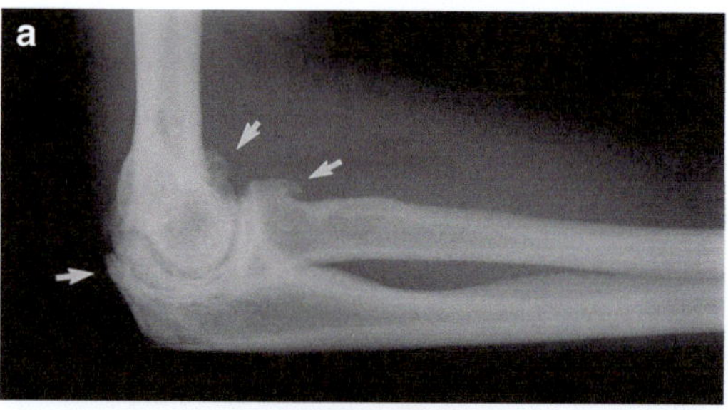

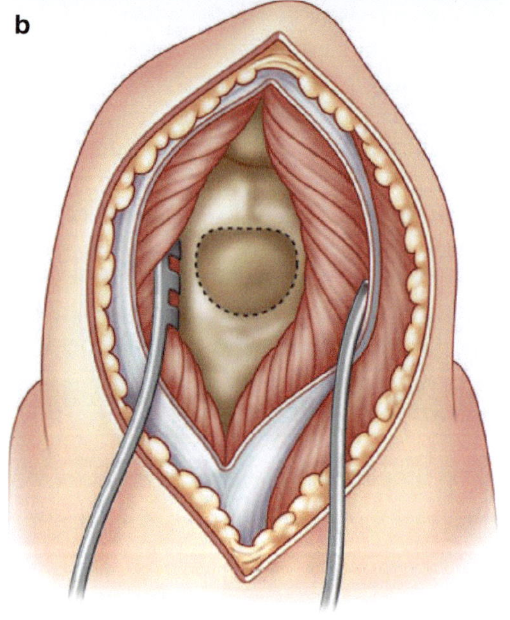

Fig. 8.3 (**a**) Lateral radiograph with *arrows* showing osteophytes at tip of olecranon and around radial head and loose body anteriorly. (**b**) Schematic representation of a triceps split approach to the posterior aspect of the elbow and the resultant fenestration in the olecranon fossa membrane. (**c**) Pre- and postoperative radiographs of a patient, who underwent the OK procedure, note the fenestration in the olecranon fossa

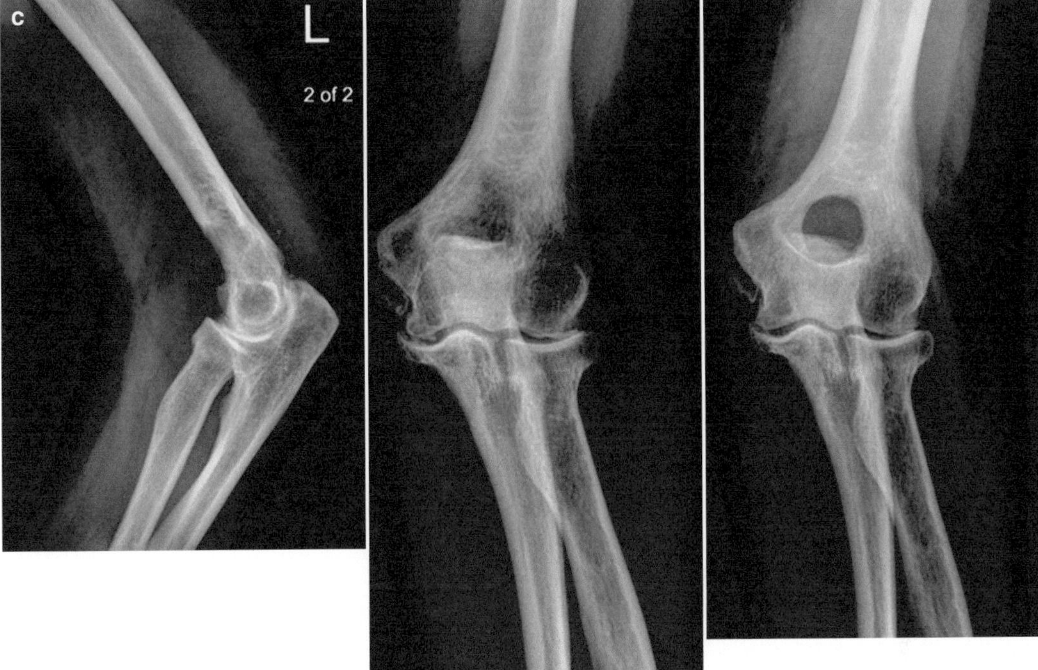

Fig. 8.3 (continued)

shown to be effective, there was slightly more improvement in the range of motion seen in open surgery. No patient-perceived difference in outcome was noted with the two techniques. Prognostic factors for a good outcome include symptoms for less than 2 years, considerable pre-operative pain or cubital tunnel syndrome. The absence of preoperative locking was associated with a significantly increased chance of a poor outcome, whilst a history of trauma, the preoperative range of movement and radiographic appearances did not predict outcome [28].

Complications of elbow arthroscopy include permanent but more commonly transient nerve injury with reports being as high as 14 % [14, 15, 24, 29]. A combined knowledge of the relevant neuroanatomy and correct choice of instrumentation in elbow arthroscopy should minimise this risk, but it is also important that only appropriately trained and experienced elbow arthroscopists undertake the procedure. The risk of deep infection following elbow arthroscopy is low (0.8 %) [30], although ongoing drainage and superficial infection rates are slightly higher [30].

Myositis ossificans [31] has also been reported but rates are low.

Complications following open debridement include ulnar nerve irritation or injury, anterior interosseous nerve injury, superficial infection, myositis ossificans and triceps rupture. The reported reoperation rate is 8 % [32].

Inflammatory Arthritis

Indications

Disease-modifying medication has had a huge effect on the medical management of rheumatoid arthritis and significantly slowed the rate of progression of the disease. Consequently, severe joint destruction and joint deformity is less common, and the need for surgical intervention has reduced. Surgical treatment is required when patients continue to suffer with joint pain despite optimum medical management; synovectomy and total elbow arthroplasty are the mainstays of operative management, and the aims of surgical management are to debulk the disease, regain elbow motion and provide pain relief.

Surgical Techniques

Synovectomy

Synovectomy for rheumatoid arthritis was originally described as an open procedure though more commonly it is now being performed arthroscopically. We perform synovectomy in patients with Larsen grade I and II disease. Traditionally, through an open approach, the radial head was excised; however, our current practice is to leave it in situ if there is no pain with associated prono-supination of the forearm. Excision of the radial head results in increased load transmission through the ulnar compartment of the elbow, with resultant degenerative changes and poorer clinical outcomes then if the radial head is retained. In addition, the valgus overload stretches the soft tissues making unlinked total elbow replacement technically more difficult.

When indicated we perform an arthroscopic synovectomy. The patient is positioned as previously described. We initially use an antero-medial portal for viewing and a lateral working portal. These portals are then reversed using a switching stick in order to allow a complete synovectomy of the anterior compartment. If radio-capitellar symptoms are present, we do a radial head excision [33] (Fig. 8.4). This is undertaken using a barrel burr in combination with rotation of the forearm to access all areas of the articular surface. The surgeon must always be aware that the posterior interosseous nerve lies directly anterior to the resection site, and therefore, great care is required during the procedure. The posterior compartment is then viewed and a posterior debridement and synovectomy performed. Elbow arthroscopy is contraindicated if there has been a previous anterior ulnar nerve transposition.

Open synovectomy can be undertaken through an extended lateral Kocher's approach to the anterior aspect of the elbow and by lifting the triceps to gain access to the posterior compartment

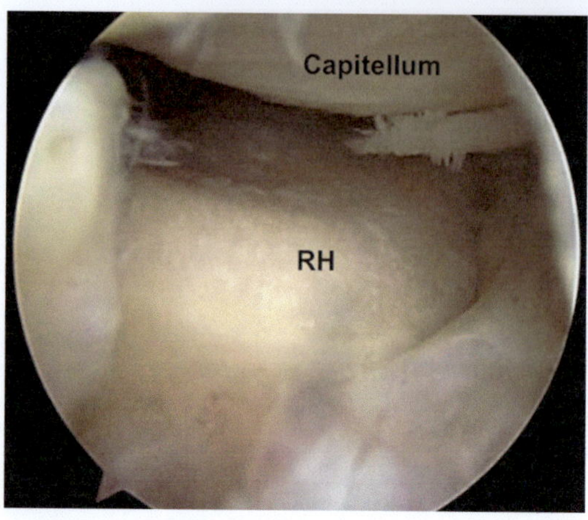

Fig. 8.4 Arthroscopic view of the lateral compartment of the elbow from the anteromedial portal. There is significant loss of radial head cartilage with pain on forearm rotation. Patient was treated with radial head (*RH*) excision

of the joint from the lateral side. Capsulectomy, synovectomy and debridement of the joint can be performed, and if required, the radial head can be excised or replaced. We perform a radial head replacement in younger individuals with radiocapitellar pain, and in patients who have pistoning of the radius proximally to prevent the development of an "Essex-Lopresti" lesion.

If a radial head replacement is not required, surgery is performed as a day case. Postoperatively patients are encouraged to actively use the elbow within the confines of comfort. If extensive surgery is performed, an axillary block is provided to facilitate continuous passive motion of the joint for 2–3 days.

Interposition Arthroplasty

We do not routinely perform interposition arthroplasty for patients with rheumatoid arthritis, but it can be undertaken in the same fashion as described for posttraumatic arthritis. Total elbow arthroplasty is now more commonly used as the treatment for rheumatoid patients with severe elbow disease.

Total Elbow Replacement

Total elbow replacement is the mainstay of treatment for rheumatoid patients with severe pain or elbow instability. Replacement arthroplasty provides reliable pain relief, with good functional outcomes and survivorship.

Initial total elbow replacement designs were fixed hinge joints that failed early with the tip of the humeral component migrating anteriorly as the axis of the implant moved posteriorly. This mode of failure reflects the posteriorly directed forces across the elbow joint in flexion and extension. More recently linked, unlinked and modular (implants that can be inserted as unlinked or linked prostheses depending on the findings at surgery) designs have provided better results. Linked prostheses incorporate a sloppy hinge to allow rotational varus and valgus motion between the humeral and ulnar components. This reduces bone-cement interface loading and reduces aseptic loosening of the implants. In addition it avoids the potential complication of component dislocation.

We favour the semi-constrained linked Coonrad-Morrey prosthesis, which is probably the most successful linked elbow arthroplasty currently available. Surgery is performed with patients in the lateral decubitus position and with a high arm tourniquet. A posteromedial skin incision is used and subcutaneous flaps are raised to the mid-lateral line both medially and laterally. The ulnar nerve is decompressed in situ and left in its bed rather than transposed. The triceps splitting Shahane-Stanley approach to the elbow is utilised to gain access to the joint. A thorough synovectomy is performed and the radial head is excised. Bony preparation of the humerus and ulna is performed as per the manufacturer guidelines. Trial implantation is performed to ensure correct alignment is achieved and to be certain that there is no pistoning of the components during flexion and extension of the elbow. If this is present, the axis of rotation is incorrect and adjustments to the implant position are required. It is also important to check that there is no evidence of impingement during flexion and extension, as this can result in rapid aseptic loosening of the components and early failure. A cement restrictor is placed in the humerus and the definitive components are cemented in situ. Careful reconstruction of the triceps mechanism is essential prior to skin closure. Figure 8.5 shows preoperative and postoperative images of a patient with rheumatoid arthritis who underwent a Coonrad-Morrey total elbow arthroplasty.

Postoperatively an above elbow plaster of Paris backslab is placed with the elbow in maximum extension for a period of 48 h to allow soft tissue swelling to settle. A lighter dressing is then applied, and patients are encouraged to perform gentle active range of motion exercises.

Results and Complications

Synovectomy with radial head excision has proven successful in short-term studies, though the results are not maintained at longer-term follow-up. Rymaszewski [34] demonstrated a common pattern of deterioration after initial good outcomes. He noted that 70 % of patients were initially pain-free following open synovectomy and radial head excision, but at 6 years this had fallen to only 45 %. The altered biomechanics following radial head excision may explain the deterioration as the ulnohumeral joint becomes diseased. Similarly, the outcomes following arthroscopic synovectomy are not maintained. Lee and Morrey [35] reported good or excellent outcomes dropped from 93 to 57 % over 42 months. However, in combination with good medical therapy using disease-modifying drugs, the recurrence of symptoms is low, and synovectomy with preservation of the radial head should be considered a good initial option for patients with early rheumatoid disease.

Total elbow replacement is best suited for low-demand rheumatoid patients. Good results have been published with linked prostheses: 87.7 % implant survival at a mean of 13.5 years using the GSB prosthesis [36] and 92.4 % survival at 10–15 year follow-up of the Coonrad-Morrey prosthesis [37]. Gill and Morrey [37] reported a mean postoperative range of movement of 28–131° of elbow flexion, and 97 % of patients had little or no pain. Unlinked prostheses have also been reported to show satisfactory results. Qureshi

Fig. 8.5 (**a**) Anteroposterior and lateral radiographs of a patient with rheumatoid arthritis affecting the elbow. (**b**) Postoperative radiographs following insertion of a Coonrad-Morrey total elbow arthroplasty

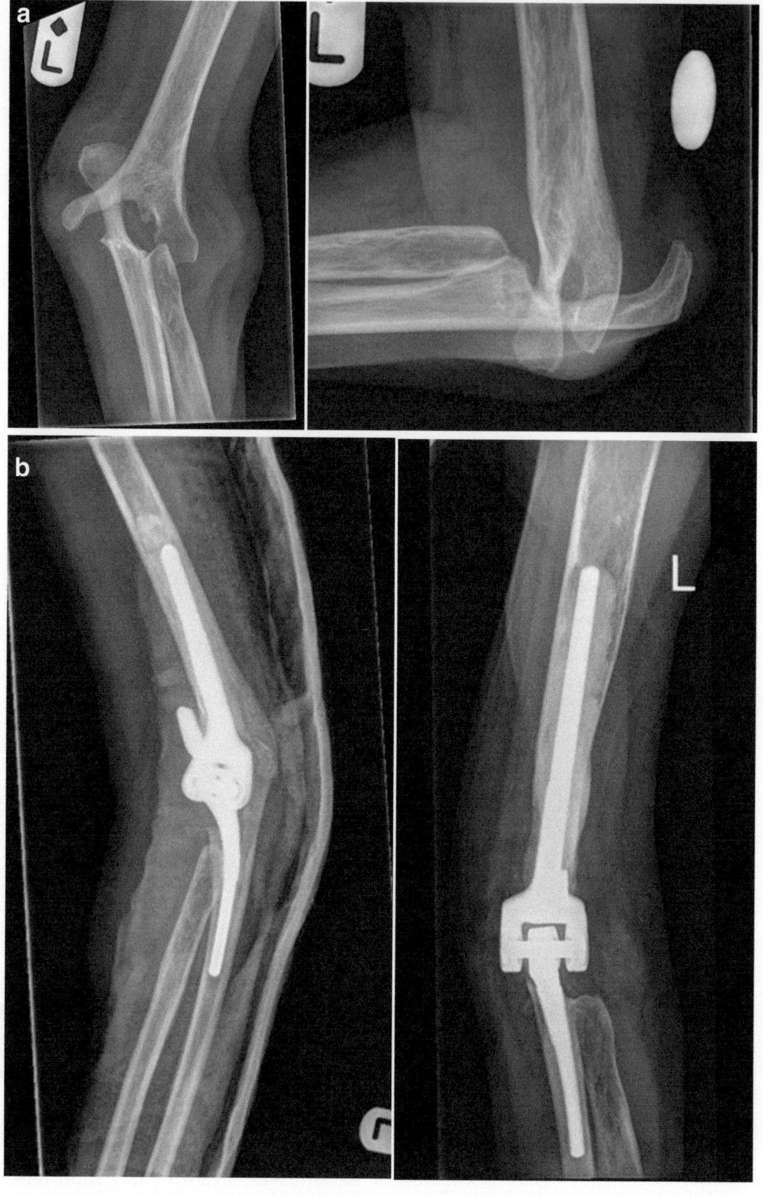

et al. [38] reported good long-term results of the Kudo prosthesis in rheumatoid patients, with an average MEP score of 82 at a mean of 11.9 years, and the estimated survival of the prosthesis at 12 years according to Kaplan-Meier survival analysis was 74 %. Little et al. [39] compared three elbow prosthesis and found similar results in outcome and 5-year survival rates, with revision and radiographic signs of loosening as the end points (85 and 81 % for the Souter-Strathclyde implant, 93 and 82 % for the Kudo implant and 90 and 86 % for the Coonrad-Morrey implant).

The complications of total elbow replacement have been well documented and include periprosthetic fracture, dislocation or instability of unlinked prostheses (Fig. 8.6a), infection, aseptic loosening (Fig. 8.6b), ulnar neuropathy and triceps insufficiency.

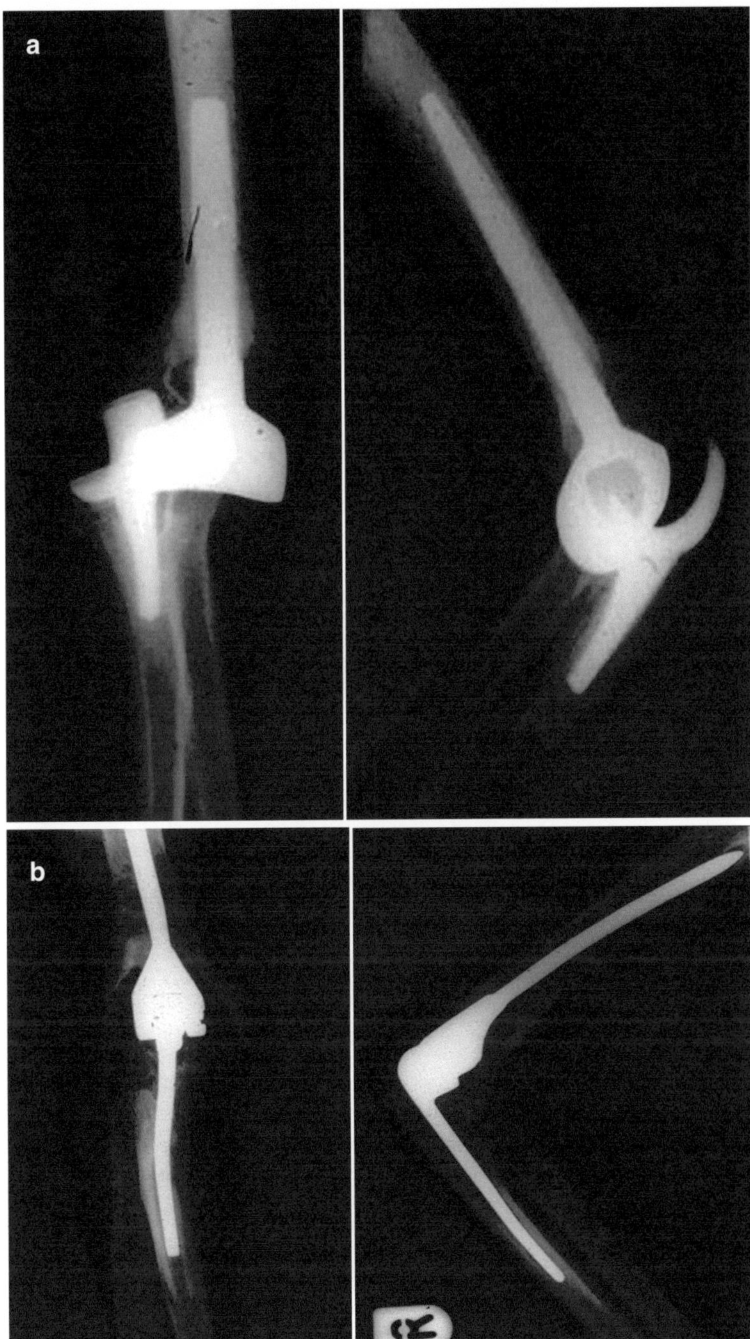

Fig. 8.6 Complications of elbow arthroplasty. (**a**) Dislocated unconstrained Kudo total elbow replacement. (**b**) Aseptic loosening of a Stanmore linked total elbow replacement

Conclusion

Elbow arthritis is characterised by loss of elbow motion and pain. It can be classified as predominantly posttraumatic, degenerative or inflammatory. The mainstay of treatment for early disease is nonoperative although when the disease process progresses, a variety of surgical options exist. Operative management can often be challenging, and the procedure of choice should be matched to the type of elbow arthritis, the individual patient's symptoms and their functional demands.

References

1. Ortner DJ. Description and classification of degenerative bone changes in the distal joint surfaces of the humerus. Am J Phys Anthropol. 1968;28:139–55.
2. Silman AJ, Hochberg MC. Epidemiology of the rheumatic diseases. Oxford: Oxford University Press; 1993.
3. Stanley D. Prevalence and etiology of symptomatic elbow osteoarthritis. J Shoulder Elbow Surg. 1994;3(6):386–9.
4. Kashiwagi D. Intra-articular changes of the osteoarthritis elbow, especially about the fossa olecrani. J Jpn Orthop Assoc 1978;52:1367–82.
5. Kim SJ, Shin SJ. Arthroscopic treatment for limitation of motion of the elbow. Clin Orthop Relat Res. 2000;375:140–8.
6. Nguyen D, Proper SIW, MacDermid JC, et al. Functional outcomes of arthroscopic capsular release of the elbow. Arthroscopy. 2006;8:842–9.
7. Shahane SA, Stanley D. A posterior approach to the elbow joint. J Bone Joint Surg Br. 1999;81(6):1020–2.
8. Pooley J. Unicompartmental elbow replacement: development of a lateral replacement elbow (LRE) arthroplasty. Tech Shoulder Elbow Surg. 2007;8:204–12.
9. Nolla J, Ring D, Lozano-Calderon S, Jupiter JB. Interposition arthroplasty of the elbow with hinged external fixation for post-traumatic arthritis. J Shoulder Elbow Surg. 2008;17(3):459–64.
10. Larson AN, Morrey BF. Interposition arthroplasty with an Achilles tendon allograft as a salvage procedure for the elbow. J Bone Joint Surg Am. 2008;90(12):2714–23.
11. Larson AN, Adams RA, Morrey BF. Revision interposition arthroplasty of the elbow. J Bone Joint Surg Br. 2010;92(9):1273–7.
12. Blaine TA, Adams R, Morrey BF. Total elbow arthroplasty after interposition arthroplasty for elbow arthritis. J Bone Joint Surg Am. 2005;87:286–92.
13. Koller H, Kolb K, Assuncao A, Kolb W, Holz U. The fate of elbow arthrodesis: indications, techniques, and outcome in fourteen patients. J Shoulder Elbow Surg. 2008;17(2):293–306.
14. Kelly EW, Bryce R, Coghlan J, Simon B. Arthroscopic debridement without radial head excision of the osteoarthritic elbow. Arthroscopy. 2007;23:151.
15. Krishnan SG, Harkins DC, Pennington SD, Harrison DK, Burkhead WZ. Arthroscopic ulnohumeral arthroplasty for degenerative arthritis of the elbow in patients under 50 years of age. J Shoulder Elbow Surg. 2007;16:443.
16. Antuña SA, Morrey BF, Adams RA, O'Driscoll SW. Ulnohumeral arthroplasty for primary degenerative arthritis of the elbow: long-term outcome and complications. J Bone Joint Surg. 2002;84-A:2168–73.
17. Morrey BF. Primary degenerative arthritis of the elbow. Treatment by ulnohumeral arthroplasty. J Bone Joint Surg. 1992;74-B:409–13.
18. Sarris I, Riano FA, Goebel F, Goitz RJ, Sotereanos DG. Ulnohumeral arthroplasty: results in primary degenerative arthritis of the elbow. Clin Orthop Relat Res. 2004;420:190–3.
19. Stanley D, Winson IG. A surgical approach to the elbow. J Bone Joint Surg Br. 1990;72:728–9.
20. Kashiwagi D. Osteoarthritis of the elbow joint. Intraarticular changes and the special operative procedure, Outerbridge-Kashiwagi method O-K method. In: Kashiwagi D, editor. The elbow joint. Proceedings of the international congress, Japan. Amsterdam: Elsevier; 1985. p. 177–88.
21. Tsuge K, Mizuseki T. Debridement arthroplasty for advanced primary osteoarthritis of the elbow. Results of a new technique used for 29 elbows. J Bone Joint Surg Br. 1994;76:641–6.
22. Adams JE, Wolff 3rd LH, Merten SM, et al. Osteoarthritis of the elbow: results of arthroscopic osteophytes resection and capsulectomy. J Shoulder Elbow Surg. 2008;17:126–31.
23. Ogilvie-Harris DJ, Gordon R, MacKay M. Arthroscopic treatment for posterior impingement in degenerative arthritis of the elbow. Arthroscopy. 1995;11:437–43.
24. Redden JF, Stanley D. Arthroscopic fenestration of the olecranon fossa in the treatment of osteoarthritis of the elbow. Arthroscopy. 1993;9:14–6.
25. O'Driscoll SW. Arthroscopic treatment for osteoarthritis of the elbow. Orthop Clin North Am. 1995;26:691–706.
26. Minami M, Kato S, Kashiwagi D. Outerbridge–Kashiwagi method for arthroplasty of osteoarthritis of the elbow. 44 elbows followed for 8–16 years. J Orthop Sci. 1996;1:11.
27. Cohen AP, Redden JF, Stanley D. Treatment of osteoarthritis of the elbow: a comparison of open and arthroscopic debridement. Arthroscopy. 2000;16:701–6.
28. Forster MC, Clark DI, Lunn PG. Elbow osteoarthritis: prognostic indicators in ulnohumeral debridement – the Outerbridge–Kashiwagi procedure. J Shoulder Elbow Surg. 2001;10:557–60.
29. McLaughlin II RE, Savoie III FH, Field LD, Ramsey JR. Arthroscopic treatment of the arthritic elbow due to primary radiocapitellar arthritis. Arthroscopy. 2006;22:63–9.
30. Kelly EW, Morrey BF, O'Driscoll SW. Complications of elbow arthroscopy. J Bone Joint Surg Am. 2001;83-A(1):25–34.
31. Gofton WT, King GJ. Heterotopic ossification following elbow arthroscopy. Arthroscopy. 2001;17(E2):1–5.
32. Adla DN, Stanley D. Primary elbow osteoarthritis: an updated review. Shoulder Elbow. 2011;3:41–8.
33. Menth-Chiari WA, Ruch DS, Poehling GG. Arthroscopic excision of the radial head: clinical outcome in 12 patients with post-traumatic arthritis after fracture of the radial head or rheumatoid arthritis. Arthroscopy. 2001;17(9):918–23.

34. Rymaszewski LA, Mackay I, Amis AA, Miller JH. Long-term effects of excision of the radial head in rheumatoid arthritis. J Bone Joint Surg Br. 1984;66(1):109–13.
35. Lee BP, Morrey BF. Arthroscopic synovectomy of the elbow for rheumatoid arthritis. A prospective study. J Bone Joint Surg Br. 1997;79(5):770–2.
36. Gschwend N, Scheier NH, Baehler AR. Long-term results of the GSB III elbow arthroplasty. J Bone Joint Surg Br. 1999;81(6):1005–12.
37. Gill DR, Morrey BF. The Coonrad-Morrey total elbow arthroplasty in patients who have rheumatoid arthritis. A ten to fifteen-year follow-up study. J Bone Joint Surg Am. 1998;80(9):1327–35.
38. Qureshi F, Draviaraj KP, Stanley D. The Kudo 5 total elbow replacement in the treatment of the rheumatoid elbow: results at a minimum of ten years. J Bone Joint Surg Br. 2010;92(10):1416–21.
39. Little CP, Graham AJ, Karatzas G, Woods DA, Carr AJ. Outcomes of total elbow arthroplasty for rheumatoid arthritis: comparative study of three implants. J Bone Joint Surg Am. 2005;87(11):2439–48.

Tendon Injuries

Bryant Ho and Guido Marra

Abstract

Tendon injuries are one of the most common reasons for consultation in an elbow clinic and are prevalent among young patients with high expectations and sport-related activities. Biceps tendon injuries affect active middle-aged males and can be very disabling in patients with high physical demands. Clinical features of this injury and the current management strategies are presented. Tendon augmentation techniques are also described for symptomatic chronic cases. Triceps tendon injuries are rare and frequently misdiagnosed. Key aspects in the diagnosis and treatment are presented, including the use of grafting techniques for chronic cases.

Keywords

Triceps tendon injuries • Biceps tendon injury • Complications

The Problem

Tendon injuries remain one of the most frequent indications that patient with elbow disorders seeks medical attention. These injuries may be related to sports or specific occupational activities. Tendinopathies around the elbow tend to be caused by degeneration of the tendinous fibers leading to tendinosis that weakens the tendon instead of inflammation. While these injuries as a group do not cause profound disabilities, they do significantly impact daily function. Many patients suffer elbow pain for long periods of time, without proper categorization of its nature, as it may occur with anterior elbow pain secondary to distal biceps tendon problems or medial epicondylitis. Prompt diagnosis is critical to the management of these disorders. The majority of patients with pain attributed to lateral or medial epicondylitis will get better over time without surgical intervention. Patients with distal biceps or triceps problems, on the other hand, quite commonly require operative treatment. This chapter will

B. Ho, MD
Department of Orthopaedic Surgery, Northwestern University, 201 E. Huron, Chicago, IL 60611, USA

Department of Orthopaedic Surgery, Northwestern University, Feinberg School of Medicine,
676 N. St. Clair, Suite 1350, Chicago, IL 60611, USA
e-mail: bryant.s.ho@gmail.com

G. Marra, MD (✉)
Department of Orthopaedic Surgery, Northwestern University, Feinberg School of Medicine,
676 N. St. Clair, Suite 1350, Chicago, IL 60611, USA
e-mail: gmarra@nmff.org

S. Antuña, R. Barco (eds.), *Essentials in Elbow Surgery*,
DOI 10.1007/978-1-4471-4625-4_9, © Springer-Verlag London 2014

review the most frequent tendon injuries seen in the elbow and their management.

Biceps Tendon Injuries

Epidemiology

Distal biceps tendon ruptures are rare injuries with an incidence of 1.2 per 100,000 people per year [1]. They typically occur in the dominant arm of men between the ages of 40 and 60 [2]. Injury is typically caused by forced extension of the arm with the elbow at 90° of flexion. The tendon typically avulses off the radial tuberosity insertion, although ruptures can also occur at the musculotendinous junction or more rarely within the tendinous substance.

The biceps tendon consists of two insertions: the long head tendon attaches proximally on the radial tuberosity, while the short head attaches distally and serves as the origin of the lacertus fibrosis. The tendon has a ribbonlike insertion on the ulnar side of the radial tuberosity that functions like a pulley to increase the mechanical advantage of the biceps musculotendinous unit [3].

Distal biceps tendon ruptures likely occur secondary to tendon degeneration. Microscopic evaluation of the ruptured tendon shows hypoxic degenerative tendinopathy, mucoid degenerative changes, tendolipomatosis, and calcifying tendinopathy [4]. Cadaveric studies show a watershed hypovascular zone in the distal biceps tendon just proximal to the tendinous insertion that may be predisposed to rupture. This portion of the distal biceps tendon is 2 cm in length and lies between the branches of the brachial artery that supply the proximal tendon and the branches of the posterior interosseous recurrent artery that supply the distal insertion and may explain the typical location of ruptures near the radial tuberosity [5].

Patient Workup

Clinical Exam

Patients typically report a sharp, tearing sensation in their arm with intense pain that transitions

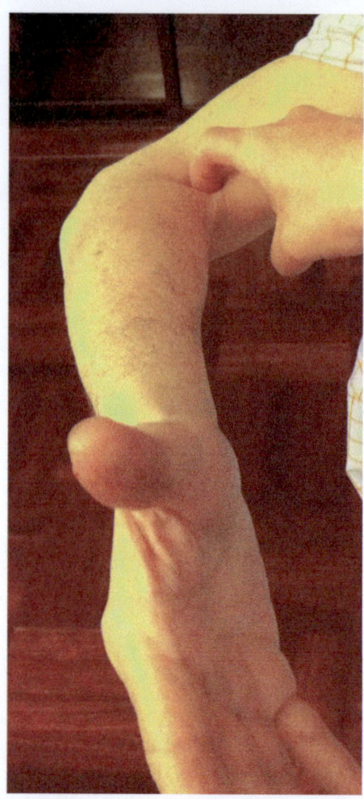

Fig. 9.1 Hook test: With the shoulder in 90° of abduction, the elbow flexed to 90°, and the hand fully supinated, when the biceps tendon is intact, the examiner's index finger can "hook" the tendon between its lateral border and the skin

to a dull ache that can last for weeks. Physical exam usually demonstrates a visual and palpable defect in the antecubital fossa with tenderness to palpation. After a few days, ecchymosis is usually present distal to the flexion crease of the elbow and tends to predominate along the ulnar aspect of the proximal forearm. Resisted flexion of the arm causes the muscle belly to further retract proximally, accentuating the deformity.

The hook test is a highly sensitive and specific test for complete distal biceps tendon tears [6]. It is performed with the elbow in 90° of flexion with the index finger sweeping from medial to lateral. In a patient with a normal intact tendon, the index finger is able to "hook" the biceps tendon (Fig. 9.1).

Patients with only partial tendon ruptures often have anterior elbow pain that radiates to the biceps. They may have a normal hook test, but often have pain with performance of the maneuver. Additionally, partial distal biceps tears can have pain with direct palpation at the

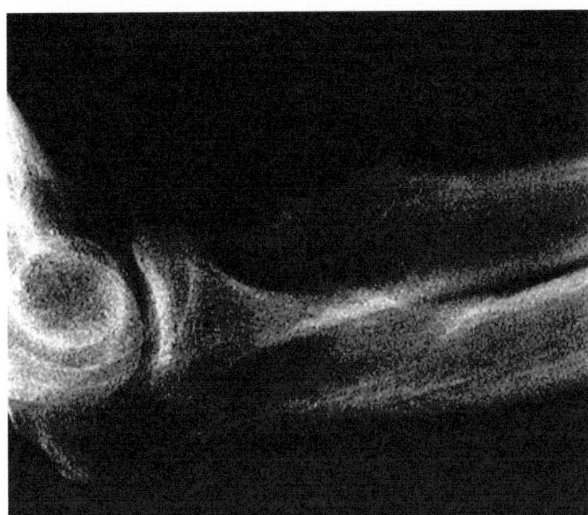

Fig. 9.2 Lateral radiograph of the elbow demonstrating irregularity of the radial tuberosity

radial tuberosity and pain with resistive forearm supination.

Imaging

The diagnosis of an acute, complete tear of the distal biceps tendon should be made based on clinical exam exclusively. However, plain radiographs may show enlargement or irregularity of the radial tuberosity or less commonly a bony avulsion (Fig. 9.2). When the hook test is normal and a partial tear or tendinosis is suspected, MRI is the study of choice. MRI can also help define the degree of tendon retraction of the rupture in both acute and chronic cases. In cases of chronic anterior elbow pain where distal biceps tendinosis is suspected, MRI can show intratendinous signal intensity, tendon defects or detachment, tendon swelling or thickening, or abnormal tendon contour.

Indications

Nonoperative treatment is an option in patients with complete distal biceps tendon ruptures, but is complicated by activity-related pain and weakness. Patients with distal biceps tendon ruptures show decreased strength in elbow flexion and forearm supination. Peak strength is decreased by 30 % in flexion and 50 % in supination with no changes in fatigue rates [7]. Nonoperative management should only be considered for elderly, low activity patients. However, Freeman et al. showed acceptable results with nonoperative treatment with 7 % decreased elbow flexion and 27 % decreased supination at a mean of 3-year follow-up [8].

Patients with chronic distal biceps tendon ruptures can be treated operatively if they continue to have disability associated with activity-related pain and weakness. Chronic tendon ruptures are associated with proximal tendon retraction and scar tissue that may prevent anatomic repair. Preoperative planning should include alternative graft options such as semitendinosus autograft or allograft to extend the tendon length. For patients with chronic tendon ruptures with only pain-related symptoms, a tenodesis of the distal biceps to the brachialis can be considered. While providing pain relief, this option will not improve strength.

Acute partial tendon ruptures can be treated nonoperatively initially with a period of rest, followed by physical therapy. Patients with continued pain and weakness despite nonoperative treatment are managed operatively. Patients with chronic anterior pain found to have distal biceps tendinosis should initially be treated nonoperatively with rest and NSAIDs followed by physical therapy. Patients who have failed conservative management for 3–6 months may be candidates for surgical debridement and reinsertion of the biceps tendon. Reported cases make no distinction between surgical repair for partial biceps tendon ruptures from acute trauma or chronic tendinosis, but show good results. Kelly et al. reported seven of eight patients returning to their previous level of activity with mean American Shoulder and Elbow Surgeons score of 96 [9].

Surgical Technique

Acute Complete Distal Biceps Tears

In managing acute distal biceps tendon ruptures, the operative surgeon has two major choices in surgical management: operative approach and tendon fixation. A number of studies have evaluated the merits of these choices, which have demonstrated their efficacy.

Approach

Acute complete tendon ruptures can be treated surgical with either a single incision or dual incisions. Grewal et al. recently reported no differences in functional outcome, strength, and range of motion between the single- and dual-incision techniques [10].

Single Incision

The single-incision technique is performed through an anterior approach. A longitudinal incision is made paralleling the ulnar border of the brachioradialis. The lateral antebrachial cutaneous nerve is identified and protected as it exits the antecubital fossa between the biceps and the brachialis. The interval between brachioradialis and the pronator teres is developed to the level of the lacertus fibrosis. The recurrent branch of the radial artery is ligated to prevent postoperative hematoma, and the posterior interosseous nerve (PIN) is protected by fully supinating the arm. Care must be taken with lateral retraction as it placed the PIN at risk.

The biceps tendon is typically in this interval. The tendon stump is debrided to healthy tendon, and locking nonabsorbable sutures are placed in the tendon. The methods for tendon fixation are described below.

Dual Incision

To decrease the risk of neurologic injury to PIN with the single-incision technique, Boyd and Anderson developed a dual-incision approach, which also offers decreased risk of damage to the lateral antebrachial cutaneous nerve [11]. This technique was later modified by Dr. Morrey [12]. A 3-cm transverse incision is made just distal to the flexion crease of the elbow (Fig. 9.3). Care is taken to avoid injury to the lateral antebrachial cutaneous nerve that is at risk in the radial aspect of the incision. The fascia of the antecubital fossa is open, and the biceps tendon is present beneath this layer. Occasionally, the tendon is retracted proximally and lies beneath the biceps muscle and brachialis. The tendon stump is debrided to

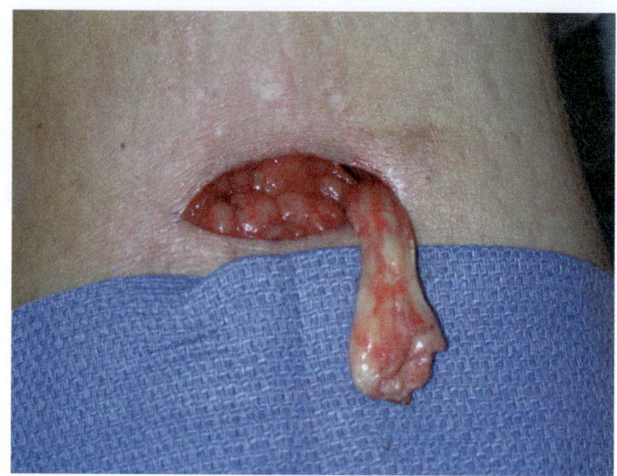

Fig. 9.3 A 3-cm transverse incision is made distal to the flexion crease of the elbow. Care must be taken to avoid injury to the lateral antebrachial cutaneous nerve. The tendon is usually found beneath the antecubital fascial layer

healthy tendon, and locking nonabsorbable sutures are placed in the tendon. The methods for tendon fixation are described below.

A second longitudinal incision is made over the radial tuberosity. The extensor fascia is identified and split along its fibers exposing the extensor musculature. The extensors are split exposing the underlying supinator. With the forearm in full pronation, the supinator is divided to expose the bare radial tuberosity (Fig. 9.4). The tendon is passed from the anterior incision to the lateral incision with the use of a tendon passer. The tendon is fixed to the radial tuberosity using one of the techniques described below.

Tendon Fixation

There are a variety of techniques for distal biceps tendon fixation, including bone tunnels, suture anchor, interosseous screw fixation, and suspensory cortical button. Numerous biomechanical studies have been published comparing the biomechanical properties of these options. All have demonstrated sufficient strength to allow for the successful surgical management of distal biceps rupture.

Bone Tunnels

A trough is created over the radial aspect of the bicipital tuberosity, which is 1–1.5 cm in length. Three drill holes are created 5 mm from the radial aspect of the trough, and passing sutures are

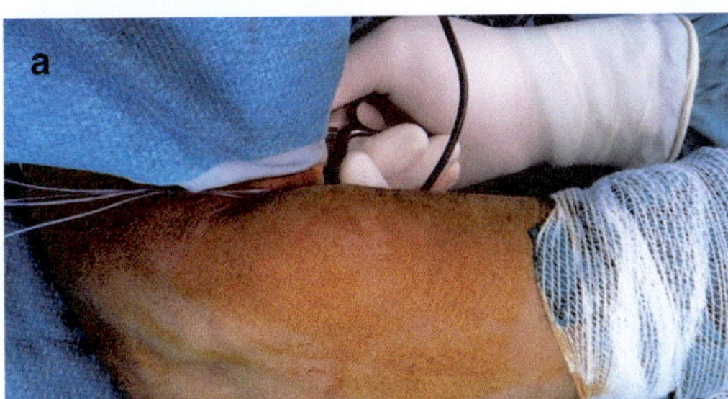

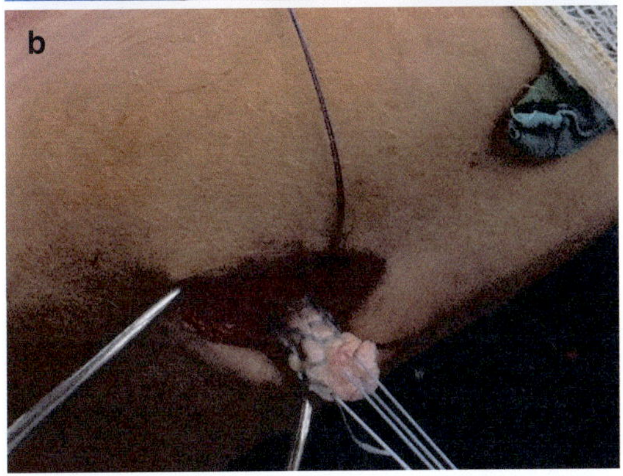

Fig. 9.4 (**a**) Exposure of the radial tuberosity is made through a second lateral incision made where the tip of the forceps protrudes from the anterior incision. To avoid injury to the PIN, the forearm should be placed in full pronation during this exposure. (**b**) The tendon is shuttled from anterior to posterolateral to bed fixed to the radial tuberosity

placed from the drill holes to the trough. The previously placed sutures in the distal biceps tendon are then shuttled through the trough to the drill holes. The tendon is reduced, and the sutures are tied over a bone bridge. The major advantage of this approach is the ease of recreating the radial and distal insertion site of the biceps tendon. Meticulous closure of all fascial layers is performed.

Suture Anchors

Suture anchor fixation can be performed through either exposure. The radial tuberosity is debrided with a curette to remove residual tendon remnant and to create a healthy healing surface. A suture anchor is first placed distally, and one of the suture limbs is placed in locked fashion into the biceps tendon. A second, more proximal suture anchor is then placed to recreate the biceps tendinous footprint, and a suture limb is placed in locked fashion into the biceps tendon. The avoidance of drilling through the dorsal cortex of the radius greatly reduces the risk of PIN injury. The tendon is reduced, and the sutures are tied. Meticulous closure of all fascial layers is performed.

Interference Screw

Interosseous fixation with an interference screw can similarly be done through the anterior approach. The center of the tuberosity is drilled and reamed. One suture limb of the locking nonabsorbable sutures sewn through the distal biceps tendon is passed through the interference screw. With the tendon reduced in the bone tunnel, the screw is inserted and the remaining suture limbs are tied. The advantage of this approach is ease of exposure although distal and radial placement of the biceps tendon is difficult in most cases due to exposure.

Suspensory Cortical Button

Suspensory cortical button fixation is performed through a dual-incision approach. After exposure of the radial tuberosity through an anterior approach, a 4.3-mm drill hole through the anterior cortex of the ulnar tuberosity exits the dorsal cortex. A nonabsorbable suture is then sewn through the distal biceps in a locking fashion and then passed through the cortical button, leaving a 2–3-mm gap between the distal tendon and the button to allow passage of the button through the bone tunnel. The elbow is placed in supination, and a beath pin is used to pass the suture and button through the bone tunnel and through the skin on the dorsal surface of the forearm. The suture is then tension and tied. Fluoroscopy is used to confirm the button positioning.

The suspensory cortical button can also be used in conjunction with interosseous fixation through an interference screw. This provides enough mechanical strength to allow for aggressive rehabilitation with active range of motion exercises at 2–3 weeks [13]. Postoperatively, patients are begun on immediate passive range of motion exercises. At 3 weeks, gravity-assisted flexion and extension are started with progression to light strengthening at 8 weeks and heavy strengthening at 12 weeks. Unrestricted activity and heavy lifting is not allowed until 5 months postoperatively.

Partial Distal Biceps Tears

The surgical technique of repair of partial tendon tears can be performed through a single lateral approach. Partial biceps tendon ruptures typically occur at the radial insertion of the tuberosity. The lateral incision is centered over the radial tuberosity. The fascia of the forearm extensors is opened, and the extensor musculature is divided to the level of the supinator. With the forearm in full pronation, the fibers of the supinator are spilt to expose the distal biceps tendon insertion on the radial tuberosity. A traction suture is placed in the biceps tendon, and the remaining tendon is released from the tuberosity. The distal biceps tendon is debrided of all degenerative tendon tissue. Grasping sutures are places in the biceps tendon. The tendon is then secured to the radial tuberosity using any of the techniques described below for complete rupture.

Postoperatively, the rehabilitation protocol is the same as in complete distal biceps repairs.

Chronic Complete Distal Biceps Tears

Chronic ruptures are challenging due to the degree of proximal tendon retraction and scar tissue. It is important to evaluate the integrity of the lacertus fibrosis. When this structure is intact, it prevents significant biceps tendon retraction, which may necessitate the use of allograft or autograft [14]. Additionally, the quality of the tendon should be evaluated both preoperatively and intraoperatively.

An extensile anterior incision is necessary to locate and mobilize the distal tendon stump. The radial nerve and lateral antebrachial cutaneous nerve should be identified and protected. If it is not possible to reduce the tendon to the

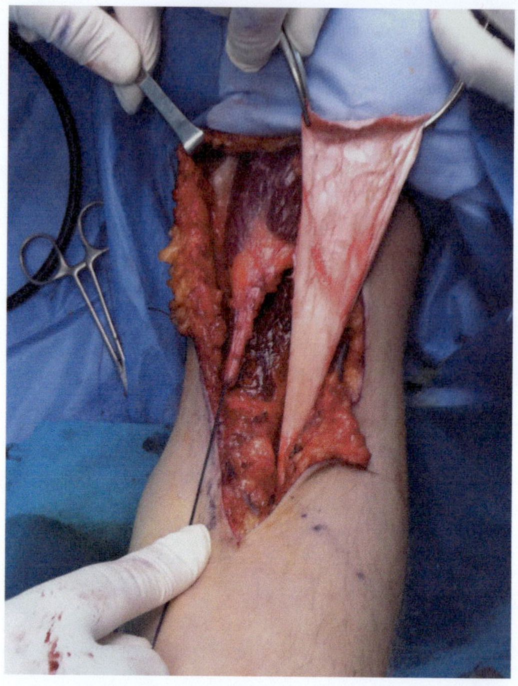

Fig. 9.5 Chronic distal biceps tear repaired with an Achilles allograft. After the distal tendon is fixed to the radial tuberosity with a bone tunnel technique, the proximal allograft tendon is sutured to the native biceps with the appropriate tension placing the elbow in 45° of flexion

tuberosity, an interpositional graft is required. A semitendinosus autograft is sutured through the proximal muscle belly and anchored in the tuberosity in the same fashion as an acute rupture [15]. Alternatively, an Achilles allograft can also be used and sewn circumferentially around the proximal muscle belly [16] (Fig. 9.5). Reconstruction with a combination of fascia lata autograft with synthetic augmentation as well as flexor carpi radialis autograft has been described with good results [17, 18]. To avoid over lengthening, the tendon reconstruction reduction should be performed in 60° of elbow flexion.

Postoperatively, patients are protected in a hinged flexion-assist splint with a 90° extension block until 6 weeks, when active range of motion exercises is begun. Strengthening exercises are started at 12 weeks postoperatively, and unrestricted activity and heavy lifting are not allowed until 6 months postoperatively.

Results

Reported results for distal biceps tendon repairs have been excellent. Morrey et al. showed 97 % strength with elbow flexion and 95 % strength in supination compared to the contralateral extremity in patients treated with bone tunnel fixation [19]. Karunakar et al. found decreased endurance in 38 % of patients in supination and 33 % of patients in elbow flexion with 19 % of patients showing decreased supination and 5 % of patients showing decreased elbow flexion [20]. Although previous studies showed increased subjective fatigue and decreased endurance, Nesterenko et al. found no differences between the injured and uninjured limbs with testing of muscle fatigability [7].

More recently, Balabaud et al. found 100 % satisfaction and full elbow and forearm range of motion in nine patients treated with suture anchor repair [21]. When suture anchor was compared to bone tunnel fixation, El-Hawary et al. found 11° of increased flexion with faster strength recovery in the suture anchor group, with no differences in strength or supination [22]. With suspensory cortical button fixation, Peeters et al. found 80 % strength with elbow flexion and 91 % strength for supination with average Mayo Elbow Performance score of 94 [23].

Biomechanical studies show that cortical button fixation provides the highest peak load failure at 400 N compared to 381 N with suture anchor, 310 N with bone tunnel, and 232 N with interference screw [24]. However, cyclical loading produces displacement of the tendon repair between 2.15 and 3.55 mm depending on the fixation type. This is less likely to compromise tendon-bone apposition and healing with cortical button, interference screw, or bone tunnel fixation due to the tendon stump buried in the tuberosity. However, this may be a concern with suture anchor fixation, and postoperative activity should be more conservative.

Based on the results found in these studies, we could conclude that no method of fixation is better than the other. The surgeon, based on expertise, patient characteristics, and financial issues, should make the choice of tendon fixation method.

Complications

The main complications of distal biceps tendon repair consist of nerve injury, heterotopic ossification (HO), and biceps tendon re-ruptures.

The most common complication from distal biceps tendon repair is paresthesia of the lateral antebrachial cutaneous nerve that usually spontaneously resolves, although permanent damage has been reported [25]. This is due to neuropraxia from aggressive retraction and is more commonly seen with the single-incision approach [10].

Injury to the PIN has been reported in up to 5 % of cases, although most are similarly from neuropraxia and resolve [11, 26]. The dual-incision approach was developed by Boyd and Anderson to decrease the risk of PIN injury. Cadaveric studies of the dual-incision approach by Links et al. show that PIN compression occurs during surgical exposure with the forearm in maximum pronation due to compression of the PIN beneath the arcade of Frohse and the supinator [27].

HO is another frequently reported complication that can progress to proximal radioulnar synostosis. The risk of HO is increased with the dual-incision technique, with a reported prevalence of 5–10 % [12, 28, 29]. A modified muscle-splitting approach that avoids the ulna may help decrease the risk of HO. Patients with HO reported an average loss of 9° of pronation [30]. Grewal et al. recently found heterotopic ossification rates of only 2 %, with only minimal calcification and no range of motion deficits. This may be secondary to their postoperative use of indomethacin, which should be given postoperatively in all distal biceps tendon repairs for HO prophylaxis [10].

Re-rupture of distal biceps tendon repairs is extremely rare and is most likely due to poor patient compliance with flexion and supination restrictions in the immediate postoperative period [31]. However, other possible factors that may risk tendon re-rupture include excessive tendon tension, inadequate fixation, and poor tendon quality.

Persistent anterior elbow pain also occurs in patients treated with a dual-incision technique, although it is more common in patients with delayed repair [12].

Triceps Tendon Tears

Indications

Distal triceps tendon ruptures are extremely rare, representing less than 1 % of upper extremity tendon injuries [32]. They are most commonly associated with anabolic steroid use and weight lifting [33]. Other risk factors include renal insufficiency [34], hyperparathyroidism [35], osteogenesis imperfecta [36], local corticosteroid injections [37], and olecranon bursitis [38]. It can be seen in all adult age groups and affects both men and women at a ratio of 2:3.

The superficial triceps insertion has three components: the lateral aspect, the medial aspect, and the central triceps tendon [39]. The deep insertion of the triceps tendon is covered by muscle and inserts directly into the olecranon. The superficial lateral triceps aspect is continuous with the fascia of the anconeus and antebrachial fascia. The superficial medial aspect of the triceps tendon inserts on the medial aspect of the olecranon and is histologically confluent with the central tendon. In triceps tendon ruptures, the lateral triceps expansion is often intact and can provide partial elbow extension [40]. Distal triceps tendon ruptures commonly occur at the central tendinous insertion on the olecranon. Less commonly, they have been reported to occur at the myotendinous junction or within the muscle belly [41, 42].

Partial tears involving less than 50 % of the triceps tendon can be treated nonoperatively with satisfactory results [43]. Conservative treatment includes a short period of immobilization followed by progressive muscle strengthening. Partial tears involving greater than 50 % of the tendon are generally treated surgically except in older, low functioning, and debilitated patients.

Patient Workup

Clinical Exam

The mechanism of distal triceps tendon ruptures most commonly involves eccentric loading of the triceps tendon, such as during weight lifting or a fall on to an outstretched hand. Less common causes include lacerations and high-energy trauma such as motor vehicle collisions or fall from height.

Patients can present with swelling, pain, and ecchymosis over their posterior elbow. A defect just proximal to the olecranon can often be palpated (Fig. 9.6). However, partial tears, body habitus, and swelling in the acute setting may prevent palpation of a defect.

Inability to extend the elbow against resistance confirms a complete distal tendon rupture. However, in the setting of a complete tendon rupture, active extension of the elbow may be retained through the function of the lateral triceps expansion. Therefore, the presence of active

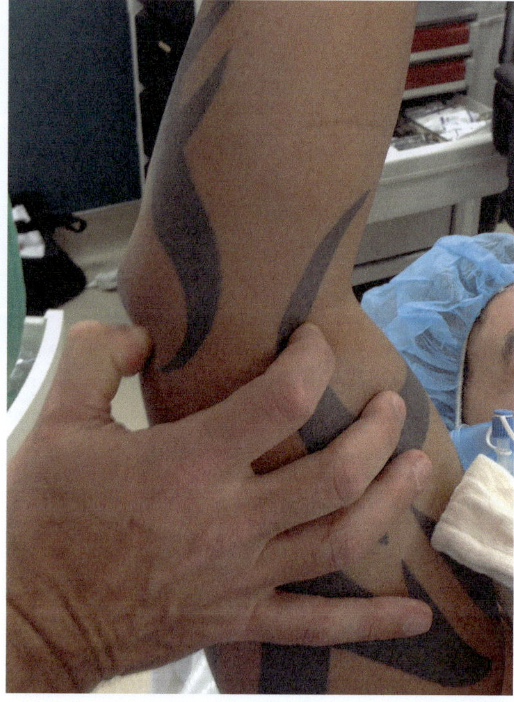

Fig. 9.6 With acute complete triceps tendon tears, a palpable defect can often be felt proximal to the triceps insertion on the olecranon

extension does not rule out a tendon rupture. A modification of the Thompson test used for Achilles tendon ruptures may be used to evaluate for triceps tendon ruptures.

Imaging

Imaging begins with plain radiographs, which may show an osseous avulsion off the olecranon, known as a "flake sign." Differentiating between a partial versus a complete tear is best done with MRI or ultrasound. On MRI, the triceps is best visualized on sagittal images. Partial ruptures show a small fluid-filled defect within the triceps tendons where complete ruptures show a large fluid-filled gap between the triceps tendon and the olecranon process [44]. Ultrasound can also diagnose as well as differentiate between complete and partial tears, although the utility of ultrasound is technician dependent [45].

Surgical Technique

Acute Tendon Tears

Typically partial triceps ruptures can be managed conservatively with immobilization in 30° of flexion for approximately 6 weeks [46]. However, large partial tears and high-functioning individuals are candidates for early surgical intervention.

Acute triceps tendon ruptures should be repaired within 2 weeks to prevent retraction and scarring of the tendon. The surgical technique involves an incision just lateral to the prominence of the olecranon. Skin flaps are carefully elevated, and the triceps tendon is exposed (Fig. 9.7a). The degenerative tendon edges are freshened, and the olecranon insertion is debrided of any remaining tendon fragments. The tendon is reduced to determine the proximal and distal extent of the triceps insertion. Nonabsorbable sutures are placed through the distal tendon using either a Krackow

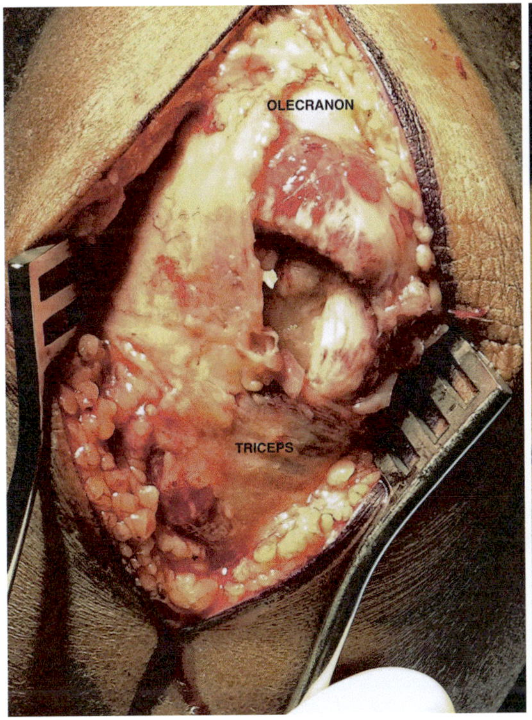

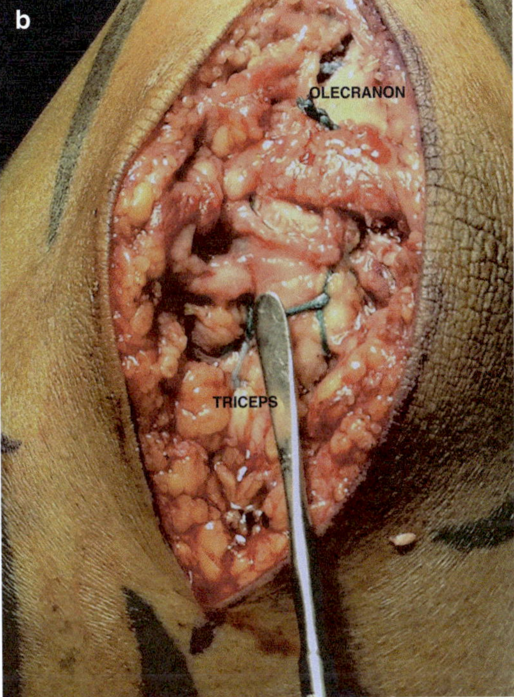

Fig. 9.7 (**a**) Exposure of a triceps tear notes the intact superficial lateral expansion of the triceps tendon. Sutures are placed in at the proximal and distal insertion of the triceps tendon utilizing a Krackow tendon grasping suture. Bone tunnels are drilled in the olecranon in a cruciate configuration to allow for reduction of the triceps tendon on the olecranon. (**b**) Pull-sutures are placed in each tunnel to shuttle the tendon grasping sutures. The sutures are shuttles through the appropriate tunnel, and the tendon is reduced and tied completing the repair

or Bunnell technique. Four transosseous tunnels are drilled in the proximal ulna in a cruciate configuration. The sutures are shuttled through the appropriate tunnel and tied after the tendon is anatomically reduced (Fig. 9.7b).

The wounds are closed, and the arm is immobilized in 40° of flexion. Patients are placed in a hinged brace, which is locked for 4–6 weeks. During this time, passive extension with gravity is allowed with no active motion in compliant patients. Isometric strengthening is started at 6 weeks in extension with gentle active range of motion. Resistive strengthening is started at 3 months.

Alternatively, Yeh et al. have described an anatomic repair involving both a proximal and a distal row of fixation using suture anchors. This restores the anatomic footprint of the triceps tendon insertion, which usually spans approximately 466 mm^2 of the surface of the olecranon. In cadaver studies, anatomic repair showed decreased fraying and intratendinous rupture as well as decreased displacement of the tendon repair when compared to a simple transosseous

cruciate or suture anchor repair [47]. However, there was no statistically significant difference in load at yield or peak load.

Chronic Tendon Tears

Distal triceps tendon ruptures are often misdiagnosed, with studies showing up to 50 % of these injuries are missed on initial presentation [48]. Delayed presentation of these injuries are challenging to repair primarily secondary to retraction and scarring of the tendon. Chronic tendon ruptures often require augmentation procedures to reinforce the repair. These include autologous or allogenic tendon grafts, forearm fascial flaps, a triceps turndown flap, or an anconeus slide [49]. Hamstring allograft or autograft is commonly used for augmentation. The semitendinosus tendon is woven through the distal triceps tendon with fixation through an olecranon transosseous bone tunnel. The surgical management of chronic insufficiency includes also the use of Achilles tendon allograft with augmentation with a triceps-anconeus rotational myoplasty as described by Celli et al. [50] (Fig. 9.8).

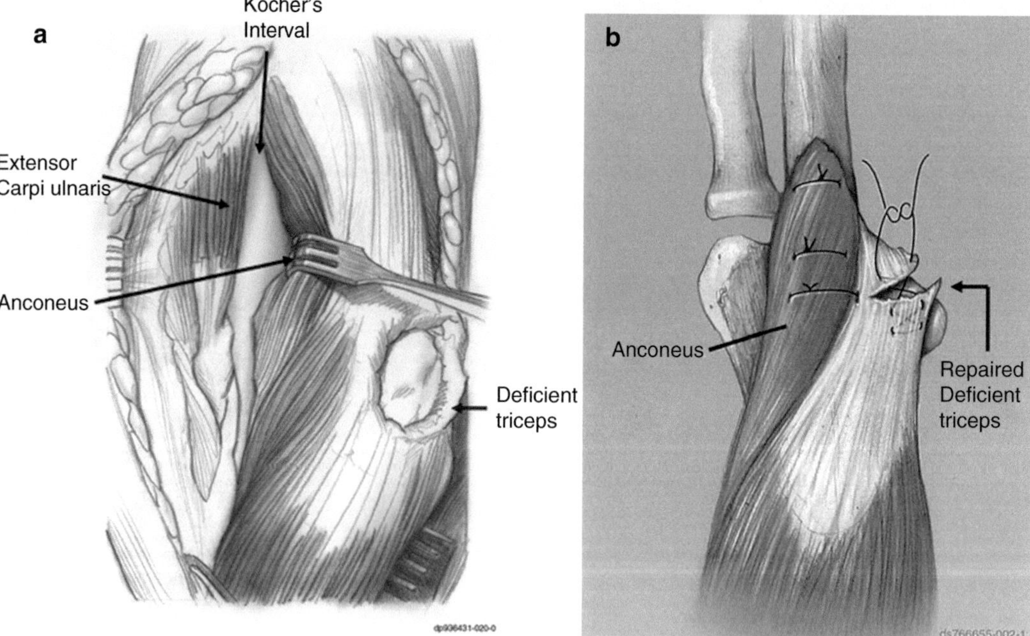

Fig. 9.8 (**a**) To perform a triceps-anconeus myoplasty, Kocher interval is open, and the anconeus is elevated off of the lateral aspect of the ulna and rotated medially, keeping the lateral expansion of the triceps tendon intact with the anconeus. (**b**) The myoplasty is positioned over the prominence of the olecranon and secured through bone tunnels

Chronic triceps insufficiency can also be seen following triceps reflecting exposures of the elbow as a result of lack of healing or partial healing. The prevalence rates reported in the literature following total elbow arthroplasty performed with either the triceps splitting approach or the Bryan-Morrey triceps elevating approach are between 1 and 29 % [51–55]. Celli et al. found triceps insufficiency in 2 % of patients following total elbow arthroplasty with good to excellent results following repair or reconstruction of the triceps tendon in 88 % of these patients [50].

Results and Complications

The results of both primary repair of acute triceps tendon ruptures and reconstruction of chronic ruptures are good. Van Riet found a 21 % re-rupture rate with 82 % peak strength and 99 % endurance when compared to the contralateral side [48]. There were no re-ruptures in reconstructed chronic triceps tendon ruptures, and patients were found to have 66 % peak strength and 92 % endurance.

The results of partial tendon tears show that they may be treated conservatively or surgically with good results. A study of triceps tendon ruptures in the NFL showed that 6 out of 10 players treated nonoperatively were able to return to play without weakness or pain. Three players had delayed surgical repair due to residual weakness and pain, and one player sustained a complete rupture on returning to play. Of the 11 players that were treated operatively, all returned to play without weakness or pain with one player sustaining a re-rupture requiring revision 6 weeks postoperatively during rehabilitation [56].

Re-ruptures are rare and usually result from a traumatic fall in the setting of complete recovery following original repair. Revision reconstructions of these patients were found by van Riet et al. to be functionally comparable to their original repair [48]. Other potential postoperative complications include flexion contractures and olecranon bursitis from wire suturing.

Lateral Epicondylitis

Indications

Lateral epicondylitis, also known as tennis elbow, affects between 1 and 3 % of adults each year, most commonly between the ages 30 and 50 years [57]. More specifically, lateral epicondylitis refers to a tendinosis of the musculotendinous structures which arise from the lateral epicondyle. This includes the extensor carpi radialis longus (ECRL), extensor carpi radialis brevis (ECRB), extensor digitorum communis (EDC), and extensor carpi ulnaris (ECU). The origin of the ECRB is most commonly affected, with rare involvement of the remaining extensor origins.

The name lateral epicondylitis is a misnomer that suggests an inflammatory condition. Microscopic analysis shows no inflammatory cells. Instead, there are degenerative changes that include fibroblast tissue, vascular invasion, and unstructured collagen, collectively termed "angiofibroblastic tendinosis" [58].

The mechanism of lateral epicondylitis results from repetitive wrist extension and alternating forearm supination and pronation [59]. Risk factors include overexertion with repetitive tasks, racquet sports, and manual labor [60]. The ECRB has been shown to be electrically active with stress of the elbow in flexion, extension, varus, and valgus. This supports the hypothesis that repetitive stressful use of the elbow leads to the degeneration of the ECRB origin [61].

Studies show that approximately 80 % of patients have improvement of their symptoms within 1 year without any treatment [62, 63]. However, even with conservative treatment, 26 % of patients have recurrence of their symptoms, and 40 % of patients have continued minor discomfort [64].

Initial treatment consists of oral NSAIDs and rest from repetitive use of the affected extremity. After resolution of the initial pain, attention should focus on altering the activities that lead to the development of the condition. This could include altering faulty sporting technique or training regiments to diminish the chance for recurrent symptoms. In racket sports, an alteration in equipment may be needed, including the use of force dissipating material on the racket grip, reducing frame rigidity, and an evaluation of string tension.

Physical therapy should focus on strengthening the wrist extensors through eccentric exercises, creating muscle hypertrophy of the musculotendinous unit that increases tensile strength. A systematic review by Raman et al. showed moderate evidence of benefit in isotonic eccentric therapy exercises and only weak evidence supporting the use of isokinetic and isometric exercises [65].

Steroid injections are another option if NSAIDs and therapy fail. They provide improved pain relief in the acute period within 6 weeks, but show no difference from other non-surgical treatment modalities at follow-up at 3–12 months [63, 66]. Altay et al. found no difference in patients injected with lidocaine and steroids compared to only lidocaine at 1 year [67]. The "pepper" technique of injecting steroids by scoring the osteotendinous junction multiple times with the needle during the injection to promote healing leads to decreased strength and DASH scores when compared to a single-injection technique and should therefore be avoided [68].

Platelet-rich plasma (PRP) injections have shown promising results at short-term follow-up. Peerbooms et al. found satisfactory results in 73 % of patients with PRP injections compared to 49 % in steroid injections at 1 year [69].

Several authors have recommended a number of other treatment modalities, such as low-intensity ultrasound or extracorporeal shock wave therapy. However, these treatments show little benefit over the natural history of the disease [70, 71].

Surgical management of lateral epicondylitis is reserved for patients with persistent debilitating pain despite at least 3–6 months of aggressive nonoperative modalities. There is no substantial evidence that conservative treatment yields clinical improvements beyond 3 months after the initiation of symptoms [72].

Surgical Technique

Open

The surgical technique involves a 3-cm incision that lies just anterior to the prominence of the lateral epicondyle (Fig. 9.9). The skin and subcutaneous tissue are dissected to the extensor fascia.

The interval between the ECRL and the extensor aponeurosis (EA) is identified and incised (Fig. 9.10). Retraction of this interval allows exposure of the ECRB origin. The diseased tendon appears as a dull greyish tendon, which may show signs of fibrillation. It is excised to healthy tendon tissue. An arthrotomy may be performed during an open procedure to examine the radio-capitellar joint for intra-articular pathology, which can be found in 11–44 % of patients [73, 74].

If the diseased tissue extends into the EA, firm reattachment of the EA to the lateral epicondyle is required with the use of suture anchors or bone tunnels. The interval between the ECRL and EA is then closed followed by routine skin closure.

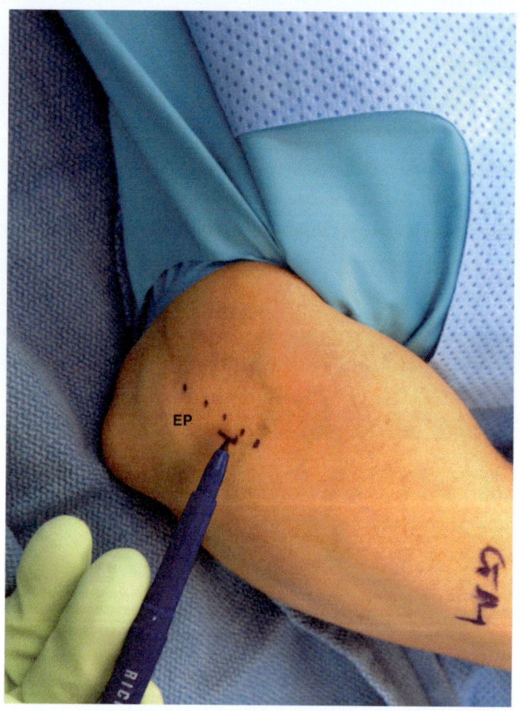

Fig. 9.9 The skin incision for open repair of lateral epicondylitis extends distal from the lateral epicondyle for 3 cm

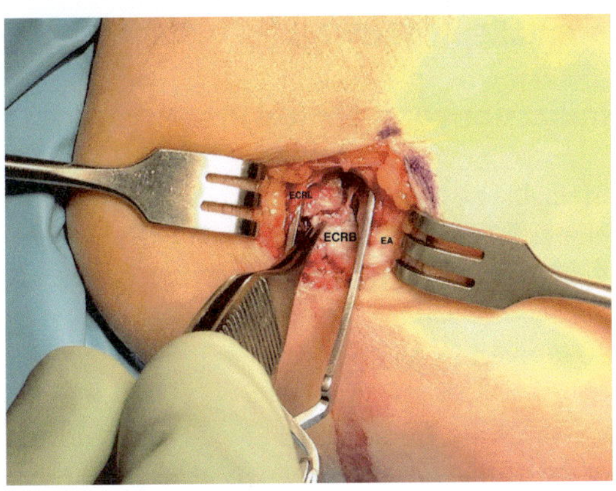

Fig. 9.10 The interval between the ECRL and EA is identified. The underlying diseased EBRB tendon appears dullish gray. It should be excised to healthy tendon

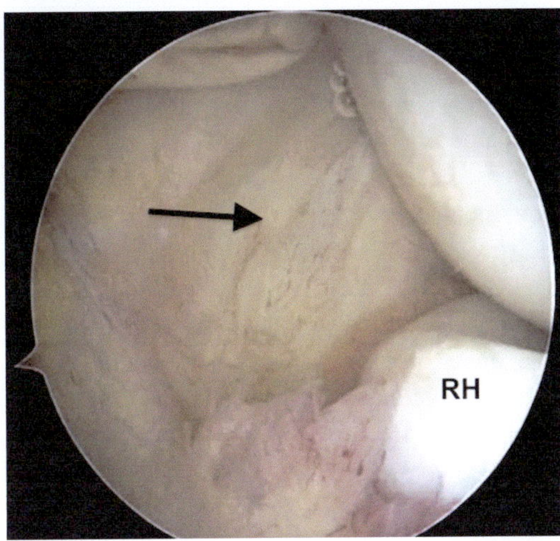

Fig. 9.11 Arthroscopic view of a patient with lateral epicondylitis showing fraying of the capsule overlying the ECRB (*arrow*). Debridement of the tendon should not go behind the line bisecting the anterior part of the radial head, to avoid damage to the lateral collateral ligament

Percutaneous

Percutaneous treatment of lateral epicondylitis is aimed at lengthening the ECRB tendon as opposed to debridement of degenerative tissue.

Release of the ECRB tendon is performed through a small incision over the midpoint of the lateral epicondyle at the ECRB origin. The arm is flexed to protect the radial nerve, and a percutaneous release is performed at the point of maximal tenderness. Release is aided by performing a Mill's manipulation. This consists of forced wrist and finger flexion with the forearm in pronation. This serves to stretch the common extensors.

Other procedures that may be performed include ECRB lengthening through a Z-plasty at the distal musculotendinous junction, which was initially shown to have a success rate close to 100 % by Garden, but subsequent studies showed persistent pain and recurrence in up to 80 % of patients [75, 76]. Denervation of the epicondylar region with decompression of the posterior interosseous nerve can also be done, with Wilhelm showing good results in 90 % of cases [77].

Arthroscopy

Arthroscopic debridement of the ECRB tendon has gained significant popularity over the past decade. Benefits over an open procedure include preservation of the common extensor origin, accelerated postoperative rehabilitation and return to work, and the ability to simultaneously address any possible intra-articular pathology.

Visualization is established through an anterior medial portal with instrumentation directed through a superior anterolateral portal. The degenerative capsule and ECRB tendon are then debrided, with care to remain deep to the ECRL tendon (Fig. 9.11).

To avoid damage to the lateral elbow stabilizers including the lateral collateral ligament (LCL), it is important to stay superior to the superior half of the capitellum. The major advantage of an arthroscopic approach is the ability to perform a detailed evaluation of the radiocapitellar articulation, the proximal radioulnar joint, and possible radial pica bands. Additional debridement of these areas can be performed based on intraoperative findings.

Results

Results for operative intervention are favorable. Long-term follow-up after an open procedure showed 40 % of patients had persistent pain at 6 weeks, decreasing to 24 % at 1 year and 9 % at 5 years [78]. Arthroscopic intervention resulted in improvement 93–100 % patients at 2 years [79–81]. However, 38 % of patients had persistent pain, with 10 % of patients experiencing pain with everyday activity [79]. Percutaneous release has been shown to result in marginal improvement compared to an open procedure, with 30 % decreased pain at 3 weeks and 4 % decreased at 1 year compared to an open procedure [82]. However, no statistical difference was found between open, arthroscopic, and percutaneous intervention by Szabo et al., with higher success rates in open and arthroscopic procedures compared to percutaneous despite longer duration of symptoms [74].

Complications

Posterolateral rotatory instability (PLRI) can result from excessive debridement extending into the lateral capsuloligamentous complex. As noted above, care must to avoid debridement below the level of the capitellum. However, PLRI can predate or occur concomitantly with lateral epicondylitis, making it an important consideration in the preoperative workup and treatment of lateral elbow pain [83]. Multiple cortisone injections have been identified as an iatrogenic cause of PLRI in patients with lateral epicondylitis.

The posterior cutaneous nerve of the forearm crosses 1.5 cm anterior to the lateral epicondyle and is at risk during an open incision. Damage to this nerve may result in numbness or a painful neuroma.

Conclusions

Lateral epicondylitis is a common ailment of the elbow, which most frequently responds to nonoperative management and modification of precipitating activity. Both open and arthroscopic debridements successfully improve chronic symptoms in recalcitrant cases. Avoidance of complication requires careful avoidance of iatrogenic injury to capsuloligamentous and neural structures.

Medial Epicondylitis

Indications and Clinical Presentation

Medial epicondylitis, also known as golfer's elbow, is much less common than lateral epicondylitis, occurring 7–20 times less [84]. It typically occurs between the ages of 30 and 50 years with no sex predilection, and incidence has been shown to be 4.5 % in repetitive workers [85]. Like lateral epicondylitis, medial epicondylitis is a tendinosis of the medial musculotendinous structures. These structures collectively referred to as the flexor-pronator mass include the pronator teres (PT), flexor carpi radialis (FCR), palmaris longus (PL), flexor digitorum superficialis (FDS), and flexor carpi ulnaris (FCU). The medial conjoined tendon (MCT) serves as a common intramuscular insertion on the medial epicondyle for the flexor-pronator group. It attaches on the anterior inferior aspect of the medial epicondyle and extends distally into the forearm for 12 cm. The MCT is a central component to the development of symptoms through attritional lesions.

The mechanism of medial epicondylitis results from repeated motion at the elbow and wrist. Repetitive motion during wrist flexion and forearm pronation results in stress and degeneration of the MCT, most commonly PT and FCR. Microscopic analysis shows degenerative changes including fibroblast tissue, vascular invasion, and unstructured collagen, collectively termed "angiofibroblastic tendinosis" [58].

Ulnar neuropathy is seen in approximately 50 % of patients with medial epicondylitis and has prognostic implication on surgical management. Gabel et al. classified patients based on the presence or absence of ulnar nerve symptoms (Table 9.1). Successful management of this condition requires careful evaluation of the ulnar nerve and treatment of both conditions when they exist [86].

The mainstay of treatment in the initial acute period is nonsurgical. Treatment includes use of oral NSAIDs and rest to decrease any acute tendinous inflammation in the surrounding tissue and allow time for tendon healing. After

Table 9.1 Classification of medial epicondylitis

Type IA	Medial epicondylitis with no associated ulnar nerve symptoms
Type IB	Medial epicondylitis with mild associated ulnar nerve symptoms
Type II	Medial epicondylitis with moderate to severe associated ulnar nerve symptoms (deficits seen on physical exam or evidence of denervation on electromyogram)

resolution of the initial pain and inflammation, nonsurgical treatment focuses on activity modification and rehabilitation to decrease any residual pain and prevent recurrence. In active patients involved in sports such as golf, baseball, or tennis that create valgus stress at the elbow, proper equipment and mechanics are emphasized.

Steroid injections are another option if NSAIDs and therapy fail. They provide improved pain relief in the acute period within 6 weeks, but show no difference from other nonsurgical treatment modalities at follow-up at 6 weeks or 12 months [87]. Other modalities such as low-intensity ultrasound and extracorporeal shock wave therapy have shown little or no improvement benefit [70, 71]. Nonoperative treatment is fairly successful, with 26 % of patients with recurrent symptoms and 40 % of patients with prolonged minor discomfort [84].

Surgical treatment is reserved for patients that have a clear diagnosis and that have persistent debilitating pain despite at least 3 months of aggressive nonoperative modalities. There is no evidence that conservative treatment yields improvements beyond 3 months after the initiation of symptoms [72].

Surgical Technique

Open

The surgical technique involves a 3-cm incision which extends distally from a point just anterior to the medial epicondyle. Care must be taken to avoid iatrogenic injury to the medial antebrachial cutaneous nerve (MACN), which is consistently in the surgical field.

The superficial flexor-pronator fascia is split distally. The underlying muscle is elevated exposing the underlying MCT. Identification of the anterior oblique ligament (AOL) prevents iatrogenic injury. Gray or fibrillated tissue is identified and surgically excised. The medial epicondyle is then decorticated with a curette or rongeur. The flexor-pronator mass is reattached through primary repair, bone tunnels, or suture anchors as indicated by the tendon defect created. If concomitant ulnar neuropathy requires surgical management, this is best performed with submuscular transposition.

Postoperatively, the arm is immobilized for 2 weeks. Active range of motion is then instated to regain motion. Flexor-pronator strengthening and stretching is started at 6 weeks. Sporting activity is avoided until pain-free full strength is achieved.

Arthroscopy

Debridement of the flexor-pronator mass can also be performed arthroscopically. The theoretical benefits over an open procedure include preservation of the flexor-pronator origin, accelerated postoperative rehabilitation and return to work, and the ability to simultaneously address any possible intra-articular pathology. Visualization is established through a lateral portal with instrumentation through a medial portal. Zonno et al. describe using a switching stick to establish a second medial portal that is more posterior and medial to provide improved inspection of the medial aspect of the elbow joint [88]. The degenerative capsule and flexor-pronator tendon is debrided until the MCL is visualized, which lies just distal to PT and FCR. This is followed by decortication or the medial epicondyle. Further clinical series will be required to determine the viability of this surgical option.

Results

Vangsness and Jobe showed excellent results in 35 patients with medial epicondylitis after open debridement. Patients had improvement of elbow function from 38 to 98 % of normal with excellent or good results in 97 % of patients and no limitations in 86 % of patients [89].

Gabel et al. found similar results, with good or excellent results 87 % of patients at 7 year follow-up [86]. They found excellent results in the type IA and IB groups, with more guarded prognosis in the type II group. The authors attributed the residual symptoms primarily as a result of lack of response to the surgical management of ulnar neuropathy.

Cadaver studies by Zonno et al. [88]. show that arthroscopic treatment of medial epicondylitis can be safety performed with low risk of injury to the ulnar nerve or the MCL. Mean distance between debridement and the ulnar nerve was 20.8 mm, and mean distance to the anterior bundle of the MCL was 8.3 mm.

Complications

Complications following the surgical management of medial epicondylitis are rare. Neurologic complications include iatrogenic injury to MACN or persistent ulnar nerve symptoms. Careful identification of the MACN is required to prevent this complication. If the MACN is injured with a resultant neuroma, it can be placed in the brachialis muscle belly. Residual ulnar nerve symptoms are best managed with submuscular transposition. The most important aspect of managing this disorder is proper evaluation and management of the ulnar nerve. Patients need to be informed of the change in prognosis when present and that the management of the ulnar neuropathy when present will dictate a successful outcome.

A series of 35 cases by Vangsness and Jobe showed no injuries. Their only complications were a case of ulnar nerve irritation that resolved after ulnar nerve transposition and a postoperative hematoma that resolved with aspiration [89].

Iatrogenic instability is a rare complication most frequently occurring as a result of injury to the AOL. This can be successfully managed with ligament reconstruction.

References

1. Safran MR, Graham SM. Distal biceps tendon ruptures: incidence, demographics, and the effect of smoking. Clin Orthop Relat Res. 2002;404:275–83.
2. Agins HJ, Chess JL, Hoekstra DV, Teitge RA. Rupture of the distal insertion of the biceps brachii tendon. Clin Orthop Relat Res. 1988;234:34–8.
3. Mazzocca AD, Cohen M, Berkson E, et al. The anatomy of the bicipital tuberosity and distal biceps tendon. J Shoulder Elbow Surg. 2007;16:122–7.
4. Kannus P, Jozsa L. Histopathological changes preceding spontaneous rupture of a tendon. A controlled study of 891 patients. J Bone Joint Surg Am. 1991;73:1507–25.
5. Seiler 3rd JG, Parker LM, Chamberland PD, Sherbourne GM, Carpenter WA. The distal biceps tendon. Two potential mechanisms involved in its rupture: arterial supply and mechanical impingement. J Shoulder Elbow Surg. 1995;4:149–56.
6. O'Driscoll SW, Goncalves LB, Dietz P. The hook test for distal biceps tendon avulsion. Am J Sports Med. 2007;35:1865–9.
7. Nesterenko S, Domire ZJ, Morrey BF, Sanchez-Sotelo J. Elbow strength and endurance in patients with a ruptured distal biceps tendon. J Shoulder Elbow Surg. 2010;19:184–9.
8. Freeman CR, McCormick KR, Mahoney D, Baratz M, Lubahn JD. Nonoperative treatment of distal biceps tendon ruptures compared with a historical control group. J Bone Joint Surg Am. 2009;91:2329–34.
9. Kelly EW, Steinmann S, O'Driscoll SW. Surgical treatment of partial distal biceps tendon ruptures through a single posterior incision. J Shoulder Elbow Surg. 2003;12:456–61.
10. Grewal R, Athwal GS, Macdermid JC. Single versus double-incision technique for the repair of acute distal biceps tendon ruptures: a randomized clinical trial. Orthopedics. 2012;35:698–9.
11. Boyd H, Anderson L. A method for reinsertion of the distal biceps brachii tendon. J Bone Joint Surg. 1961;43:1041–3.
12. Kelly EW, Morrey BF, O'Driscoll SW. Complications of repair of the distal biceps tendon with the modified two-incision technique. J Bone Joint Surg Am. 2000;82-A:1575–81.
13. Heinzelmann AD, Savoie 3rd FH, Ramsey JR, Field LD, Mazzocca AD. A combined technique for distal biceps repair using a soft tissue button and biotenodesis interference screw. Am J Sports Med. 2009;37:989–94.
14. Hamer MJ, Caputo AE. Operative treatment of chronic distal biceps tendon ruptures. Sports Med Arthrosc Rev. 2008;16:143–7.
15. Wiley WB, Noble JS, Dulaney TD, Bell RH, Noble DD. Late reconstruction of chronic distal biceps tendon ruptures with a semitendinosus autograft technique. J Shoulder Elbow Surg. 2006;15:440–4.

16. Darlis NA, Sotereanos DG. Distal biceps tendon reconstruction in chronic ruptures. J Shoulder Elbow Surg. 2006;15:614–9.

17. Kaplan FT, Rokito AS, Birdzell MG, Zuckerman JD. Reconstruction of chronic distal biceps tendon rupture with use of fascia lata combined with a ligament augmentation device: a report of 3 cases. J Shoulder Elbow Surg. 2002;11:633–6.

18. Levy HJ, Mashoof AA, Morgan D. Repair of chronic ruptures of the distal biceps tendon using flexor carpi radialis tendon graft. Am J Sports Med. 2000;28:538–40.

19. Morrey BF, Askew LJ, An KN, Dobyns JH. Rupture of the distal tendon of the biceps brachii. A biomechanical study. J Bone Joint Surg Am. 1985;67:418–21.

20. Karunakar MA, Cha P, Stern PJ. Distal biceps ruptures. A followup of Boyd and Anderson repair. Clin Orthop Relat Res. 1999;363:100–7.

21. Balabaud L, Ruiz C, Nonnenmacher J, Seynaeve P, Kehr P, Rapp E. Repair of distal biceps tendon ruptures using a suture anchor and an anterior approach. J Hand Surg Br. 2004;29:178–82.

22. El-Hawary R, Macdermid JC, Faber KJ, Patterson SD, King GJ. Distal biceps tendon repair: comparison of surgical techniques. J Hand Surg. 2003;28:496–502.

23. Peeters T, Ching-Soon NG, Jansen N, Sneyers C, Declercq G, Verstreken F. Functional outcome after repair of distal biceps tendon ruptures using the endobutton technique. J Shoulder Elbow Surg. 2009;18:283–7.

24. Mazzocca AD, Burton KJ, Romeo AA, Santangelo S, Adams DA, Arciero RA. Biomechanical evaluation of 4 techniques of distal biceps brachii tendon repair. Am J Sports Med. 2007;35:252–8.

25. Meherin J, Kilgore E. The treatment of ruptures of the distal biceps brachii tendon. Am J Surg. 1960;99:636–40.

26. Hovelius L, Josefsson G. Rupture of the distal biceps tendon. Report of five cases. Acta Orthop Scand. 1977;48:280–2.

27. Links AC, Graunke KS, Wahl C, Green 3rd JR, Matsen 3rd FA. Pronation can increase the pressure on the posterior interosseous nerve under the arcade of Frohse: a possible mechanism of palsy after two-incision repair for distal biceps rupture – clinical experience and a cadaveric investigation. J Shoulder Elbow Surg. 2009;18:64–8.

28. Failla JM, Amadio PC, Morrey BF, Beckenbaugh RD. Proximal radioulnar synostosis after repair of distal biceps brachii rupture by the two-incision technique. Report of four cases. Clin Orthop Relat Res. 1990;253:133–6.

29. Bisson L, Moyer M, Lanighan K, Marzo J. Complications associated with repair of a distal biceps rupture using the modified two-incision technique. J Shoulder Elbow Surg. 2008;17:67S–71.

30. Wysocki RW, Cohen MS. Radioulnar heterotopic ossification after distal biceps tendon repair: results following surgical resection. J Hand Surg. 2007;32:1230–6.

31. Katolik LI, Fernandez J, Cohen MS. Acute failure of distal biceps reconstruction: a case report. J Shoulder Elbow Surg. 2007;16:e10–2.

32. Anzel SH, Covey KW, Weiner AD, Lipscomb PR. Disruption of muscles and tendons; an analysis of 1, 014 cases. Surgery. 1959;45:406–14.

33. Sollender JL, Rayan GM, Barden GA. Triceps tendon rupture in weight lifters. J Shoulder Elbow Surg. 1998;7:151–3.

34. Mankin HJ. Rickets, osteomalacia, and renal osteodystrophy. Part II. J Bone Joint Surg Am. 1974;56:352–86.

35. Preston FS, Adicoff A. Hyperparathyroidism with avulsion of three major tendons. Report of a case. N Engl J Med. 1962;266:968–71.

36. Match RM, Corrylos EV. Bilateral avulsion fracture of the triceps tendon insertion from skiing with osteogenesis imperfecta tarda. A case report. Am J Sports Med. 1983;11:99–102.

37. Lambert MI, St Clair Gibson A, Noakes TD. Rupture of the triceps tendon associated with steroid injections. Am J Sports Med. 1995;23:778.

38. Clayton ML, Thirupathi RG. Rupture of the triceps tendon with olecranon bursitis. A case report with a new method of repair. Clin Orthop Relat Res. 1984;184:183–5.

39. Keener JD, Chafik D, Kim HM, Galatz LM, Yamaguchi K. Insertional anatomy of the triceps brachii tendon. J Shoulder Elbow Surg. 2010;19:399–405.

40. Gabel GT, Zwahlen B, Morrey BF. Surgical management of the extensor mechanism of the elbow. Instr Course Lect. 1998;47:151–6.

41. Wagner JR, Cooney WP. Rupture of the triceps muscle at the musculotendinous junction: a case report. J Hand Surg. 1997;22:341–3.

42. O'Driscoll SW. Intramuscular triceps rupture. Can J Surg. 1992;35:203–7.

43. Vidal AF, Drakos MC, Allen AA. Biceps tendon and triceps tendon injuries. Clin Sports Med. 2004;23:707–22, xi.

44. Kijowski R, Tuite M, Sanford M. Magnetic resonance imaging of the elbow. Part II: Abnormalities of the ligaments, tendons, and nerves. Skeletal Radiol. 2005;34:1–18.

45. Tagliafico A, Gandolfo N, Michaud J, Perez MM, Palmieri F, Martinoli C. Ultrasound demonstration of distal triceps tendon tears. Eur J Radiol. 2012;81:1207–10.

46. Farrar 3rd EL, Lippert 3rd FG. Avulsion of the triceps tendon. Clin Orthop Relat Res. 1981;161:242–6.

47. Yeh PC, Stephens KT, Solovyova O, et al. The distal triceps tendon footprint and a biomechanical analysis of 3 repair techniques. Am J Sports Med. 2010;38:1025–33.

48. van Riet RP, Morrey BF, Ho E, O'Driscoll SW. Surgical treatment of distal triceps ruptures. J Bone Joint Surg Am. 2003;85-A:1961–7.

49. Sanchez-Sotelo J, Morrey BF. Surgical techniques for reconstruction of chronic insufficiency of the triceps.

Rotation flap using anconeus and tendo achillis allograft. J Bone Joint Surg Br. 2002;84:1116–20.

50. Celli A, Arash A, Adams RA, Morrey BF. Triceps insufficiency following total elbow arthroplasty. J Bone Joint Surg Am. 2005;87:1957–64.

51. Pierce TD, Herndon JH. The triceps preserving approach to total elbow arthroplasty. Clin Orthop Relat Res. 1998;354:144–52.

52. Morrey BF, Bryan RS, Dobyns JH, Linscheid RL. Total elbow arthroplasty. A five-year experience at the Mayo Clinic. J Bone Joint Surg Am. 1981;63:1050–63.

53. Hildebrand KA, Patterson SD, Regan WD, MacDermid JC, King GJ. Functional outcome of semiconstrained total elbow arthroplasty. J Bone Joint Surg Am. 2000;82-A:1379–86.

54. Gill DR, Morrey BF. The Coonrad-Morrey total elbow arthroplasty in patients who have rheumatoid arthritis. A ten to fifteen-year follow-up study. J Bone Joint Surg Am. 1998;80:1327–35.

55. Morrey BF, Adams RA. Semiconstrained arthroplasty for the treatment of rheumatoid arthritis of the elbow. J Bone Joint Surg Am. 1992;74:479–90.

56. Mair SD, Isbell WM, Gill TJ, Schlegel TF, Hawkins RJ. Triceps tendon ruptures in professional football players. Am J Sports Med. 2004;32:431–4.

57. Verhaar JA. Tennis elbow. Anatomical, epidemiological and therapeutic aspects. Int Orthop. 1994;18:263–7.

58. Kraushaar BS, Nirschl RP. Tendinosis of the elbow (tennis elbow). Clinical features and findings of histological, immunohistochemical, and electron microscopy studies. J Bone Joint Surg Am. 1999;81:259–78.

59. Goldie I. Epicondylitis lateralis humeri (epicondylalgia or tennis elbow). A pathogenetical study. Acta Chir Scand Suppl. 1964;57(Suppl 339):1+.

60. Haahr JP, Andersen JH. Physical and psychosocial risk factors for lateral epicondylitis: a population based case-referent study. Occup Environ Med. 2003;60:322–9.

61. Funk DA, An KN, Morrey BF, Daube JR. Electromyographic analysis of muscles across the elbow joint. J Orthop Res. 1987;5:529–38.

62. Haahr JP, Andersen JH. Prognostic factors in lateral epicondylitis: a randomized trial with one-year follow-up in 266 new cases treated with minimal occupational intervention or the usual approach in general practice. Rheumatology (Oxford). 2003;42:1216–25.

63. Hart LE. Corticosteroid injections, physiotherapy, or a wait-and-see policy for lateral epicondylitis? Clin J Sport Med. 2002;12:403–4.

64. Binder AI, Hazleman BL. Lateral humeral epicondylitis – a study of natural history and the effect of conservative therapy. Br J Rheumatol. 1983;22:73–6.

65. Raman J, MacDermid JC, Grewal R. Effectiveness of different methods of resistance exercises in lateral epicondylosis – a systematic review. J Hand Ther 2012;25:5–25; quiz 6.

66. Lewis M, Hay EM, Paterson SM, Croft P. Local steroid injections for tennis elbow: does the pain get worse before it gets better? Results from a randomized controlled trial. Clin J Pain. 2005;21:330–4.

67. Altay T, Gunal I, Ozturk H. Local injection treatment for lateral epicondylitis. Clin Orthop Relat Res. 2002;398:127–30.

68. Bellapianta J, Swartz F, Lisella J, Czajka J, Neff R, Uhl R. Randomized prospective evaluation of injection techniques for the treatment of lateral epicondylitis. Orthopedics. 2011;34:e708–12.

69. Peerbooms JC, Sluimer J, Bruijn DJ, Gosens T. Positive effect of an autologous platelet concentrate in lateral epicondylitis in a double-blind randomized controlled trial: platelet-rich plasma versus corticosteroid injection with a 1-year follow-up. Am J Sports Med. 2010;38:255–62.

70. D'Vaz AP, Ostor AJ, Speed CA, et al. Pulsed low-intensity ultrasound therapy for chronic lateral epicondylitis: a randomized controlled trial. Rheumatology (Oxford). 2006;45:566–70.

71. Haake M, Konig IR, Decker T, Riedel C, Buch M, Muller HH. Extracorporeal shock wave therapy in the treatment of lateral epicondylitis: a randomized multicenter trial. J Bone Joint Surg Am. 2002;84-A:1982–91.

72. Bisset L, Paungmali A, Vicenzino B, Beller E. A systematic review and meta-analysis of clinical trials on physical interventions for lateral epicondylalgia. Br J Sports Med. 2005;39:411–22; discussion 22.

73. Nirschl RP, Pettrone FA. Tennis elbow. The surgical treatment of lateral epicondylitis. J Bone Joint Surg Am. 1979;61:832–9.

74. Szabo SJ, Savoie 3rd FH, Field LD, Ramsey JR, Hosemann CD. Tendinosis of the extensor carpi radialis brevis: an evaluation of three methods of operative treatment. J Shoulder Elbow Surg. 2006;15:721–7.

75. Garden RS. Tennis Elbow. J Bone Joint Surg. 1961;43B:100–6.

76. Carroll RE, Jorgensen EC. Evaluation of the Garden procedure for lateral epicondylitis. Clin Orthop Relat Res. 1968;60:201–4.

77. Wilhelm A. Tennis elbow: treatment of resistant cases by denervation. J Hand Surg Br. 1996;21:523–33.

78. Verhaar J, Walenkamp G, Kester A, van Mameren H, van der Linden T. Lateral extensor release for tennis elbow. A prospective long-term follow-up study. J Bone Joint Surg Am. 1993;75:1034–43.

79. Baker Jr CL, Murphy KP, Gottlob CA, Curd DT. Arthroscopic classification and treatment of lateral epicondylitis: two-year clinical results. J Shoulder Elbow Surg. 2000;9:475–82.

80. Owens BD, Murphy KP, Kuklo TR. Arthroscopic release for lateral epicondylitis. Arthroscopy. 2001;17:582–7.

81. Mullett H, Sprague M, Brown G, Hausman M. Arthroscopic treatment of lateral epicondylitis: clinical and cadaveric studies. Clin Orthop Relat Res. 2005;439:123–8.

82. Buchbinder R, Johnston RV, Barnsley L, Assendelft WJ, Bell SN, Smidt N. Surgery for lateral elbow pain. Cochrane Database Syst Rev. 2011;(3):CD003525.

83. Kalainov DM, Cohen MS. Posterolateral rotatory instability of the elbow in association with lateral epicondylitis. A report of three cases. J Bone Joint Surg Am. 2005;87:1120–5.
84. Leach RE, Miller JK. Lateral and medial epicondylitis of the elbow. Clin Sports Med. 1987;6:259–72.
85. Descatha A, Leclerc A, Chastang JF, Roquelaure Y. Medial epicondylitis in occupational settings: prevalence, incidence and associated risk factors. J Occup Environ Med. 2003;45:993–1001.
86. Gabel GT, Morrey BF. Operative treatment of medical epicondylitis. Influence of concomitant ulnar neuropathy at the elbow. J Bone Joint Surg Am. 1995;77:1065–9.
87. Stahl S, Kaufman T. The efficacy of an injection of steroids for medial epicondylitis. A prospective study of sixty elbows. J Bone Joint Surg Am. 1997;79:1648–52.
88. Zonno A, Manuel J, Merrell G, Ramos P, Akelman E, DaSilva MF. Arthroscopic technique for medial epicondylitis: technique and safety analysis. Arthroscopy. 2010;26:610–6.
89. Vangsness Jr CT, Jobe FW. Surgical treatment of medial epicondylitis. Results in 35 elbows. J Bone Joint Surg Br. 1991;73:409–11.

Index

S. Antuña, R. Barco (eds.), *Essentials in Elbow Surgery*,
DOI 10.1007/978-1-4471-4625-4, © Springer-Verlag London 2014

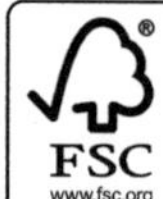

If you have any concerns about our products,
you can contact us on
ProductSafety@springernature.com

In case Publisher is established outside the EU,
the EU authorized representative is:
Springer Nature Customer Service Center GmbH
Europaplatz 3, 69115 Heidelberg, Germany

Printed by Libri Plureos GmbH
in Hamburg, Germany